*Provided
compliments of*

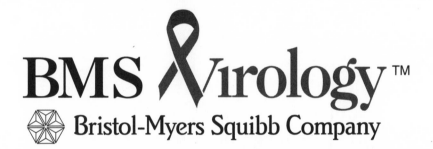

OTHER WORKS BY RONALD BAYER AND GERALD M. OPPENHEIMER

By Ronald Bayer
Homosexuality and American Psychiatry: The Politics of Diagnosis
Private Acts, Social Consequences: AIDS and the Politics of Public Health

Edited or Co-edited by Ronald Bayer
In Search of Equity: Health Needs and the Health Care System
The Health and Safety of Workers: The Politics of Professional Responsibility
AIDS in the Industrialized Democracies: Passions, Politics, and Policies
Blood Feuds: AIDS, Blood, and the Politics of a Medical Disaster

Edited by Ronald Bayer and Gerald M. Oppenheimer
Confronting Drug Policy

AIDS *DOCTORS*

Voices from the Epidemic

Ronald Bayer
and Gerald M. Oppenheimer

OXFORD

UNIVERSITY PRESS

Oxford   New York
Auckland   Bangkok   Buenos Aires
Cape Town   Chennai   Dar es Salaam   Delhi   Hong Kong
Istanbul   Karachi   Kolkata   Kuala Lumpur   Madrid
Melbourne   Mexico City   Mumbai   Nairobi   São Paulo
Shanghai   Singapore   Taipei   Tokyo   Toronto

and an associated company in Berlin

First published by Oxford University Press, Inc.., 2000
First issued as an Oxford University Press paperback, 2002
198 Madison Avenue, New York, New York 10016
www.oup.com

Oxford is a registered trademark of Oxford University Press

Library of Congress Cataloging-in-Publication Data
Bayer, Ronald.
AIDS doctors: voices from the epidemic: an oral history/
Ronald Bayer, Gerald M. Oppenheimer.
p.   cm.
ISBN 0–19–512681–5 (cloth); ISBN 0-19-515239-5 (pbk)
1. AIDS (Disease)—United States—History.
2. Oral history.   3. AIDS (Disease)—United States—Biography.
I. Oppenheimer, Gerald M.   II. Title.
RA644.A25 B387 2000
616.97'92'00973—dc21   00–020913

9 8 7 6 5 4 3 2
Printed in the United States of America
on acid-free paper

To the Memory of
Jonathan Mann and Tom Stoddard
and for
Jane Alexander and
Anne and Julia Stone Oppenheimer

CONTENTS

Acknowledgments

The effort to create an oral history archive incurs many debts along the way. Above all, we owe our deepest appreciation to the AIDS doctors who agreed to be interviewed and who shared with us their memories in a spirit of remarkable candor. Most, although not all, appear in this book, but even those who are not cited directly taught us much, and we are grateful to them. They are Donald Abrams, Donald Armstrong, Arnaud Bastien, Robert Bolan, Carol Brosgart, Jerry Cade, Leonard Calabrese, James Campbell, Lisa Capaldini, Richard Chaisson, Mardge Cohen, Robert Cohen, Marcus Conant, Molly Cooke, Deborah Cotton, Judith Currier, Larry Drew, Waafa El-Sadr, Margaret Fischl, Stephen Follansbee, Gerald Friedland, Alvin Friedman-Kien, Donna Futterman, Eric Goosby, Michael Gottlieb, Jerome Groopman, Howard Grossman, Ronald Grossman, Hunter Handsfield, Margaret Heagarty, Margaret Hilgartner, Martin Hirsch, Harry Hollander, King Holmes, Elizabeth Kass, Donald Kotler, Sheldon Landesman, Jeffrey Laurence, Alexandra Levine, Harvey Makadon, Peter Mansell, Ken Mayer, John Mazzullo, Hermann Mendez, Donna Mildvan, Howard Minkoff, Janet Mitchell, James Oleske, Joseph O'Neill, Stosh Ostrow, William Owen, Robert Redfield, Arye Rubinstein, Neil Schram, Gwendolyn Scott, Robert Scott, Peter Seitzman, Peter Selwyn, Victoria Sharp, Renslow Sherer, Fred Siegal, Joseph Sonnabend, John Stansell, Barbara Starrett, Gabriel (Ramon) Torres, William Valenti, Charles van der Horst, Anita Vaughn, Paul Volberding, Joyce Wallace, Joel Weisman, Dan William, Constance Wofsy, Peter Wolfe, David Wright, and Abigail Zuger.

An oral history project also takes money. The Royal Marks Foundation offered sustained support, for which we thank the foundation and its board. We were supported along the way by a number of other foundations and public sources. The first to provide assistance, and without which our attempts would never have taken off, was the National Library of Medicine. In addition, the Public Health Service's Office of Minority Health and the AIDS Education and Training Center Program as well as the Mathilde and Arthur Krim Foundation offered us funding at key moments in our project. Also, Ronald Bayer's effort was supported by NIMH Grant K05M401376-01 and Gerald Oppenheimer's by two grants from the Research Foundation of the City University of New York, 6-67238 and 6-68526, and a CUNY Sabbatical Fellowship.

We came to this project with only the barest understanding of how to organize and create an oral history archive. Ronald Grele and Mary Marshall Clark of the Columbia University Oral History Office taught us with patience. And when the laborious tasks associated with such an effort had to be executed, their devoted staff—including David Hopson, Michelle Montgomery, and David Skey—not only approached their jobs with care, but also were quick to respond to our every request.

Catherine Stayton, our talented and indomitable research assistant, helped set up our interviews and expertly prepared background material on each of the doctors. We were very lucky to have her during the first years of this project. We also want to thank Gregory Weinberg, who expertly interviewed two physicians when our schedule was bursting at the seams. James Colgrove came to us at the very end but provided a uniquely critical eye.

Jane Alexander, Anne Stone Oppenheimer, Carol Levine, Ronald Grele, Mary Marshall Clark, and Howard Markel carefully read an earlier draft of our manuscript and offered important criticism to us; Peter Ginna, our editor at Oxford University Press, read the manuscript not once but several times to better guide our revisions. Cheryl Healton provided us with institutional support at the Joseph L. Mailman School of Public Health at Columbia University. We thank them all.

Finally, we wish to express our admiration to Lela Cooper, who transcribed virtually all the interviews and who prepared the manuscript with such exceptional skill that a "thank you" can be but a pale reflection of what we feel.

AIDS DOCTORS

Introduction
LOOKING BACKWARD

The year 2000 is a remarkable moment to look back on AIDS in America. Almost 20 years have passed since the first cases that signaled the epidemic's onset were reported by federal health officials. The years were filled with great suffering, especially in gay communities where young men in the prime of life fell victim. Simultaneously in some cities, later in others, that suffering was experienced in the poor African-American and Latino neighborhoods where intravenous drug use served to fuel the spread of HIV (human immunodeficiency virus) infection. Drug users infected each other and, in turn, infected their sexual partners and their babies. Over the course of the epidemic years, more than 400,000 men, women, and children died. It was this terrible world of AIDS-related suffering that framed the lives of doctors who came to care for those who were afflicted. This book is about their experiences and their memories.

Striking therapeutic achievements—the discovery of powerful antiviral drugs—in the past five years have radically transformed the threat posed by AIDS (acquired immunodeficiency syndrome). People infected with HIV live longer before they develop symptoms of AIDS. Those who become sick can have their illnesses controlled, thus prolonging their lives. Death, which so marked the epidemic, is no longer a constant presence. While infection continues to spread and individuals continue to fall ill and succumb, the sense of crisis has abated. Memories of what it was like to confront a grim, disfiguring, contagious, and lethal threat at a time when medicine was all but powerless have already begun to fade.

In this oral history, we have sought to capture an important perspective on the epidemic's course before it is lost, to preserve the memory of a long and dreadful period for those who may come to look back, uncomprehendingly, on what it was to be a doctor caring for those afflicted by AIDS in the epidemic's first two decades.

Like all epidemics, AIDS brought in its wake great fear and consternation—fear of contagion and fear of death. That those most at risk were gay, drug users, Black and Latino, only added to the sense of dread, contributing to the desire to establish boundaries and maintain distance. Physicians and the medical institutions within which they worked were not immune to such impulses. Six years into the epidemic, a spate of reports began to appear in the media detailing the decisions of a number of doctors not to treat AIDS patients. In Milwaukee, a surgeon stated bluntly, "I've got to be selfish. It's an incurable disease that's uniformly fatal, and I'm constantly at risk for getting it. I've got to think about myself. I've got to think about my family. That responsibility is greater than to the patient."[1] In New Jersey, a heart surgeon went further, asserting that doctors had a duty to those with whom they worked *not* to operate on people infected with HIV because it would expose colleagues to an unacceptable risk. For him the choice was "not a matter of medical ethics or irrational fear" but an appropriate response to the danger of blood-borne contamination.[2]

These statements, which so boldly rejected conventional assumptions about the duty of doctors to the sick, were all the more striking because they were made publicly, without shame. They suggested a rupture of the moral ties that bound healers to those who needed them. And, of course, such candid rejections of the duty to treat represented but the tip of the iceberg. There were many who said privately what a small number would say publicly, many who acted with stealth, without giving voice to their decisions.

Surveys of doctors, residents, and medical students showed the breadth of this response to AIDS. In the mid- and late 1980s, substantial numbers of physicians indicated that they believed they had no ethical obligation to care for patients with HIV infection.[3] A study of primary care practitioners found that half would not care for such patients if given a choice.[4] As late as 1990, a national survey of doctors revealed that only 24 percent believed that office-based practitioners should be legally required to provide care to individuals with HIV infection.[5]

This was not, however, the first occasion when doctors had turned their backs on the sick. The history of medicine is punctuated with accounts of refusals to treat patients in times of epidemic. Three centuries before AIDS, in *Journal of the Plague Year*, Daniel Defoe recorded the antagonism felt for fleeing physicians during an outbreak in London: "Great was the reproach thrown on those physicians who left their patients during the sickness—they were called deserters."[6] There were, of course, others—those who stayed behind to face the risks. In the mid-20th century, there was a special ward at New York's Bellevue Hospital for doctors who had contracted tuberculosis, largely from their patients.

This book is about American doctors who chose to care for patients with AIDS. They came to the new disease for a host of reasons: shared sexual orientation with their gay patients, a political commitment to providing care to the despised, a deep interest in the mysteries of infectious disease, the desire to confront and tame an awful natural threat. But whatever drew these doctors to AIDS, they had to respond to a set of profound challenges. Trained to cure and imbued with an ethos of medical optimism, they had to acknowledge their own therapeutic impotence in the 1980s. Protected from the contagions that had routinely threatened doctors in an earlier era, they had to confront their own fears of an unknown infectious agent. Unaccustomed to witnessing the death of patients before old age, they encountered death in patients often no older than they were. It was in that context that they met and came to know patients who were often despised because of their sexuality, their drug use, their race, or their class.

As they forged identities in the face of the AIDS epidemic, doctors found their professional lives transformed. Some were compelled to deal with the stigma their patients bore, the anger and indifference of colleagues and hospital authorities. Others discovered success and precocious fame. Often their private lives were touched in remarkable ways. The AIDS epidemic had taken hold, making these doctors witness to a public passion that would mark the last two decades of the 20th century.

Our decision to write this book was made in the early 1990s. Three physicians invited to a meeting sponsored by the Centers for Disease Control (CDC) in Atlanta—one of the innumerable sessions that punctuated the lives of AIDS doctors—shared a dinner and began to reminisce about their lives as AIDS doctors, about how they had been yanked from the routines of medicine when the epidemic emerged. Gradually, the conversation shifted from the professional to the personal. Sometimes with levity, sometimes darkly, they spoke about how AIDS work had affected their relationships to their wives and their children, had changed them in ways big and small. Their tales—like war stories exchanged by soldiers—were at once vibrant and idiosyncratic. As that conversation among professional friends unfolded (prodded along by one of us), it became clear that their stories reflected dimensions of the epidemic's history that had been left untold.

These colleagues and those like them would write a great deal, as their scientific and clinical commitments required. But most would never write about themselves, about how those epidemiological events had so shaped their lives. Certainly, they would never write with the candor they showed when speaking. We wanted to capture the vividness and emotion of their oral accounts.

But why, we have been asked, a book only about doctors? After all, there have been others—nurses, social workers, counselors—who have cared for patients with AIDS and who might have provided perspectives every bit as critical to understanding what it was to be a caregiver in the epidemic's midst. We believe they deserve an analysis of their own experience of the epidemic. But the question posed to us also reflects, at least in part, an antagonism to the current dominance of physicians in the provision of health care, a fear that focusing on doctors and the challenges they faced could only serve to bolster the status of those already too powerful, at the expense of others.

In a review of Margaret Edson's *W;t*, an emotionally riveting play about an English professor dying of ovarian cancer, Abigail Zuger, a doctor in this volume, wrote in the *New York Times*, "Sixty years ago Paul Muni, as Louis Pasteur, and Ronald Colman, as the fictionalized Arrowsmith, thrilled and inspired their audiences. Now the pendulum has swung round: It is patients who are the heroes while doctors have receded into sketchy caricatures, like the foolish depraved medics Molière created three centuries ago."[7] We were interested in neither romanticized depiction nor caricature but in the possibility of understanding the complex response of doctors faced by a fierce threat to the public health and the lives of their patients. By restricting our attention to doctors, we thought we would be best positioned to see them at both their most heroic and less exalted moments, as they struggled to understand an emerging medical threat for which they were utterly unprepared and which challenged their very understanding of what it was to be a doctor. We believed that our focus would open up the possibility of seeing doctors as varied, as differing even while faced with a common enemy. Professional training, ethnicity, gender, and sexual orientation each shaped their responses. Warts and all, these physicians were, as Abigail Zuger notes of the physicians in *W;t*, "rooting" for their patients. It was just that they had no choice, as one doctor told us, but to root for a team that always lost.

A few doctors have written biographical accounts of their professional lives. When they have done so, they most typically have written about their patients. The best of such efforts have permitted those patients to come to life for the nonprofessional reader and have often revealed something about the doctors as well, but almost always in the interstices of the patients' stories. Those AIDS doctors who have written about their experiences, have largely followed the same pattern. Abraham Verghese's *My Own Country*[8] and Peter Selwyn's *Surviving the Fall*[9] tell frankly personal stories of their authors' encounters with the AIDS epidemic, but they are exceptions. Other books, like Daniel Baxter's *The Least of These, My Brethren*,[10] Jerome Groopman's *The Measure of Our Days*,[11] and Abigail Zuger's *Strong Shadows*,[12] adhere to the tradition of focusing on patients. Our goal in this volume was to move doctors' lives to the foreground, where their fears, hopes, disappointments, needs, and experiences could be viewed directly. We wanted our work to serve as a collective memoir, a biography in which the lives of the first generation of AIDS doctors would emerge. Ultimately, we believed that our goals could best be served by embarking on the creation of an oral history archive of doctors and AIDS. (A brief methodological note on the creation of the oral history archive is found in Appendix 1.) Our book could then draw on the record of memories thus collected.

Who were the doctors whose memories form the heart of this book? We interviewed 76 doctors, all of whom had been involved in caring for AIDS patients since the earliest years of the epidemic. (Brief biographies of these physicians are provided in Appendix 2.) They came primarily from the two coasts, where AIDS first exploded. Thirty-nine were from New York, Newark, Boston, Washington, and Baltimore. Twenty were from the San Francisco Bay area and Los Angeles. The remainder came from Miami, Atlanta, Cleveland, Chicago, Seattle, Las Vegas, Rochester, Austin, and Houston. They were strikingly young. While a few had long-established careers by the time of the AIDS epidemic, many others were just completing their medical education and training. Sixty percent were younger than 35 in 1981, the epidemic's first year. Like most physicians, those we interviewed were overwhelmingly—90 percent—white. Just less than half were Jewish. Unlike physicians in general, the AIDS doctors included a significant number of women—3 in 10—and a dramatic representation of gay men and lesbians—about 40 percent. Of the 22 office-based doctors, all but seven were gay or lesbian with primarily gay practices.

What doctors could offer varied with their experiences and personalities. Most wanted the interviews to work. After all, here was an opportunity to preserve for posterity their own understanding of what had happened in the AIDS epidemic, to make their unique contributions known. A few regretted, at first, agreeing to be interviewed, only to become thoroughly involved in the process. A very few, although submitting to the interview, were begrudging of the questions allowed and of the information shared. But all physicians, in addition to their professional knowledge, brought personal conceptions of the history of AIDS infused with their memories and emotions, along with an autobiographical sense of self.

We did not undertake this project—the creation of an oral archive and the writing of this book—primarily to gather additional facts about the epidemic's history. Our central aim was to use the oral narrative to do what it does best: to tap each speaker's subjective sense of events and to elicit the *meaning* that he or she found in them. Seventy-six narratives provided us with a spectrum of meanings regarding discrete moments, such as the discovery of AZT, the first antiretroviral drug, as well as the long saga of therapeutic impotence. These narratives came from doctors whose names are known internationally as well as from others known only within the communities in which they practiced. A few came from those known only to their patients. We wove these voices with our own into a tapestry, creating a textured account of the epidemic years.

We are reminded by Alessandro Portelli, a prominent Italian oral historian, that "oral sources tell us not just what people did, but what they wanted to do, what they believed they were doing, and what they now think they did."[13] In their interviews, the doctors reflected on an epidemic that powerfully churned established medical expectations and values, and on their continuous struggle to come to terms with what happened during the tumultuous AIDS era of the 1980s and 1990s. They recalled how the meanings they imputed to past events altered over time as new experiences pressed themselves onto their consciousness and as they themselves gained in knowledge, authority, and years. Capturing these changing outlooks and meanings is at the heart of our interviews. It is also central to the oral history enterprise. How to treat these evocative memories of and reflections on the experience of AIDS was an issue to which we turned as we thought about the writing of this book.

Initially we envisioned that the book would, in a conventional way, provide an account of doctors and AIDS, citing portions of our interviews in the same way that we might quote from published texts and other documentary material. But as we reviewed the transcripts of our encounters, as we recalled the extraordinary experience of listening to those with whom we met, it became clear to us that the book we wanted to compile had to be different. While we decided to impose a narrative structure on the text, pride of place would be given over to the voices of those we had interviewed.

On the last page of *The Plague*, Albert Camus's allegory of the city of Oran's encounter with bubonic plague, Dr. Bernard Rieux, his central figure, resolves to compile a chronicle so that he should not be one of those who held their peace but should bear witness in favor of those plague-stricken people and of . . . all who, while unable to be saints, but refusing to bow down to pestilence, strive their utmost to be healers.[14]

In undertaking to create an oral history archive and then to write this book, we too became witnesses, not only to the suffering of those who were affected by AIDS but to the efforts of those who sought to care for them as well. When we began our work, we both believed that a stance of critical distance was essential if we were to preserve the objectivity so important to careful social and historical analysis. But as we conducted our interviews—and experienced what felt like an extraordinary privilege of having those with whom we met open their lives to us—we found ourselves drawn closer to the AIDS doctors than we had anticipated. As we read and reread the transcripts of our interviews, we reexperienced a sense of deep respect and even affection for those who had talked with us about their lives in the epidemic. In a way, then, like Camus's Dr. Rieux, we had learned that "in a time of pestilence . . . there are more things to admire in men than to despise." If we lost some distance, we gained from a sense of immediacy.

Our account is not, however, a hagiography; the doctors brought together for this book are, after all, healers, not saints. Some are selfless, others self-serving. Yet, whatever they brought to AIDS, what is so striking is that their ordinary lives were transformed, became bigger, precisely because of their involvement with a medical challenge none could ever have imagined. Their accounts touch us deeply just because they are so human and say so much about suffering, despair, hope, and courage. At a moment when medicine is in the throes of a profound transformation, dominated by a relentless drive for efficiency and profit, when huge bureaucratic enterprises increasingly intrude into clinical practice, recounting the stories of doctors and AIDS captures an enduring dimension of the human encounter with disease.

1
DISCOVERY AND COMMITMENT

In the period October 1980–May 1981, 5 young
men, all active homosexuals, were treated for
biopsy-confirmed *Pneumocystis carinii* pneumonia
at 3 different hospitals in Los Angeles, California.
Two of the patients died. . . . *Pneumocystis* pneumonia in the United States is almost exclusively
limited to severely immunosuppressed patients.
The occurrence of *Pneumocystis* in these 5 previously healthy individuals without a clinically apparent underlying immunodeficiency is unusual.
The fact that these patients were all homosexuals suggests an association between some aspect
of a homosexual lifestyle or disease acquired
through sexual contact and *Pneumocystis* pneumonia in this population.

Morbidity and Mortality Weekly Report,
June 5, 1981

First Cases

Epidemics do not announce themselves but enter on cat's paws. The first
cases came before the official start of the AIDS epidemic in June 1981,
before the new disease had a name. They came in the form of strange,
inexplicable, and untreatable conditions in young men, women, and children. These initial encounters, in the late 1970s, left physicians perplexed, sometimes disturbed. Only gradually, as they told their colleagues
about what they had seen and began to hear about other cases, did the
realization begin to take hold that something unusual and worrisome
was occurring.

Donna Mildvan, chief of Infectious Disease at Beth Israel Hospital on Manhattan's Lower East Side, had been studying sexually transmitted intestinal infections in gay men since the mid-1970s. Her initial interest in the subject was piqued by an unusual, puzzling case of protozoal infection, "unheard of" in a patient with no travel history. She and her colleague Dan William, a gay physician working on sexually transmitted diseases at New York City's Department of Health, assembled a cohort of sexually active gay men to study enteric diseases. In the late 1970s, Mildvan noticed lymphadenopathy or swollen lymph glands in a number of them. Neither she nor other doctors she consulted could make a diagnosis. Lymph node biopsies came back negative. Here was another medical mystery, one that Mildvan set aside for want of sufficient data. In 1980, an event occurred that only heightened her perplexity.

In June of 1980 a German patient was admitted to Beth Israel. He'd been a chef in Haiti for three years. Of course, nobody at the time understood the significance of that, least of all myself. He came in with bloody diarrhea and a low white blood count. Then he was in and out of the hospital with the stormiest, most chronic, most perplexing course that one can imagine. We treated him with steroids, and both the bloody diarrhea and white count responded. We thought he had Crohn's disease or maybe ulcerative colitis. But then all his symptoms recurred in three weeks, and he developed salmonella. Now we thought he had gay bowel syndrome. Every week he had a new diagnosis, because every week he was back in the hospital with something new. I had exhausted all the diagnoses on my list. So it meant that my list was too short, and I had to spend more time in the library. I spent his entire course in the library.

Then he developed encephalitis, an extremely rare complication. He started to become cognitively impaired and began losing vision in one eye. Routine cultures were negative. Finally, a colleague, Dr. Usha Mathur, suggested we culture his eye fluid for viruses. This was unheard of in those days. So we got the ophthalmologists to biopsy the patient's vitreous and sent the specimen to Dr. Ilya Spigland's virology laboratory at Montefiore. Six weeks later, lo and behold, it grew out cytomegalovirus. What on earth was this? Back to the library! There may have been two reports in severely immunocompromised patients of cytomegalovirus retinitis, but they had all grown at autopsy. This was the first case where the virus grew from the eye *during life*. We were totally bewildered. Why should he have this? What do you do for it? There was no treatment. We tried a few drugs, but nothing changed.

He died in December. I can't even begin to tell you what an awful experience it was. You don't lose a 33-year-old patient. We agonized over it. Agonized over it all the time.

Two weeks later, a nurse was admitted to Beth Israel with an aggressive case of *Pneumocystis carinii* pneumonia (PCP), a condition known to be associated with a compromised immune system. He died soon after; an autopsy showed that he was infected with cytomegalovirus.

After the second case, there was no question in anybody's mind. This was a new disease. It was in gay men. This was the fatal form of it. We had just seen two people die. The lymphadenopathy was the early stage of it. Just like that, it all came together in a flash.

In January 1981, Mildvan met with Dan William to share her suspicions. He responded by informing her of devastating news:

"Donna, you're not going to believe what I have to tell you. Three patients of mine have Kaposi's sarcoma. Gay men. For no reason." And that, too, is a disease of immunocompromise. All the color drained from his face, and we were both speechless. We really saw the whole thing written out before us. We couldn't have dreamt that it would be of these proportions. But we knew we were scared. We were really scared.

In the same month, Dr. Alvin Friedman-Kien, already a well-established dermatologist and virologist at New York University's Medical Center, examined a gay man whose diagnosis had eluded physicians at another local hospital. The results of the patient's laboratory tests were entirely contrary to Friedman-Kien's experience and expectations.

He had enlarged lymph nodes, he had fever, weight loss, large spleen; and incidentally he had some brownish purple spots on his lower extremities which were ignored by all the physicians who were taking care of him. They removed his spleen, did lymph node biopsies and liver biopsies with no finalized diagnosis. And he was discharged; but he said to me, when he finally came to see me, "nobody would look at my feet, at this rash on my feet." They were faint, they were purple-lavender, they looked like bruises. In any case, I did a biopsy and quite surprisingly it came back as Kaposi's sarcoma. . . . It didn't look typical, because prior to that man I had only seen maybe seven or eight cases of classical Kaposi's sarcoma, usually in elderly men of Eastern European or Mediterranean origin, mostly Eastern European Jews from Russia, and they developed their disease in the fifth or sixth decade of life. They had purple sores on the lower extremities and the longevity was 10 to 15 years. Most of these men would die of causes other than KS. But then, not two weeks later, I saw another man, an actor, who was perfectly healthy and he just had pink-purple spots on his face, and he couldn't cover them up with makeup anymore.

Kaposi's sarcoma (KS), a cancer of the walls of blood vessels, is a rare disease in the United States. To see two new cases within two weeks was very unusual. To find the disease, typically seen in the elderly, in two young men was more than unusual. It required investigation. Friedman-Kien contacted colleagues and a newly formed group of gay doctors who treated gay men, Physicians for Human Rights, inquiring if any of its members had patients with Kaposi's sarcoma. Within four weeks, he knew of 20 cases in the New York City area. A call to Marcus Conant, a dermatologist in San Francisco, who was to become a national figure in the fight against AIDS, eventually alerted him to six more cases, all gay men. Friedman-Kien also phoned the Centers for Disease Control (CDC), telling them, "I had all these gay men who had Kaposi's sarcoma, and many of them had amebiases or giardia [the gay bowel syndrome], and perhaps this is due to that." He also began to plan an article on his Kaposi's sarcoma cases for *Morbidity and Mortality Weekly Report*, the then little-known publication of the Centers for Disease Control.

Marcus Conant had been disturbed and mystified by Friedman-Kien's call. Conant was a dermatologist with a large private practice and a strong research and clinical interest in genital herpes. A long-time resident of the Castro, the city's gay district, he was concerned about diseases that affected his community. He had already been informed that one of his former residents had a gay patient in his mid-30s with Kaposi's sarcoma.

[It was a case of] Kaposi's sarcoma of the mouth. Now Kaposi's sarcoma in those days, in 1981, was so rare that the average dermatologist was expected to diagnose one case in his career, okay? It was the kind of thing that you saw at a meeting. It was so rare that the average dermatologist [only] read about it.

Joyce Wallace, a doctor in private practice in Greenwich Village, was caught short when she heard a diagnosis of Kaposi's sarcoma for the first time. "Kaposi's sarcoma? What's that?"

A day after his conversation with Alvin Friedman-Kien, Conant, as scheduled, gave grand rounds at the medical school of the University of California, San Francisco (UCSF).

[I] reviewed not only herpes simplex, but all the different herpes viruses that were known, and when I reviewed cytomegalovirus and [the] hypothesis that it was the cause of Kaposi's sarcoma in Africa, I mentioned the cases that were being seen in San Francisco and New York. Marion Salzberger (who was the dean of American dermatology at that time) said: "This is not some new manifestation of an old disease. Homosexuality has been here for at least as long as Alexander the Great, and we haven't seen this before. What you're seeing is a new disease." And, as fate would have it, he was absolutely correct. But what happened immediately was other doctors in the community started saying, "Wait, I've got one of these cases too," and within a week or two, we started getting phone calls from doctors who had a case in their practice.

As the first cases began to appear, it was not always apparent to clinicians that a complaint or symptom was indicative of something graver. The new disease was difficult to diagnose. Stephen Follansbee, a young infectious disease fellow in San Francisco, witnessed a patient demand a hospital admission while around him clinicians could not appreciate the seriousness of his malady.

There was a patient at UCSF who got admitted to the hospital because he threw a temper tantrum in the hallway of the gastroenterology clinic. He said, "I'm sick. I need to be in the hospital," and didn't feel he was being listened to, and so basically lay down and pounded the floor, and they admitted him; and as part of his workup for diarrhea [he] had a chest X ray, which showed pneumonia and went on to being diagnosed, after open lung surgery, to have *Pneumocystis*. And one of the pulmonary fellows said to me, "You know, there are some people in New York who are seeing this also."

It was the uncertainty about what symptoms might mean and their implications for particular patients that provided the context for the set

15

of seemingly bizarre instructions given to Abigail Zuger, who had just graduated from medical school and was beginning her residency at New York's Bellevue Hospital.

I admitted a guy with pneumonia in the middle of the night. He was very sick and breathing quickly. And I was very tired. My resident, who was keeping an eye on me, said that I had to wheel him over for a very, very good chest X ray, because he was an unmarried man and there was some kind of pneumonia going around among unmarried men. I thought, "This is it; she's finally cracked! I have to get out of here. These people are crazy." She didn't know PCP, or if she did she couldn't think of the name. But that was clearly on her mind, and I wheeled the guy over for an X ray.

But *Pneumocystis* pneumonia and Kaposi's sarcoma, terrible as they were, were not the only manifestations of the new disease. They were often accompanied by other illnesses, also difficult to diagnose but devastating in their consequences. Constance Wofsy, who would help to shape the AIDS program at San Francisco General Hospital, was completing the last year of an infectious disease fellowship at the hospital when she saw her first AIDS case in March 1981. For her, there was the striking realization that in treating *Pneumocystis* pneumonia, she had missed the presence of an infection in the brain.

[My] first experience was a 24-year-old gay white man who was in the neurology service for a brain tumor, and he'd had two biopsies without confirming the diagnosis. [He] developed a pneumonia after about three weeks in the hospital, ultimately got a bronchoscopy, and I remember that the pathology department hadn't done a stain for *Pneumocystis* in so many years that they had to sort of reconstruct it. So they did a silver stain and found that he had *Pneumocystis*. The patient was discharged from the hospital. I called [him] about four months later; he had stopped taking his treatment for *Pneumocystis,* as he would have at the end of three or four weeks, and his brain lesions had come back. It's an embarrassment now, but he had toxoplasmosis in his brain. He'd always had [it], and it's astounding to think how many specialties and studies he went through without anyone considering toxoplasmosis in his brain. I think he died about nine months later.

In Los Angeles, Jerome Groopman's first case was a young man whose pneumonia was accompanied by a ravaging herpes infection, at that time difficult to contain and treat.

[He] was known as Queenie, because he called himself Queenie. He was a very sad person, probably 18 years old. He was a street prostitute with bleached blond hair. He was found to have *Pneumocystis*. He then developed a severe invasive perianal herpes simplex which was so aggressive and so hard to control that it required surgical intervention. So the surgeons were going in there, chopping away large chunks of his buttocks and thighs. It was really gruesome. And ultimately he died.

Donald Abrams, who had joined Marcus Conant at the Kaposi's Sarcoma Clinic that Conant had established at the University of California, San Francisco, was similarly stymied by this new disease.

One of my patients developed this awful diarrhea that was like nothing I'd ever seen. We kept on looking in his stools for an organism, and there was nothing there. Then somebody came up to me from Pathology or Microbiology and said, "Your patient has cryptosporidium." And I said, "What's that?" And they said, "It's an animal parasite."

For Donald Kotler, a gastroenterologist at St. Luke's Hospital on the edge of Harlem, severe diarrhea in a gay man who was wasting away before his eyes only took on clinical meaning once the patient developed *Pneumocystis* as well.

A consult [came] out of nowhere from a person whom I know, and why he would have called me for this case I don't know. He was a 37-year-old man, the assistant principal of a school for troubled children, with bad diarrhea and lots of weight loss. I did an incredibly intensive workup, sort of gave it the best of 1981 medicine and came up with bizarre stuff—like a small intestine that looked like a tropical stew, that looked like diffuse intestinal damage. . . . It turns out he was from Seattle, and his mother was friends with a very famous gastroenterologist, Sy Rubin, went to the same *schul*. It was a bad GI problem, bad nutritional problem, and then *Pneumocystis* pneumonia. And it was only after we diagnosed the *Pneu-*

mocystis pneumonia that a colleague came to me and said that he'd been hearing about some disease going on in California, something going on in New York, that in fact it was in the gay community, and it could turn out to be something really bad.

Recognizing an Epidemic

Although cases of *Pneumocystis* had begun to appear on both coasts, it fell to Michael Gottlieb, a 33-year-old immunologist at UCLA, to bring together the first series that would, when published, mark the official start of the epidemic. In December 1980, as a recently hired assistant professor, Gottlieb was informed by one of his immunology fellows about a gay man with thrush and a low white blood count. Gottlieb immediately detected that "there was something medically interesting about him. He *smelled* like an immune deficiency. You don't get a mouth full of candida without being immune deficient." The man's disclosure of his homosexuality also impressed Gottlieb. "He was on the telephone to a friend one day when we were in the room, and he said to his friend, sort of in jest, 'Hey, yeah, Bruce, the doctors here tell me I am one sick queen!' And we all chuckled because we had very minimal knowledge of the gay community. We weren't familiar with this kind of self-deprecating humor."

On returning from the patient's room, Gottlieb encountered a colleague who was "beginning to fool around with some of the antibodies to T-cell subsets which had just become available as a research tool." At his suggestion, they examined the patient's blood "and found that this man's T-cells were all messed up, that he had virtually no helper T-cells—CD4 cells—and that his CD8 cells, the suppressor cells, were very high."

Soon thereafter, Gottlieb received a call from the chief of rheumatology at Wadsworth VA Hospital in West Los Angeles. He had examined a couple of very sick men, sent to him by Joel Weisman and his colleague, gay physicians with a largely gay practice. Having heard about Gottlieb's patient, he believed that "something interesting" was occurring and wanted to arrange a meeting. Weisman and his partner had already begun to notice unusual diseases in their patients by 1979.

When you go from relatively healthy people with single system disease—somebody would come in with gonorrhea or diarrhea— [to] seeing multisystem problems, the lymphadenopathies with the fevers, with the funguses, with the rashes [it is striking]. My belief was that you don't have a whole group of people go from having a few problems to a lot of problems. It scared me and I don't scare that easily.

By October 1980, Weisman and his partner had two patients who were very sick with similar conditions: chronic fevers, swollen lymph nodes, diarrhea, and thrush. After Gottlieb and Weisman met in January 1981, Gottlieb tested the T-cells of Weisman's patients and "found the same, now typical, abnormality."

Gottlieb soon had a fourth and a fifth case, all gay men. The fourth case came to Gottlieb through a former student, who was now the CDC Epidemic Intelligence Officer in Los Angeles. Michael Gottlieb phoned him to warn him:

"Something's up. It's in gay men and I think it may have something to do with cytomegalovirus; why don't you see what you can find out?" He said, "Yeah, I'll get right on it." And he went up to the sixth floor of the county health department building, and there was an isolate of cytomegalovirus growing in culture that had been taken from an autopsy of a young man. He decided to look into the case. And he called me the next day and said, "I've reviewed the record. The case is a little more complicated in that the patient had Hodgkin's Disease 10 years ago and gotten radiation therapy. That might be a predisposing factor for immune deficiency, but he was also gay and he had *Pneumocystis.*"

Ultimately, all the cases developed *Pneumocystis carinii* pneumonia. The final case, case number five, came from a Beverly Hills internist who had heard about Gottlieb's experience. Soon thereafter, Gottlieb and the CDC officer began to write up their cases.

[We] met in his apartment and we sat down and we sketched out what became the *Morbidity and Mortality Weekly Report* (*MMWR*) of June 5, 1981 that reported five patients, all gay men, and it was called "*Pneumocystis* Pneumonia, Los Angeles."

But what was to become a landmark report went largely unnoticed. Carol Brosgart, a public health doctor in Oakland, California, recalled reading about the five young men and asking herself, What's the malignancy? What's going on here? This is incredible. Probably more representative were the remarks of Neil Schram, a kidney specialist in Los Angeles who would become an AIDS treater and political activist:

> Understand, most physicians were absolutely disconnected from the *MMWR*. That was a publication that the CDC put out for the public health people. I had never heard of the CDC; I'd never heard of public health doctors.

His remarks were echoed by Stosh Ostrow, a physician in private practice in Atlanta, who observed, "I wasn't reading the *MMWR* back then; who read the *MMWR*?"

Like physicians, most of the press failed to pick up the *MMWR* story. Two West Coast papers, the *Los Angeles Times* and the *San Francisco Chronicle*, and the Associated Press ran short pieces on the CDC's report. Only when a second *MMWR* appeared on July 3—Alvin Friedman-Kien's description of Kaposi's sarcoma in 26 gay men in New York City and California—was media interest aroused. National Public Radio, the Cable News Network, and the Associated Press ran stories; so did the *New York Times,* with a column-long article headlined "Rare Cancer Seen in 41 Homosexuals." The next day, July 4, 1981, the *Washington Post* followed suit.[1]

At New York Hospital/Cornell Medical Center, an oncologist interested in viral causes of cancer and viral immunology recalled Gottlieb's article in the *MMWR*, then noted the almost complete absence of press coverage in its wake. On vacation in Maine, Jeffrey Laurence read the July 3 *New York Times* report on Kaposi's sarcoma and thought, "God, now it's come out." Returning to Manhattan the following day, he began to field calls from gay friends worried about the new gay cancer.

Epidemic Fears

The official early history of AIDS could be told with the headlines of five articles in *Morbidity and Mortality Weekly Report* that appeared subsequent to those published in June and July 1981:

- July 9, 1982. Opportunistic Infections and Kaposi's Sarcoma Among Haitians in the United States.[2]
- July 16, 1982. *Pneumocystis Carinii* Pneumonia Among Persons with Hemophilia A.[3]

- December 10, 1982. Possible Transfusion Acquired Immune Deficiency Syndrome (AIDS)—California.[4]
- December 17, 1982. Unexplained Immunodeficiency and Opportunistic Infections in Infants.[5]
- January 7, 1983. Immunodeficiency Among Female Sexual Partners of Males with Acquired Immune Deficiency Syndrome (AIDS)—New York.[6]

In that 18-month period, the contours of the epidemic as a sexually transmitted, blood-borne disease were made clear, although the extent of infection in the gay and drug-using population would not be known until the viral agent responsible for AIDS was discovered and a blood test developed.

But the landmark reports in *MMWR* tell only the public part of the story; they do not capture the extent to which those who first encountered patients with AIDS struggled with the epidemiological significance of their clinical experiences, or the extent to which their growing fears of a potentially catastrophic spread of the new disease met with resistance from colleagues. Even those who would commit themselves to AIDS work had no reason to believe initially that a grim clinical picture would produce a grave social burden.

Treating patients with Kaposi's sarcoma in Los Angeles, Jerome Groopman thought, "This was possibly just an isolated occurrence in certain areas and would probably be a relatively unusual disease." Never having seen an AIDS patient, Neil Schram heard about the new disease at a conference organized by the gay doctors' organization, Bay Area Physicians for Human Rights (BAPHR): "I remember thinking, That's peculiar. It can't mean anything." Fourteen years later, recalling that period, Schram noted sardonically: "I was insightful at the time." Even as late as 1984, when many had become seized with anxiety, infectious disease specialist Stephen Follansbee recalled:

I think there was certainly the idea that this was a flash in the pan, that this was going to come and go and would die out. I can remember sometime around '83, maybe '84, when we thought actually that cases were dropping off. . . . So therefore this was dying out, and that this was some sort of an epidemic phenomenon that is reproducible in other epidemics where the most vulnerable people get it and die and everyone else develops immunity. That little window of optimism didn't last long.

An error in clinical judgment by many hemophilia specialists had tragic significance for those with bleeding disorders and profound professional consequences for those who had treated them with clotting factor. Margaret Hilgartner, a pioneer who had helped to usher in what some had called "the golden years" of hemophilia treatment, recalled the early response to the first reports of AIDS in those with hemophilia A, the severest form of the disorder:

> Even though this might be the same disease that the gays had, the discussion kept coming into the conversation: Was this going to be like hepatitis? Because if we had 72 percent [infected with hepatitis B], and some clinics had even higher percentages and were surviving, would these patients then survive? Was it going to be as lethal? And if it wasn't going to be lethal like it appeared to be in the gays, did we really have to inform the patients to the same degree and worry about them?

The reluctance to acknowledge the extent to which AIDS would take on epidemic proportions was not unique to the world of hemophilia. Those who already believed that a menacing new disease was taking hold faced what, from the perspective of a few short years later, would seem like sheer blindness. Donna Mildvan, who acknowledged her own failure to recognize AIDS in an intravenous drug user because he wasn't gay, was nevertheless troubled by the resistance she witnessed.

> Everybody was resistant in stages . . . or maybe believed it and couldn't deal with it. I don't know. But it was like nothing was going away; nothing was untrue of our worst fears, and they were just growing, because there would be new fears and new implications, and new populations were getting drawn into this to the point that it had gotten very very awful. . . . The reality was a lot worse than anybody would have ever dreamt.

Dan William, who had worked with Mildvan, was especially concerned about the extent to which the new disease would spread among gay men.

> The anxiety of those early years was palpable. It was very, very much greater than you can describe, because people like Donna and myself, and I think other physicians recognized the potential for the devastation that eventually could ensue. . . . I had very

strong feelings about it, and many people didn't want to believe it. If you listen to Jim Curran [head of the CDC's AIDS Program] in the early days of the epidemic, he always used to end on an optimistic basis, that epidemics come, and they go, so we may be at the peak, we may not; maybe this is just a little quirk. Keep calm, and don't be too upset. It was beyond frightening. . . . Realizing early on that this is probably sexually transmitted, that it's sexually transmitted the same way as hepatitis B, that the prevalence of hepatitis B in the gay community [may be 40 percent], and the end result is death or disability, you're talking about a major disaster. . . . History is full of situations like AIDS; it's really not unique. I mean it's our own holocaust. . . . And [in] every holocaust there were warnings. There was Crystal Night in Germany.

For many gay men, a lifestyle involving the broad acceptance of multiple sexual partners and the thrill of sexual abandon was part of a precious and newly won freedom. To be told this freedom was implicated in a life-threatening disease was especially disturbing, even oppressive. To counsel restraint was tantamount to a rejection of their liberation. In looking back to the first years of the AIDS epidemic, William Owen, a founding member of the gay doctors organization, BAPHR, was especially concerned to place gay anxieties in historical perspective and to provide a justification for those who were circumspect in their warnings about sex.

It's very easy to look through the retrospectoscope, but the fact of the matter is that this was a group of people who for many years had been repressed in terms of their sexuality. And for the first time in the mid-'70s and after Stonewall in '69, with the dawning of the gay revolution, people really felt the ability to express themselves sexually, like they couldn't do before; and in some ways it's like a kid in a candy store. They suddenly had the ability to do something that they were previously restricted from doing; so sometimes they go a little bit too far and have too many contacts. . . . Basically the kind of diseases that we saw people coming in for were essentially treatable diseases. The gonorrhea was treatable; syphilis was treatable. Giardiasis, shigella infections, they were all treatable things. If doctors were to have come out then [by warning about the dangers of an exuberant sexuality], they would have been seen as some sort of fringe element aligned with either the church or the state or the psychiatric profession, all of whom were not held in very high esteem. And so I think our voices would not have been listened to anyway.

While BAPHR did ultimately issue guidelines on sexual risk reduction in 1983, the reaction of many to those who sought to sound the tocsin was dismay. As an openly gay physician, Dan William was especially troubled.

I can remember very vividly; I was scared and anxious and afraid. Not for my own personal safety but for the health of the community. And 95 percent of people were pooh-poohing it. . . . Any kind of intrusion on sexual behavior was looked at as an intrusion upon one's gayness, and that got in the way. And in those early years . . . I got into a little bit of hot water with the community for implying that people had to consider making changes and altering behavior to lessen the probability of transmission of this illness which we did not understand at all.

Joseph Sonnabend, whose professional work had involved caring for gay men in New York and who had been especially concerned with sexually transmitted diseases (STDs), suspected that AIDS was the consequence of an immunologic overload, of too many STDs. Although he was skeptical of the notion of contagion, his thesis led to the same behavioral recommendation: radically reduced sexual exposure. The reaction to his urgings was often dismissive. Fifteen years later, he still evidenced a kind of sad perplexity. "I thought I was being of help, but . . . I was being vilified. [I] didn't understand it."

It was the same for Larry Drew in San Francisco, who had been invited to speak in early 1983 by Lea Belli, the wife of attorney Melvin Belli, at their home.

They had a monstrous house on Pacific Avenue, probably the biggest house I'd ever been in, and they devoted the entire upper floor to basically an auditorium, and [I] and three or four others spoke to the group. These were all gay men. [I said] that it was transmissible; that the bathhouse lifestyle was liable to be very important in the transmission. . . . You would have hoped that the reaction was, "Well, gee, thanks for coming and helping us understand this," but the reaction [was], "You're just trying to take away the one recreational activity that we have. You guys all have your golf clubs and tennis clubs, and what have you, and we have the bathhouses. It's just a plot by the straights to screw us again."

But it wasn't just the nonphysician members of the gay community who found the cautionary messages of risk reduction in the face of AIDS difficult to accept. So too did some gay doctors. Even as some like Dan William struggled to convey a message of caution, others continued to embrace denial. Stosh Ostrow describes what may have been the first national conference on AIDS in 1983, a meeting sponsored by the American Association of Physicians for Human Rights and the National Gay and Lesbian Health Education Fund. It was, he recalls, a "horrible meeting."

> The physicians were conservative; the others very radical. We were talking about this disease and lack of government response and blah, blah, blah, and Bernice Goodman got up and said it was a CIA plot to kill the homosexuals. . . . And it was very, very strange, now looking back on it, that we were talking about this disease that was killing people, and [we] knew at that point that it was sexually transmitted but didn't clearly know that we had a responsibility to behave differently. I can remember having sex with another physician there and using Phisohex as a lubricant, thinking, well, it's antibacterial, maybe it'll help. Never considered the idea of a condom.

The focus on gay men made it difficult to recognize that AIDS was also occurring in men who were not exclusively homosexual. In Oakland, California, just across the bay from San Francisco, where the epidemic was taking hold among gay men, Carol Brosgart's first case at a public health clinic for sexually transmitted diseases was bisexual.

> He was a young Black man who said he was bisexual. He was quite poor; he was clearly a prostitute and very open about that. He looked like he had bunches of grapes in each groin and up in the neck and under the arms, just massive lymphadenopathy. The oncologist at the time at the county hospital was very homophobic, so I finally got the surgical resident to do a biopsy on him. And I remember getting a call, and he said, "This is so weird; we got the biopsy results back. The pathologist says it's something called Kaposi's sarcoma." And right after the first report was the second re-

port of KS in the 26 men in New York, San Francisco, and Los Angeles. He said, "But it's so weird, because it's like this gay cancer." And I go, "But Steve, he's bisexual," and he says, "Yeah, but this is only in gay men!" He understood there was this new problem, but it had to be in gay men.

In the Bronx, in the summer of 1981, Gerald Friedland, an infectious disease doctor who had recently arrived from Harvard, was asked to consult on three cases, all young men admitted to Montefiore Hospital with *Pneumocystis* pneumonia. In his 15 years as an infectious disease specialist in Africa, the Middle East, and the United States, these were the first cases of PCP he had ever seen—and his first AIDS cases. Well informed about the recent reports of *Pneumocystis* and KS, he automatically assumed that the patients he was to examine were gay men.

People were talking about these cases, but it was in gay men. So we said to these guys, "You're a gay man, you must be a gay man, come on, admit it." And one guy had an earring.

When the patients still denied being gay, Friedland watched them for further clues and finally established that they were drug users, as they claimed. "I watched to see who visited them, and it was wives and girl-friends and children. It wasn't other gay men. So it look[ed] like it's the same weird disease that doesn't yet have a name, but they're not gay men."

It was not until January 1983 that the CDC directly addressed the issue of the risk to which female partners of men with AIDS were exposed. For Gerald Friedland and his colleagues in the Bronx, recognition of heterosexual transmission of AIDS came sooner.

We had a few male patients who had female partners. The female partners were not drug users, so if they were at risk it was risk through sexual transmission. . . . And I had one of these sexual partners in clinic, and I'm about to examine her. I put my hands on her neck, and I feel these huge lymph nodes and [I'm thinking], "Oh, shit, she's got it, it's the end of the world." I mean, there are a limited number of gay men in the world, but many, many more heterosexuals. . . . Everything [until then] had been an embellishment, commentary, [but this] to me was a visceral documentation of the fact that it's a heterosexually transmitted disease. . . . This was dread, the end of the world.

Friedland had a dream that gave voice to his fears.

I used to have a dream. . . . Did you ever see *Wild Strawberries*? There's a scene where the old doctor's walking in a town, and there's a clock that doesn't have any hands on it, and there's a hearse that sort of drives off and a coffin falls out. It's very disturbing. So it was similar. And I was walking on Jerome Avenue [where Montefiore is], this train going overhead, and the green grocer stalls were all out, and there were a lot of cars and trucks, but there were no people. They had all died of AIDS. I remember that dream—I had the sense there was this sort of thing seeping into the population, and we knew nothing about it, and lots of people already had it and didn't know about it.

Although Friedland and others had come to recognize that AIDS could be heterosexually transmitted, there remained a reservoir of resistance to the idea. Because of his role as a military doctor, Robert Redfield was particularly interested in the possibility of such transmission and was struck by the reluctance of others to acknowledge it.

There was a meeting at Bob Gallo's lab in the fall of 1983, and I remember there were some CDC representatives, . . . and I remember getting up and presenting the fact that I had five men with AIDS. . . . And I remember saying it bothered me because three of the wives have [low T-cells counts]. And I can tell you that most people just dismissed it. And that kind of frustrated me.

When at last he was able to test for the presence of HIV, his assumption proved correct.

As we got into the cusp of '84, I started actually having viral data now from Bob's lab, so I knew I was right. And I can tell you, there was a second of excitement when . . . I was looking at this stuff. And then I was sick to my stomach. I didn't want to be right.

But even as the possibility of transmission from men to women was being established, the possibility that women could transmit disease to men met with resistance. This was especially so in New York City, where the Department of Health, concerned about damping AIDS-related hysteria, was particularly skeptical. Donald Kotler, many of whose patients came from Harlem, was struck by the Health Department's refusals to acknowledge heterosexually acquired AIDS in men.

> What does it take to realize that something is [sexually] transmissible? It's in the gay community. And then to find that it can be transmitted by needles, and it's in the IV drug community. How could it not be? And then to see a woman, and then to see a straight man. The official interpretation is that "a heterosexual man who's not an IV drug user and develops AIDS is defined as a liar." The Department of Health came when I had such a person in the hospital, and that's what they said; they said, "He's a liar. It can't be."

It was in the especially bitterly contested question of what accounted for the apparently elevated case rate of AIDS among Haitians that both official and popular resistance to recognizing the extension of the epidemic was placed into bold relief. For Sheldon Landesman, the effort to study AIDS among Haitians brought down upon him the wrath of a community he thought he had tried to help.

> The unusual thing about Haitians that we had noted was that they were neither drug users nor gay. We gently pulled the charts on 10 of these patients and reviewed their histories. Basically, we wrote up a report on heterosexual non-IV drug-using men with HIV disease and sent it down to the CDC, and it was initially published in *MMWR* and then in the *New England Journal [of Medicine]*. In the *Journal*, I believe I said something about potentially HIV or AIDS coming from Haiti to here. Within two years or so, I wasn't [a] particularly popular person within the Haitian community. There may have been a demonstration at Downstate [in Brooklyn] around the issue of AIDS and Haitians. . . . I was the focus of some irritation.

Arnaud Bastien, a Haitian-born physician who was between medical school and internship when he came to Downstate in 1988 to do research on AIDS, saw the encounter with Landesman as harsher. His parents, who were living in political exile in Brooklyn, and many members of the Haitian community were dismayed by where he had chosen to work.

> They were bothered when I came to work [at Downstate] because, to many in the community, Downstate was responsible for Haitians being a "risk group." The paper that came from [Downstate] was written by Sheldon [Landesman]. Sheldon was not looked upon

very well in the Haitian community, and, as he liked to remind me, he was hanged in effigy in front of Kings County [the municipal hospital across the street from Downstate] . . . by a small group.

Working at Jackson Memorial Hospital in Miami, Margaret Fischl encountered not only popular resistance but disbelief on the part of the CDC as well. Her first AIDS cases were among Haitians. *Pneumocystis* pneumonia, disseminated cytomegalovirus—almost unheard of until she saw it in her patients—were among the first indications of a burgeoning problem. She was aware of the literature on Kaposi's sarcoma in Uganda but was perplexed about "why on earth we were seeing [it] among those of Haitian ancestry, and what [the] connection [was] to Africa." For Fischl, these cases were crucial because at a time when so much attention was focused on the unique outcropping of disease in gay men, they were signs of heterosexual spread. But the CDC, struggling to understand the new syndrome, was dubious.

I would say the CDC was very skeptical about what we were seeing. Were we really seeing AIDS, as we subsequently came to call it? The CDC came down here and interviewed our patients, insulted our patients, got into homosexuality issues and what was really going on in Haiti, got into voodoo rituals and all sorts of things. Although I think one had to look very carefully, I was amazed at the reluctance to accept that if this virus could be transmitted among homosexual men, why couldn't it be transmitted among heterosexual men and women?

When the CDC came to accept the fact that something was placing Haitians at increased risk—that Haitians, like gay men, were a risk category—Haitians themselves rejected the stigmatizing label as a "medical calumny." And so Fischl, like Landesman, became the target of ire.

I went to a meeting, and we went there to really assist them, to say we were seeing an increased incidence. We asked them to ask themselves, look at their practices, to get involved in the research, in the Haitian and Black community. And we were called white affluent racists—and that bluntly. I was pretty appalled and shaken, because we were there for a medical reason, out of very deep concern for a disease and for patients that we were seeing. And we wanted to get them involved, and we were called white affluent racists. That simple.

The recognition that AIDS could be transmitted heterosexually emerged concomitantly with the discovery of the new disease in babies. Commenting on four cases of unexplained immunodeficiency and opportunistic infections in infants in New York, New Jersey, and California, the CDC wrote in December 1982, "Transmission of an 'AIDS agent' from mother to child, either in utero or shortly after birth, could account for the early onset of immunodeficiency in these infants." But here too those who first encountered the disease were confronted with what they took to be more than the normal level of scientific skepticism from both professional colleagues and the public health community. Gwendolyn Scott, a pediatric infectious disease specialist at Jackson Memorial, began to see her first cases of children in the same community of patients being seen by Margaret Fischl.

I saw my first children early in 1981, and they were both under six months of age. They both had mothers who were quite well, at least by appearance, and both of them were very, very sick. Both of them hadn't grown well, so that they were below weight, what we would call "failure to thrive." They were Haitian children. One child had severe oral thrush. She had continuous fever. And she later developed a sepsis, had severe complications, and died before six months of age. The other child had similar problems and she died from a gastrointestinal bleed. They never got out of the hospital. These two children bothered me, because I couldn't decide what they had. So I basically labeled these children as some kind of immune deficiency. It was something I had never seen before. So it was a mystery and an enigma.

In the Bronx, Arye Rubinstein, an Israeli-born pediatric immunologist—both a clinician and a researcher—was convinced early on that the disease he was seeing in young children was the same disease being diagnosed in gay men. But few would listen.

We caused a lot of turmoil before anyone else started even to think about pediatric AIDS. I remember [a] meeting, when I raised my hand and spoke about children. Everyone pooh-poohed it. I spoke about women, and everyone pooh-poohed it. So the general opinion I think in 1980 and '81 and '82 was that I don't know what I'm saying; this is probably another kind of immune deficiency. . . . Jim Curran came to me in the fall of '81 and said, "Arye, what am

I going to do? I'm convinced that this is pediatric AIDS, but no one in a sane mind will accept it. How do we bring it out to the public?"

In 1981, Rubinstein submitted an abstract of the first case of AIDS in a child to the American Academy of Pediatrics. It was not accepted for publication. "They just didn't find it meritorious." James Oleske's experience in Newark, New Jersey, would lead him to recognize that this disease was being transmitted from parent to child, but armed with what he took to be clear evidence that AIDS was attacking children, he found the path to professional acceptance and the publication of his findings filled with obstacles.

It was probably late in '80–'81. They called me down to the adult ID [infectious disease] clinic to say they had a drug user they just couldn't get blood on, and they wanted T cell studies. And so I drew the blood on the guy. And I looked at him, and I recognized him; and he had sort of looked at me, and I said, "I know you from somewhere." He said, "Yeah, you know, doc, don't you remember?" It was about six months ago I took care of his little girl who died, and I had to tell him his girl died of *Pneumocystis*. . . . We did the count that night, and there were no T-cells, no helper cells . . . and this guy had the syndrome.

When Oleske prepared an article based on a review of his babies with AIDS, he faced resistance from the *New England Journal of Medicine* because his cases had been discussed in a news article in the *Wall Street Journal* and had thus violated the *Journal's* rule on prepublication release.

The *New England Journal of Medicine* sent my article back. So I redid the article and sent it to *JAMA* [*Journal of the American Medical Association*], and they gave me a hard time, but a good hard time. They had seven reviewers. I think the problem was that no one wanted to believe that this was happening. There was such distaste for this disease. It was a disease of people that others didn't necessarily always like, drug users and gay men. How could this sort of filthy disease occur in children? One reviewer said, "Dr. Oleske just doesn't know how to diagnose sickle cell anemia and in his article didn't report the results of sickle cell testing." Well, as a pediatrician working in Newark I know an awful lot about sickle cell, and we did not include the sickle cell results because we didn't think it was germane. And then another guy said it was malnutrition and I just didn't know how to recognize malnutrition. And then someone said that I was confusing an epidemic in New Jersey of a primary immunodeficiency called Nezelof's syndrome, which is an inherited primary immune deficiency. And I couldn't believe they'd rather think we're having an epidemic of a primary inherited immune deficiency syndrome than what was clearly obvious to me at the time. It was frustrating, because I was seeing it. I was pretty confident I had worked it out pretty carefully, but no one wanted to believe it.

Ultimately Oleske's review of pediatric AIDS cases was published in May 1983 in *JAMA*.[7] One month later, on the second anniversary of the first report of AIDS, an update of cases in the *MMWR* included 21 infants "with opportunistic infections and unexplained cellular immunodeficiencies."[8] Still, the CDC noted that "infant cases are recorded separately because of the uncertainty in distinguishing their illnesses from previously described congenital immunodeficiency syndromes." It would be another half year before the CDC would publish its "provisional case definition for acquired immunodeficiency syndrome in children."[9]

Gay men, drug users, blood transfusion recipients, hemophiliacs, the sexual partners of those at risk, and babies born to infected mothers would all be officially diagnosed with AIDS by June 1984, three years after the first case reports. By then, 4,918 cases had been reported to the CDC; 2,221 were dead.[10] Less than a year later, in May 1985, *MMWR* announced the 10,000th case of AIDS.[11] It had taken three years for the first 5,000 cases to be reported, 10 months for the second 5,000 cases. Those escalating numbers revealed only a small part of the story. The new HIV antibody test, first available for research purposes in 1984, made clear that Gerald Friedland's fear that "this thing was seeping into the population" was all too prescient. Among gay men attending a sexually transmitted disease clinic in San Francisco, the prevalence of antibody to the virus thought to cause AIDS had gone from 1 percent in 1978 to 25 percent in 1980, a year before the first case of AIDS was reported. In 1984, when testing for undiagnosed infection became possible, 65 percent were infected. In New York City, a sample of frequent drug users had an infection rate of 87 percent. Seventy-two percent of asymptomatic hemophiliacs being treated at home had a positive antibody test response.[12]

The Roads to Commitment

As the epidemic began to spread case by case, it evoked a sense of dread and dismay. Memories of the first encounters recalled by those who would become AIDS doctors virtually always entailed vivid, appalling images. Victoria Sharp, who years later would start her professional life by directing an AIDS service for prisoners in upstate New York, was still a medical student in 1981 when she viewed a case of AIDS for the first time in Los Angeles.

> All I remember is that the patient came out of his room and was very tall and was covered with KS lesions. And there was a sort of quiet that occurred as he walked through the halls. Cedars Sinai is a hospital with a lot of movie stars, and it was almost as if a star was walking through. There was this kind of hush.

But at the same time, physicians who had encountered the new disease experienced what some would come to feel was almost an illicit sense of exhilaration. This was not conventional medicine, with its routines, its expected and predictable successes and failures, its ordinary joys and sorrows. It was thrilling as well as horrifying to recognize that a new disease had appeared on the horizon, observed Paul Volberding, who, at 31, had just been appointed to head the division of oncology at San Francisco General Hospital. As he groped for metaphors that could capture the feelings evoked by encountering AIDS in young gay men, he settled upon images of the great European explorations of the 15th and 16th centuries.

> It'll take me for the rest of my life; the energy from those first years will carry me as long as I live, I think. It was an absolutely remarkable period where every time I'd see a patient there'd be a new disease. It was like it must have felt to be an explorer and to discover America. There really is the sense of breathless excitement. It's not so hard now [in 1995], but it was hard then to talk about that because obviously the people didn't feel that they were fascinating. They felt they were sick. It was endlessly fascinating, you know, just an experience in medicine you don't ever anticipate happening. You know, you go through medicine and you expect that everything has been pretty much described and that you'll make progress, and you'll make discoveries, but they're going to be

incremental advances in areas that are pretty well outlined. But here there was no history. We were it.

When Volberding went on to create what would become the world-famous AIDS ward at San Francisco General Hospital, he would be joined by Donald Abrams. Equally young, Abrams, who had been drawn to the study of the relationship of virology and cancer, was struck by what appeared to be the emergence in rapid succession of a series of new diseases that challenged medicine's capacity to lay bare etiology, to understand pathogenesis, to cure.

All of this is sort of happening right as I'm just coming out of my training, and I didn't know what it was like to be a doctor. One could say that I was just this side of thinking that, gee, all of medicine is always like this, you're always faced with a brand new disease that you have to figure out. And, you know, I'd gone through my training during toxic shock syndrome and Legionnaire's disease, and it seemed like this was the next one of those and we were going to be the team that was going to unravel the mystery and be so much better off for all of mankind. For me it was a sense of tremendous stimulation to be faced with this mystery and to try to figure out how to get to the bottom of it. It was just a very challenging and exciting time. . . . So it seemed like every patient presented a challenge, and every patient was offering something that was unique, and you really felt like you were on the frontier and a pioneer. And I wondered, Could the practice of medicine be like this forever?

Like Abrams, Fred Siegal at New York's Mount Sinai Hospital was seized by the realization that the new disease posed questions at the frontiers of medicine—in this instance, of immunology.

Oh, it was tremendously exciting. Here we were riding the cusp of this fascinating wave of medicine and immunology. It was as if I had been created to be there for this, because I'd trained in immunology, I'd been interested in infectious diseases, I had a public health background, and here was a new epidemic under my nose! Terrible, and at the same time fascinating.

In common with so many infectious disease doctors, Gwendolyn Scott was drawn to problem solving. She too was struck by the sheer intellectual excitement of inexplicable manifestations of disease in those she encountered. But it was an excitement tempered by the realization that her babies, largely Haitian, were dying.

> Because I like to solve mysteries, I found it very intellectually stim-
> ulating because, again, of the multipresentations. You could see
> children with autoimmune disease. You could see children with low
> platelet counts. You could see children with different kinds of in-
> fections and very unusual infections, and children with lymphoid
> interstitial pneumonitis. So it was an extremely varied presentation,
> and intellectually it was very interesting and fascinating. But it was
> also very tragic. Absolutely.

To those who were beginning their careers, the excitement of the first years reflected, in part, a recognition that a new disease provided un-paralleled opportunities for advancement. Rarely do young physicians have an opportunity to describe a new syndrome and its clinical course, its implications for normal life functions. Those prospects attracted How-ard Minkoff, an obstetrician at the Downstate Medical Center in Brook-lyn, where poor African-American, Haitian, and Latino women came to deliver their babies.

> Academically it was an unclaimed niche. It was going to be an
> interesting area to explore. No one had the foggiest idea what the
> effects on pregnancy were going to be or what the effects of preg-
> nancy on the disease were going to be, or about transmission; and
> so it was clear that there was a lot of fertile ground for academic
> tilling. And I was not one, at that point in my career, to shy away
> from an opportunity.

But AIDS also provided Minkoff with an opportunity to break free of the mold of normal medicine, to experience the intellectual stimulation and spark on the cutting edge of professional life.

> Those of us from the sixties realized college was the great opening
> into the world of ideas, and medical school was an apprenticeship
> which sort of shut you back down. Here was a chance to get back
> out of that little mold and deal not only with medical issues but
> with social issues, and the medical issues were very interesting be-
> cause it was mysterious, it was an opportunity to get in on the

ground floor and try to help solve the mystery one way or the other.

Even those who were well along in their careers, like Joseph Sonnabend, whose office-based practice in Greenwich Village served primarily gay men, were aware that AIDS provided an occasion to do something extraordinary.

> When this thing became explicit I thought it was the opportunity of a lifetime. I don't know if I feel that any longer, but it seemed so at the time. . . . It's really rather horrible . . . , but it was pretty exciting too. It's not every day that you [encounter] a new disease.

Although AIDS cases would ultimately appear throughout the nation in cities large and small, it was the two coasts that bore the brunt of the epidemic in the first years. Thus it was doctors in New York, Newark, San Francisco, Los Angeles, and Miami who first came into contact with the disease. But not all those who encountered AIDS or who became aware of its existence chose to assume the responsibility of caring for those who were afflicted. Indeed, the doctors who threw themselves into AIDS were atypical. Donald Kotler had a long-standing interest in how starvation affected body mass. His initial experience with AIDS in gay men seemed to crystalize a line of scientific investigation that had intrigued him.

> I was seeing diarrhea and wasting. I was seeing 35-year-old gay men who had diarrhea and a 55-pound weight loss, to the point where [they] couldn't get out of bed and then were brought to the hospital and given to me to figure out. People came here and wasted away and died. One after another after another after another. And I'd been making nutritional assessments. And I sat and looked at the data that I had and then realized I had in some way sort of a natural course of wasting, a whole bunch of people who I had studied and then died. And eventually I got the papers from the Warsaw Ghetto, from the siege of Leningrad, and from the lethal hunger strike at Maze Prison by Bobby Sands, the IRA prisoner; and there were numbers in those papers, and the numbers weren't so different from my numbers. So a person with AIDS who wastes away and dies, dies at a body weight that's kind of the same as somebody who starves to death. So at that point, there was a unity that, to me, was a revelation.

Although scientific concerns drew him to these new patients, more vital still were his Jewish identity and the community in which he worked. His first AIDS case almost immediately evoked Holocaust associations; that event had destroyed family members and deeply affected him. Kotler recalled:

> He looked like my father. His last name was my grandmother's maiden name. That was the first of the Holocaust links. His family was from Berlin and got out of Berlin in 1939 on the last ship, came towards the United States, got diverted down to Argentina because the United States stopped accepting those people, and then eventually worked their way back up. He could have been my brother.

Further, practicing medicine in one of the epidemic's epicenters, watching the influx of people with AIDS into his hospital, he felt compelled ethically to reevaluate his professional commitments.

> I was on the fence, not knowing if I wanted to give it my full attention, because I had another agenda that I was trying to follow through. But it mushroomed, snowballed. I didn't think, after what I'd been through by the end of 1983, that I could stay in New York, stay on the West Side and say that I'm not going to take care of these people or to take care of their needs, which are after all much more than the needs of somebody who has heartburn or duodenal ulcer or a hemorrhoid or hepatitis, acute things that come and go. Their needs were so much more, so I didn't think I could do it in a half-baked way. I either had to deal with it or not.

Not surprisingly, gay physicians came to AIDS out of all proportion to their numbers in medicine. For them, there was an immediacy to the threat to their communities, friends, and lovers that drew them to providing care. The epidemic would provide the occasion for many gay doctors to establish a professional identity. They would not be like an older generation of gay physicians who had primarily treated sexually transmitted diseases—"clap doctors," "drippy cock doctors"—who worked at the margins of medicine.

Puerto Rican and gay, trained at Columbia's College of Physicians and Surgeons, Gabriel Torres was 25 years old when he began to encounter AIDS patients as a resident at St. Vincent's Hospital, a Catholic institution in New York City's Greenwich Village.

It was very shocking to see the devastation. I mean young, robust, muscular gay men from the Village literally dying with their first bout of PCP. That was something I think that motivated me to remain interested in AIDS, seeing members of my own community really suffering like that, something so unknown.

Howard Grossman was not much older. Like Torres, he worked in New York, initially at Kings County, a public hospital in Brooklyn. Grossman had planned to become a specialist in geriatrics because he believed that insufficient attention had been paid to the needs of older gay men. But AIDS drew him to the young. For him, there was no other choice.

It was what was happening to my generation of gay men. I mean, there was no place else to be. If there's a war going on all about you, you can't just turn your back on it. Although plenty of people did. I couldn't. I was [going to practice] geriatrics because I thought that it was the important place to be at the time in the early '80s, late '70s. [But with AIDS] there was a chance nobody was going to get old.

Some lesbians, for whom AIDS posed no discernible risk, were drawn to AIDS out of a sense of identification with gay men. Working in New York before returning to San Francisco, Lisa Capaldini, who would go on to develop a large AIDS practice in San Francisco's Castro district, followed the course of the epidemic on the West Coast. Like Grossman, she evoked images of war to capture the experience of hearing about the threat to those with whom she shared a homosexual orientation. She also underscored the extent to which gay men and lesbians could call upon personal experience to enhance their professional response to those who were sick and dying.

I remember really thinking about AIDS when I started working for the Office of Management and Budget [in New York]. I felt like someone who was hearing about a war in their homeland but was out of the country. . . . Having AIDS happen within my community, in a sense, was very empowering during my residency because I felt like I might be able to offer these patients something special. I didn't think it was weird if someone's partner was a man. . . . I wonder sometimes would I have gotten as involved, let's say, [if this were] an epidemic of heterosexual women; would I have the same connection as a woman? And I honestly don't know.

For a number of gay physicians, encountering AIDS forced a confrontation with their own sexuality. Fearful and closeted, many had gone through medical school unaware that any of their classmates were gay. Lacking senior mentors, older gay physicians on whom they could model themselves, they often wondered whether it was possible to be both gay and a good doctor. Witnessing the suffering of openly gay men and caring for AIDS patients could provide the occasion for coming out. Joseph O'Neill, who studied medicine at the University of California in San Francisco, was drawn to AIDS even before he fully acknowledged his own homosexuality.

What attracted me to it was the more social issues surrounding it. I was very much in the closet. I mean I'm openly gay, been out for years, but at the time I was closeted to myself and to most of the world. And so there was something, I think, that drew me to it as it was something happening to gay men. . . . How could you be a health care professional, interested in public health medicine, and be alive in the '80s and '90s and be working professionally and not be involved in this stuff?

John Mazzullo, who worked in Boston, noted that his life had been marked by indecision. His sexual identity and his professional identity were worlds apart. AIDS forced him to end that troubling separation.

In '83 I started to realize that this illness is galvanizing me because not only is it fascinating from a medical standpoint, but it's starting to fuse my gay life and my medical life in that I never wanted to be a gay doctor on Park Avenue, because I just didn't want to do hepatitis and STDs. But this was bigger than that. And then the other part of the fusion was that I was never a political person. You've not heard in my talking that I went down to Stonewall or that I went to Gay Pride marches or that I even knew what Stonewall was, because I was too closeted and too frightened and too wrapped up in my own *meshugass* [madness] to worry about the big picture. But this was a political issue. Not only could we all die from this, but they could put us in concentration camps. So I had a medical awakening and a political awakening that occurred between '82 and '84 that was just unique in my professional life.

If AIDS drew gay physicians because of the profound threat it posed to their own communities, it drew many on the Left whose political commitment made the care of the disenfranchised and despised morally compelling. For them AIDS was not simply a new disease; it was an opportunity to offer their professional services and their emotional support to gay people, drug users, undocumented aliens. It was a political act, an act of solidarity. As an older generation of medical students and doctors had gone to the South in the early days of the civil rights movement, this generation would see in AIDS a cause to be embraced.

Carol Brosgart, the daughter of Jewish immigrants to Canada who had earned a living in the *"shmatteh* [garment] business," was a self-identified radical in medical school, refusing an industry-supplied stethoscope and deeply suspicious of her pharmacology class, which she saw as providing ideological cover to the "medical-industrial complex." She was a public health physician in Oakland, California, when the epidemic began.

> I think if you were political or community minded before medicine, and you wanted to continue to do work of social value, [you worked] in community medicine or public health or neighborhood clinics. . . . I got a lot of satisfaction from taking care of people that other people had shunned. That was true of most of my patients; it wasn't just my patients with AIDS. Nobody wanted to take care of the refugees; nobody really wanted to take care of poor Blacks and Latinos; nobody was very interested in taking care of gay men; nobody was interested in taking care of prostitutes or injecting drug users. There was a lot of return; if you take care of people who other people don't want to take care of, and your patients are treated with respect, they give so much back to you, because they're so appreciative. . . . If you scratch the surface, and you look at the age group, the age group of a lot of people doing AIDS work [now] are the 40–50 somethings; and the 40–50 somethings, if you go back 30 years—"Ban the Bomb," the civil rights movement—a lot of people who found themselves in the midst of their training or coming out of their training were many of the same people who were on picket lines and voter registration and the women's movement. It's not unusual that they would gravitate and choose to take care of stigmatized people, people who have been discriminated against. So here's another social movement.

Gerald Friedland's political biography exemplified what Carol Brosgart had described. He had first studied sociology because he thought it would be linked to social activism. Instead he found "nose counting and survey taking." Ultimately he decided to go to medical school because he believed it would be possible to use medicine as a "social instrument," as a way of addressing social inequities. Friedland's service as a Peace Corps volunteer in Nigeria after graduation from medical school further radicalized him, and on returning to Boston he worked with the Medical Committee on Human Rights, the Medical Resistance Union, which supported physicians who sought to avoid military service in Vietnam, and with the Black Panther party. All of this he saw as a prelude to his work in AIDS.

[In AIDS] you're gonna get a collection of sort of aging hippies; so there's some of that, and then there's people who are younger, who would have been politically active if they had been in the sixties, because they're of that stripe. So for lots of reasons, AIDS sort of brings those people forward and actually provides an opportunity for them to express themselves in that way. So a lot of people come in with a great commitment to the work that is above and beyond the usual work commitment.

And Robert Cohen, a leftist who had gravitated to medical administration rather than direct patient care and who had taken a position overseeing the medical service at New York's Riker's Island jail, saw the care and protection of prisoners as demanding his personal attention.

I was concerned out of my ideological [perspective] that [prisoners] needed protection. I wasn't sure how much I could protect them, but I thought I had to do what I could, because I thought they were at risk from the society at large. Prisoners with AIDS were going to be way up at the top of people who were going to get hurt, if anybody was going to get hurt in this epidemic, so I thought I had a responsibility there. I worked in prisons out of a feeling that this was a population that had great medical needs and would tend not to get served, and that this was a place where there are not lots of doctors around; this is a place where I could be particularly helpful.

The route from politics to AIDS was not always so explicit, so direct. In some instances, doctors were inspired by the heroic image of medicine, the Promethean encounter between human ingenuity and the forces of nature. For Richard Chaisson, who would go to San Francisco for his residency before he became a central figure in the establishment of the AIDS service at Johns Hopkins in Baltimore, a political humanism was at the core of medicine. Like many others, he took Dr. Rieux, the protagonist in Albert Camus's *The Plague,* as a model of selfless commitment to those threatened by the forces of darkness. Nevertheless, he only gradually came to see in AIDS a way of realizing what he understood as medicine's moral imperative.

What I had always been interested in in medicine from before I went to medical school was the really age-old mythic battle of man versus microbe. And one of the books that I read that far and away influenced me to decide on medicine rather than oceanography was *The Plague.* I loved *The Plague,* and I loved that story of battling these vicious microbes and the story of trying to do good in the face of overwhelming bad, whether it's the evil of fascism or plagues, trying to do good in the face of the overwhelming odds that are external, that aren't because of bad diet or smoking or alcohol and drugs, but something outside, microbes. So I ultimately decided that infectious disease was where it was at, because you could fight the bugs, these evil bugs that come in and attack.

When I told [my advisor in medical school] I was going to go to San Francisco for my residency, he said, "Why would you want to go there? There's nothing happening in infectious diseases in San Francisco." And I went to San Francisco as AIDS occurred, and I have to say that when I went there I thought it was interesting but I didn't have any overwhelming passion for it. That changed over time, and that passion grew enormously. . . . By the time I was a third-year resident I was immersed in AIDS. Everybody was. I found it fascinating, and I really loved the patients and thought it was very compelling work. A lot of my fellow residents disliked it. They felt that it was ruining their training, or if not ruining it, it was detracting from it.

I'm interested in infectious disease. I'm interested in things that have a great burden on society. Should I go study malaria and go to India? Or should I go work on schistosomiasis and go to North Africa? Or tuberculosis and go anywhere in the Third World? But what occurred to me was that I didn't have to go anywhere, that I was surrounded by an incredible epidemic that had everything that intrigued me about medicine and that people were walking away from. So it actually gave me the opportunity to step in where other people didn't want to step in.

Coming to AIDS was not always or centrally a matter of identity politics or political commitment. In a number of instances it was the scientific challenge that provided the attraction, the way in which the new disease seemed to provide the opportunity to understand a broader set of medical questions or an underlying biological process. While such motivation could seem passionless, it sometimes led to deep and sustained interest in AIDS. Jerome Groopman's own work bridged the worlds of clinical practice and science. He was drawn to AIDS by both the suffering of those who were sick and the wonder that research could uncover. He captured the dual attraction in speaking about cancer.

> I remember the first time looking at a leukemic cell under the microscope and saying, "What a beautiful, wonderful, interesting looking, aesthetic cell." Large and convoluted and so on. It was fascinating. Biology's fascinating. The disease is the horror. And that's what AIDS is. The biology is incredible. So you have to develop an emotional distance, which you do. I wouldn't say you go into a trance state, but you do move sort of through doors. So, this morning, I'm sitting there . . . and we were talking about how leukemic cells communicate and all this new information about what's called signal transduction. It's incredible. I was thinking to myself, "What a blessing. What an opportunity to sit and listen to this kind of stuff and to participate in it." And then you go to the clinic and you see a 55-year-old woman dying of leukemia with three kids sitting around her, and you think to yourself, "What a curse, what a horrible thing."

King Holmes, a Seattle-based physician who had done much to shape the study of sexually transmitted diseases, found in AIDS an almost natural extension of his professional commitments.

> My own interest started with studies of gonococcal infection, but then evolved sort of sequentially through a series of interests that went from various aspects of gonococcal infection to nongonococcal urethritis to chlamydial infection and ureaplasma and mycoplasmas, to pelvic inflammatory disease to vaginal infection to herpes and then to other viruses, first papilloma virus and then hepatitis viruses and HIV.

For Deborah Cotton, who began her career as a physician-researcher at the National Institutes of Health, the first sign of AIDS was, almost shockingly, like a breath of fresh air. What she saw was scientific possibilities.

When I started in '78 was when everyone was saying, "It's over. It's done." There were editorials saying, "What are we going to do with these infectious disease doctors? They're going to culture each other. There's nothing. We've conquered this." And so it was sort of like, "Well, see? Not only did we have toxic shock and Legionnaire's, but now we've got this other weird thing." We were also very excited because one of the problems in doing immunology in those days was there were no natural models really of immune deficiency. When AIDS came along we thought, "Whoa, now we've got enough people with one kind of immune defect that we can really study this." And so I would say the initial reaction was elation, elation. . . . It was sad, but it didn't hit me the way it hit me when I was taking care of all these little kids with cancer who were dying. That was my issue at that time. AIDS felt very different than two-year-olds dying of horrible infections, at a time when my own kids were little. They were grown-ups; they could understand; you could explain. The worst nightmare is babies with cancer, right? God striking down your child. So it didn't get my gut.

The absence of an initial sense of tragedy was mirrored in the experience of Arye Rubinstein, who would take on the responsibility of establishing a service for very sick children at the Albert Einstein College of Medicine in the Bronx, a service that would focus on more than the scientific issues that so seized him at the start.

There was a tremendous excitement, and excitement came for two reasons. Number one, the first patients were not so sick that we had. The first patients all survived. So we didn't look at a fatal immune deficiency. And the second excitement was that everyone here in the basic science department for years was laughing at me and saying, "Ari, how can you do research on one patient? You find a common viral patient; you make an antibody and its helper T-cells; or you look at different factors. Stay in your lab! Go and start work with mice. Pull them [out of the cage] by the tail. And I said, "Yes, I'm studying this, but I want to stay with patients." When pediatric AIDS and AIDS in women came up, suddenly you can see how people started listening. Finally we have a situation in which we can unravel the mysteries of the immune system or the regulation of the immune system. So there was a tremendous excitement. This excitement somewhat abated when the first patients were dying, when we realized that this is a very consuming, energy-consuming and emotionally consuming disease.

To those who came to see in AIDS an almost limitless set of scientific possibilities, it became increasingly difficult to understand why others did not. Rockefeller University is an elite research institution in New York City with a very small clinical service. For Jeffrey Laurence, who was on the faculty working under the guidance of Dr. Henry Kunkel, a world-renowned immunologist, AIDS had the appeal of a medical mystery as well as an emotional charge. It was his friends from the theater world who were falling ill.

I couldn't understand people who were not working on this problem, but nobody else wanted to work on it. . . . Dr. Kunkel used to accuse me of working on diseases nobody got. I was working on these genetic immune deficiencies—there are a couple of hundred in the United States. Kunkel said, "You'll never get any patients. Nobody gets this disease. Why are you working on it?" And then I started working with AIDS, and he was convinced no one gets that either. This was a scientific problem; these were people who were dying; and they were friends of mine that were dying.

Not only was AIDS a disease for young doctors, but it provided unique opportunities to physicians in their postgraduate years as interns and residents. Many, as Richard Chaisson noted, resented the way in which AIDS shaped their training experience. They saw it as too limiting. They felt little or no commitment to the people who were sick, and they were frustrated by how little they could do. But it was precisely the absence of effective treatments that made AIDS so special for some doctors in training. For Judith Currier in Boston, having an engaged mentor mattered as well.

The primary care track that I was in was just a terrific opportunity. You had your own patients; you had a preceptor, but they were *your* patients; and here was this disease that nobody knew what you were supposed to do. And so I just thought this was great. I could learn about a new disease, try to figure out what to do, and try to help this patient, and . . . he was very dependent on me, and that was the incentive—that I had to figure out what to do. And he was willing to put his trust in me. But he realized nobody knew what they were doing. It didn't matter how experienced they were. During the time that I was a resident, Deborah Cotton came to the [Beth Israel Hospital] to be our AIDS clinical director, and to me she was a terrific role model. And she knew about everything that was going on, and she was very smart, and she was very good with the patients. And I wanted to be like her.

It was at the end of their residency years that some physicians were virtually drafted to take on the responsibility of establishing new AIDS services. They need not have accepted such offers, but to those who had the ambition as well as the interest in providing care to patients with AIDS these offers provided an unparalleled opportunity.

That is how Victoria Sharp's involvement began. Her efforts to get a medical degree had taken her to Belgium. She then went to Albany, New York, before going on to direct ever larger AIDS services in New York City.

[It] was spring of '87. I knew what I didn't want to do. I knew that I didn't want to go into private practice. I knew that I didn't want to see patients in terms of their ability to pay, and I'd had a really frightening experience as a chief resident. I was assigned an internal medicine clinic, and shortly into the year I realized that I really didn't like it, and that my clinic started at 1:00 and at 1:15 I'd be looking at the clock. It was so frightening to me that I couldn't even acknowledge it to myself, because I thought, Oh, my God, what have I done? I went seven years to Brussels and now four years of residency, and I don't like what I'm doing? At around that time Albany Medical Center was going through the process of becoming a designated AIDS center, and they needed a director. Now I had no experience in AIDS or administration, and I was beginning to see a lot of it as a house officer, but the new center was going to open in July—that's when I was available—and so I was made acting head of the AIDS program. The way I got into AIDS was sort of backing into it. This opportunity came along and grabbed me.

Once she had made the decision, however, her commitment intensified.

There were many people that said to me, "Why are you doing what you're doing, working with prisoners, working with AIDS?" I felt that the appropriate question would have been, "How can you do anything else except this?" This was where everything was happening in medicine in the '80s as far as I was concerned. The science, the politics. I felt like I was really on the front lines, and, again, it was completely engaging work, and I never once watched the clock.

Not all roads to AIDS entailed explicit choices. Sometimes the involvement simply seemed to take hold without conscious decision. Abigail Zuger was a resident at Bellevue Hospital in New York City in the epidemic's first years. In recounting her experience she adopted a characteristically antiheroic, sardonic tone, setting herself apart from those who saw in AIDS something more than a compelling medical challenge and who sought to imbue their involvement with AIDS care with deeper meaning.

I was actually semiconscious for most of my residency, because I don't do well without a lot of sleep. But I had absolutely no idea that I was going into HIV at that point, although there was plenty of HIV around. . . . I stayed, but not because I said to myself, Boy, this is exciting. Mostly because I said, Oh, I'm so tired. What do I do now? . . . At some point I thought, Well, I have a skill here, and that's how I still think of it really. I have a skill. . . . If you look at the spectrum of people who choose to work with AIDS patients there are a lot of dubious characters in there. A lot of people have issues of their own, and they resolve them by becoming very emotionally identified with their patients, which I don't think I've done.

The experience of doctors in locales where AIDS came later was very different. They had heard and read about the disease in New York, San Francisco, and Los Angeles, and so when they became involved in caring for AIDS patients, the shock of the first clinical encounters experienced on the coasts was absent. So, too, was the burden of dealing with a rapidly increasing caseload.

Cleveland is a city to which AIDS came late. The first case was reported in 1981. By 1985, when New York and San Francisco had already reported approximately 2,000 cases, Cleveland had only 45. Leonard Calabrese was a physician at the Cleveland Clinic when he saw his first case in 1981, a young man en route to his home in Chicago. Called to the intensive care unit because the patient appeared to have an immunological disease, Calabrese was stunned by what he saw.

At post-mortem he had no less than 11 opportunistic infections. And the whole picture of this was just heretofore strange, unusual, kind of otherworldly. I was struck by the gravity of the whole thing.

It was a year before he saw his next AIDS case. What pulled him to AIDS was not only the science—he would go on to study the rheumatological complications of AIDS—but the injustices he witnessed, as people with AIDS were subjected to acts of discrimination.

For the first few years, it was a very sterile thing. I knew it was bad, and I had feelings about it, but it was dominated by this kind of intellectual curiosity, excitement, like this was the place to be, this was the thing to do. Over time I just got pissed off. I don't want to make it sound like I'm a crimson crusader or something, but there are certain things about this that are just visceral. . . . I was always a very liberal guy, and I always kind of carried this notion of injustice.

Whether it was in New York or Cleveland, many of the doctors who took on AIDS saw their lives indelibly marked, their professional worlds transformed. Joyce Wallace, who was to throw herself into the unglamorous street scene, working with New York's prostitutes despite very significant obstacles, notes:

It was so exciting. In a way it's shameful to think back on the excitement. This disease is one of the most horrible things that has happened in this century. You know there have been other horrible things, the Holocaust, maybe World Wars I and II, but this has to be right up there with them. . . . But it was very exciting, and it became my life.

It was this fusion of life and work, and the zeal so unusual in the practice and organization of medicine, that are reflected in Constance Wofsy's characterization of those who became involved with AIDS as "gripped." Part of the triumvirate (together with Paul Volberding and Donald Abrams) who would lead the world-famous AIDS service at San Francisco General Hospital, she typified the engaged physicians about whom Zuger was so skeptical.

How gripped we were, how separate we were from everyone else who wasn't part of this thing. There were the involved and the not-involved, and they just didn't understand one another. [There was] the imperative sense that you had to do everything, that it wasn't coming from elsewhere. It was an inner "must." You must go to the school because, my God, who else is going to talk to the kids. Oh, my God, the kids need to know. You must be on this task force because maybe we can make some policy that will protect somebody. You must meet with this somebody because maybe we can get the research study done. So it was really coming, this inner sense of You must, who else will? How else will they know? Who else will do it?

But AIDS was not only a commitment and a passion; it quickly became a career, with all the demands, expectations, rewards, and ambitions of professional life. As Michael Gottlieb co-authored the first published report on what would become known as AIDS, he was euphoric. He told himself, Your job now, Michael, is to get this into print and stake your claim with having discovered something new. Joel Weisman, also a co-author, was more modest as he thought back on the report. "This wasn't the discovery of penicillin; we were chroniclers. Two weeks later, someone else would have written this."

Something of the same sentiment was expressed by Molly Cooke, a young internist working at San Francisco General Hospital, the public institution that became the heart of AIDS treatment in that city. She recalled that "in June '81, Mike Gottlieb published his paper [in the *MMWR*], and of course we said, "Why didn't we write this paper?" Donald Abrams similarly recalled a sense of opportunity lost. "I can kick myself for not having published that back in 1979, because that would have been one of the earliest identifications of a pre-AIDS condition."

How rapidly careerist thinking could emerge was revealed by the response Jerome Groopman received when he announced to his colleagues in Los Angeles that despite a promising beginning he had decided to move to Boston, a city with only a nascent epidemic.

When I decided to come back to Boston, the people at UCLA said to me, "You're crazy." I had set up a Kaposi's clinic; I had gotten funding; I was part of a big program project grant; it looked like here was the right niche for academic advancement, a typical Young Turk approach to medicine. You find a rare disease, and you study it an inch wide and a mile deep and get funded and published. "How can you go back to Boston? There's no AIDS there. There won't be any AIDS there. It's a backwater provincial town, very conservative, and you're going to lose out on all of this equity you've built up."

The Ironies of Commitment

None of the first generation of doctors who encountered AIDS could have anticipated the demands, both professional and psychological, that it would place on them. Yet for some, the training they had received or their past experiences provided the context within which even so extraordinary a disease could be made manageable. This was especially so for oncologists.

Paul Volberding's experience as an intern in Utah taught him how much he wanted to work with patients facing death.

> The most significant patient, the patient that I remember most from my internship and residency and almost the most important patient to me ever was [someone] that I took care of in one of my first weeks as an intern. [He] was a faith healer, an Assembly of God missionary, an incredible fundamentalist. . . . He had a very aggressive anaplastic thyroid cancer, was dying, was bleeding out from his bladder. . . . But his wife believed that he would be healed, that if he and she believed strongly enough and prayed hard enough that God would heal him. It was apparent to him that that was not going to happen. And at one point he took me aside and said that it was really a problem, that their belief was limiting his ability to talk to his wife during a period of time when he really needed to talk to her about his dying. And it totally transformed me in a sense, because here I was, I knew nothing, I was just an intern, and I was finding myself being treated with a level of honesty and as a very important person in this man's life. . . . He died shortly after that. Suddenly I found myself in a responsible position, and I really enjoyed that feeling. I enjoyed the honesty that can come with medicine. . . . When people face their death, as often as not, they're incredibly open and willing to share their feelings with other people. And I really enjoy that part of medicine. So that's what, as much as anything else, convinced me that the care of cancer patients is what I wanted to do.

For those who had been trained in infectious disease, the story was very different. A few—those who worked in cancer hospitals or in oncology services—were accustomed to dying patients for whom little could be done. Among them was Donald Armstrong, who had begun to work in the infectious disease service at New York's Sloan-Kettering Hospital in 1970.

> I saw everybody dying of infection or of hemorrhage, because we didn't have platelet transfusions then. And that's really how I got my first interest in infectious disease. It started with seeing these cancer patients die.

But for most who chose infectious disease, it was the capacity to diagnose and cure that presented the greatest appeal, and it was oncology that represented the kind of medicine from which they had virtually taken flight.

Early in her career, Deborah Cotton had the kind of experience that defined the outlook of her generation of infectious disease doctors.

> I loved the fact that you made people all better, and you cured them. And we would have people literally at death's door with meningitis or whatever, and you gave them the magic potion, and the next day they were saying, "What happened? I feel fine." . . . I think people went into ID [infectious disease] expressly because they either didn't have the personality to be an oncologist or, like me, they just loved the idea of curing people. We never did primary care. Infectious disease is a specialty, academically based. Virtually everybody did lab work. They'd pop out of their lab two months a year, see inpatients with interesting ID problems, and then at the end of that time, *sayonara*, they'd go back to the lab. It was a lovely academic lifestyle. [And then AIDS came along.] . . . It was just depressing. I sort of felt like, oh my God, I've turned into [an oncologist]. I've turned into somebody who goes into the room, when there's absolutely no chance of this person surviving at all, and tries to put the best face on it. . . . And we did talk in those days, ID people, more in a joking way, of "My God, we're all turning into oncologists."

Donna Mildvan forcefully underscored the abrupt change experienced by infectious disease specialists, noting, "It was such a good field for an optimist. Until [AIDS]."

For those who had begun their careers explicitly rejecting oncology, there was a palpable irony in treating dying AIDS patients. William Owen, in San Francisco, noted:

I thought about becoming a pediatrician and then when I went into pediatrics I went through a rotation in pediatric oncology, dealing with little children who had cancer. And that had to be the most devastating experience of my medical career. Back then, in the early '70s, they were just getting into the very first start of chemotherapy, but they didn't know exactly how to do it. It didn't work very well. So most of the children died, and they weren't very pleasant deaths either. After that experience I felt that I couldn't really cope with dealing with little children dying. Years later I ended up going into a field where I dealt with people who were just past being children and who were in fact dying.

For pediatricians, the clash between what they had anticipated in their medical careers and the suffering they witnessed in children with AIDS was startling. Even those who worked in hospitals where the conventional fare of well-baby care was not the routine were unprepared. Caring for poor Black children in Newark, James Oleske, who had specialized in both infectious disease and immunology, expected to treat and cure even his very sick patients.

All of us went into pediatrics, I think, because we loved kids—or certainly most of us. And certainly we didn't go into pediatrics because we wanted to take care of dying kids, except for those few who went into oncology. Infectious disease [and] immunology were exciting choice[s] for me, because in the few rare kids that got congenital immune defects I knew about this new thing, bone marrow transplantation. And in the infectious part of my life most kids had meningitis, and you gave them antibiotics, and they got well, and you saved them. And then I [began] seeing kids that I tried to save; they'd just die, poor mostly, mostly minority, from families that were pretty fractured by poverty and drug use. . . . I was scared. I was frightened by the fact that kids were sick and dying, and I didn't know why they were, and I didn't know much that I could do, and every time I tried to do something I had people saying, "You shouldn't be doing that."

Perhaps the bitterest of ironies was that encountered by physicians who had devoted themselves to the care of hemophiliacs. Margaret Hilgartner had built her long and distinguished career around the care of people with bleeding disorders. She was 58 years old when the first cases of AIDS in hemophiliacs were reported in 1982. Although she did not long remain a caregiver to those with AIDS, she bore the sorrow of having inadvertently treated her patients with lethally contaminated factor VIII concentrate, which had so recently transformed the lives of hemophiliacs.

I was one of the first people who went into . . . pediatric hematology. . . . I got interested in the patients with coagulation disorders because of a young man who I had to take care of as a medical student at Duke, who had classic hemophilia and had some teeth drawn without telling the dentist that he had hemophilia and so bled under the tongue. And it was a horrible, terrible death. . . . I vowed to myself then that I would not let another hemophiliac die a bleeding death the way he did. I'll never forget it. . . . [Then in the 1970s we developed] comprehensive treatment centers, the ability to transfuse at home, the ability to attend school or work. So whatever the patients felt they wanted to do in life, they really could. Until AIDS came along.

New Worlds

As physicians worked intimately with their patients, they found themselves exposed to new worlds, worlds to which they had previously been insensible. Heterosexual doctors had known that homosexuality existed but typically knew no one who was gay; and gay culture and mores were as foreign to them as the craters and plains of Mars. The same was true of poverty. Most AIDS treaters were politically liberal or progressive and concerned about the misery of racism and poverty. Many worked in hospitals that drew indigent patients. Previously, however, their perspective on such patients had been essentially clinical. Most white doctors, with rare exceptions like Gerald Friedland, who had practiced in Africa and in Boston's slums, lacked direct experience of how the poor lived. AIDS work, of necessity, shattered the barriers of heterosexual presumption and often forced the removal of middle-class blinders.

Before AIDS, doctors rarely took a sexual history of their patients, even when they had been taught to do so. Alvin Friedman-Kien, after diagnosing KS in a series of gay men, began making inquiries into previously proscribed areas.

I suddenly began to take sexual histories, something nobody ever taught me in medical school. Asking about one's personal sex life? I mean, I've never asked anybody those questions. Nobody, not even of a prostitute. What questions do you ask? How do you ask them?

Molly Cooke, trained during the sexual revolution of the 1970s, had learned how to take a sexual history—but rarely did so. The underlying premise in her training was that human sexuality was relatively homogeneous. The standard of sexuality assumed in sexual histories was heterosexuality. Cooke was, herself, blind to other possibilities. She confessed to being completely oblivious to the presence of homosexuality in her world, never having realized that two of her friends were gay. "My assumption that people were heterosexual was so strong; . . . it just had to do with my understanding of the world."

Jeffrey Laurence was just as unconscious of sexual orientation in his patients. Between 1977 and 1980, he saw five patients: young unmarried men with varying infections that failed to remit. "When the fourth patient was hospitalized, some of the staff actually discussed whether he was gay. But it was just something to write down in the chart; it didn't mean anything to anybody. In retrospect, probably all were gay, unnoted because sexual orientation was of almost no clinical interest." Cooke, in thinking about San Francisco General in the early 1980s, found, "My strongest recollections from this phase of experience with HIV was how much it pushed sex forward in my experience of medicine; and I think it was a common experience for heterosexual physicians."

With so many gay men presenting with AIDS or pre-AIDS symptoms—then called "AIDS-Related-Complex"—homosexuality became a visible presence, forcing itself on heterosexual doctors previously innocent of its proximity. They discovered that there were many more gay men in their world than they had ever realized.

As the epidemic legitimated sexuality as a category of medical concern, degrees of sexual activity and types of partners became clinically relevant information. This was a seismic shift from the days when Donna Mildvan, only with great trepidation, asked a patient whether he was gay, knowing that what she was doing was audacious. But gay sexual practices, once manifest, astonished and unsettled many heterosexual physicians. What they heard or saw was difficult to square with their heterosexual experience. Victoria Sharp, who chose to work closely with men in New York's prisons, was challenged by the porousness of sexual boundaries.

I think clinicians were put in a situation where they had to learn new skills in taking a history, because we were confronted with a

whole group of patients who had life stories that we were not necessarily conversant with or comfortable with. Disgusting! An example, an inmate, my first patient as an attending, takes off his
inmate clothes, and there are two breasts staring at me. I mean,
you really had to learn to become comfortable discussing topics that
normally you might not have been.

Jerome Groopman, a religiously observant Jew raised in a politically liberal, tolerant household in New York City, was nonetheless deeply disturbed by the sexual practices he heard about and the justifications offered in their defense.

When I was first exposed, in taking histories, to a lot of the sexual
practices in California, it was shocking, and it was shocking to
everyone who was previously unaware of it. But it was also sad, I
found. The politics of the gay community, at least as I understood
them, in responding to discrimination, was to affirm that all forms
of behavior could be a political statement, almost of the right to do
this. So that fist fucking or having someone urinate on you or co-
praphasia, there were those who didn't want to be critical of this.
It was hard for me to see those as political.

Paul Volberding was also amazed and distressed by what he learned.

It seemed very foreign. It seemed frankly bizarre. I'm not homophobic at all, I don't think. But I didn't know what was going on.
The idea of anonymous sexual contacts, I mean, I can sort of understand it more easily now. I absolutely could not understand that
people would do this. I remember [one of my earliest patients, who]
had a birthday in the hospital. A bunch of his friends came to cel-
ebrate his birthday and brought as a card a huge cardboard fold-up
penis, a seven- or eight-foot-tall penis that they'd all signed their
names to. And I have to say it was somewhat appalling, given my
[rural, Lutheran] background. Also, I just thought, shit, this guy is
dying of a sexually transmitted disease, and the last thing we really
need is glorifying the kind of activity that resulted in him dying. It
felt horribly, sadly ironic to me; but I remember some of these moments of, I don't understand what's going on here.

Incredulous but wry, a worldly physician in Manhattan recalled discovering a type of sexual practice unknown to him until he began to take
sexual histories.

And then there were these fisters, people who fist-fucked or fist-fornicated. I couldn't understand it. I didn't even know it existed. I wouldn't have thought it was possible. And I'd suddenly become the doctor for the Fist-Fuckers of America. There was [such] an organization. Almost everybody in that group died.

More philosophically, and with a twist of humor, Harry Hollander, director of the AIDS Clinic at Moffitt Hospital in San Francisco, described his "initiation" into gay sex.

I recall very well an administrative assistant in the emergency room at Moffitt Hospital, who subsequently died of AIDS, showing us young doctors membership cards to bathhouses, telling us about bathhouses, and it would not be an overstatement to tell you the depths of my naïveté in thinking, You did what? To whom? How many times? And yet, within a few years, I was put in the odd and uncomfortable situation of talking in great detail with gay men about those lifestyle factors. And I suppose one of the real discordances in this job was feeling as if I was placed in the role of being an expert in a type of sex that I had never engaged in and have never even seen.

Molly Cooke had a measured, somewhat more curious response to gay sexuality than did her husband, Paul Volberding. She noted that she, like many women, was less uncomfortable with homosexual sex than the men around her and more intrigued by the mechanics of gay sexuality.

There was such a strong reaction to the number of sexual partners. People were just floored. I was. I think, like a lot of women, it didn't bother me one way or the other. But seeing people's health problems so linked to their sexual histories was startling. It was like there was sex everywhere. And we were frankly fascinated by what did people do at the technical level that enabled them to have so many partners. Heterosexual sex is just not that quick.

Many physicians who discovered, through AIDS, the deep and encompassing effect of racism and poverty on their patients, were shaken, like those doctors for whom gay sexuality was a revelation. Although they might have seen poor patients in their clinics, they now perceived, as if for the first time, that poor people lived in a world unlike their own. That world was one of harsh choices, dangerous vulnerability, unimaginable violence and deprivation. A poverty that uniformly diminished the lives of these patients could not help but distort and blunt clinical efforts made on their behalf. The urban poverty of the Bronx where he worked was far from the Israel where Arye Rubinstein had grown up and the Switzerland where he received his medical training. Before AIDS, he had seen patients in his examining rooms and lab; in the early years of the epidemic, he made his first home visits.

> In the beginning, I was very naive. I went to the South Bronx, to the worst neighborhoods. I had no idea what poverty was. I had no idea what conditions these families were living in. . . . Look, I came to the United States in '72. I really was not privy to the situation of this population. So when you go into such an apartment, and you see a kid on the bare floor, with just a television set, a kid who's living with rats, has never seen the ocean, or a nice tree, or anything nice in life, I was shocked. At that time, in '84 and '85, we had volunteers who took the kids to the zoo, to the beach. And one of the kids, I'll never forget it, when this kid saw the ocean, he thought it wasn't real because he had seen it on television. He saw it only as a television picture. They're living so close to the ocean and had never seen it.

In Miami, Gwendolyn Scott, in caring for Haitian babies, found herself drawn closer to their mothers, from whom she first learned how vulnerable and impoverished they were.

> I remember women coming in and telling us they were living in abandoned cars; they had no money. Some of them were illegal aliens, and so they were afraid to go to government agencies to get things done. We had instances of families basically being deported with this very sick child, and in many instances we did intervene successfully. I can remember the mother who I must have given about five prescriptions to, and she brought them back two days later covered with a wet material and partially chewed. I asked her what happened, and she told me that the rats and mice got them. It was just story after story after story. They are not going to buy medicine if they can't give the baby a bottle of milk. . . . [I realized the plight of these families] because I was doing more primary care than prior. And these children were so sick, and they depended on myself and [my staff] to help them. There were many times when people in the clinic, myself, the other workers, would give them

money, would buy them food, would sometimes buy medications. You became involved in their lives, and you couldn't help it.

Joseph O'Neill had treated AIDS patients as a medical student and resident at San Francisco General Hospital and the University of Washington before he went to Baltimore, where he saw patients in the AIDS program at Johns Hopkins University in 1990. Politically progressive, with a strong belief in medicine as a mission as well as a career, he was stunned by the degree of destitution, violence, and racial tension he found in Baltimore. He recognized that he had crossed the bar into another world.

At Hopkins, the patient population is so different. . . . You're dealing with homeless people sleeping on warm air ducts in the streets with *Pneumocystis* pneumonia, no home to go to and waiting rooms crowded. Just the overwhelming poverty of the inner city, just the hopelessness, and then some of the strengths. I mean it's a different world; it's not a world to which I had ever been. [I'd] never experienced racism, where I'm seen as a white person primarily. I am seen as the enemy; no matter what I'm doing; I'm not trusted for great lengths of time, and some patients would never trust me. One patient, a young Black woman who [had] bad heroin and cocaine addiction, very advanced HIV disease, who was very, very depressed. Then her son was murdered. I remember that so clearly because two of my patients both had children killed that week. You know, I was sitting there thinking, really trying to understand what it would be like to have a child murdered. It wasn't until I really rolled up my sleeves and started working there that I really got the glimmer that I have of how truly horrible people's lives are in this world we have created.

As doctors watched their patients sicken and die, they discovered how many responded to AIDS in unexpected ways, contrary to stereotype. A number described the humanity and strength with which impoverished, even self-destructive individuals, faced the final indignities of their disease. In the Bronx, at Montefiore Hospital, Gerald Friedland and Marnie Callan, his social worker, organized a patient group during the early years of the epidemic. As he attended the group sessions, he discovered how impressive its participants could be.

I [listened] to these people with AIDS talk about their disease, talk about how they were treated by their families, by other people, talked about their wishes, their hopes, their aspirations, things they hadn't done in their lives. I watched them support each other. I watched them visit other people among them who were hospitalized. It was a wonderful thing.

Gwendolyn Scott spoke movingly about how families faced with the impending death of a child found sources of strength in their faith.

I think I realized what tremendous courage people have and what tremendous strength people have. And, also, many people that we have dealt with have strong religious beliefs. You see families who really rely on one another. I remember a scene in the hospital where a young child was very, very sick, about six months old, and we did not expect the child to survive. And I [will] always remember the scene of the father and the mother sitting at the bedside. The father was reading the Bible; the mother was holding the baby. And the father had his arm around the mother, and there was this muted light. It was just a touching scene, because it was a sense of faith, and, I guess, a sense of how they were working together with a belief in God to assist the child in any way they could to have a peaceful death.

Those heterosexuals who treated gay men were often moved and impressed by a group of men they had seen but never recognized before AIDS. Jerome Groopman, who had been among those deeply disturbed by the sexual practices they learned about, discovered that, as the epidemic continued, these became less relevant. As he treated and became closer to gay patients, "it was as though this curtain was being pulled aside. I was beginning to see a society with real diversity and complexity that had essentially been invisible to me."

Almost tritely, the paradox is to see the reversal of the social stereotype. Here's a group that's characterized as being a bunch of sissies and pansies and fairies and all those ridiculous things. [Yet I recall] the strength and the courage and the fortitude and the endurance of so many people that I've taken care of, who in many ways, don't have the defined classical family supports that I think I have. It's unbelievable. I've also seen how friendship and relationships replace family when family no longer functions.

Treating a crippling and disfiguring disease, doctors were witness to despair, terror and suffering, the reduction of the human spirit as desperate patients clung to life. All of that was to be expected. What was surprising, even uplifting, was how some individuals could confront the most awful circumstances with courage. Leonard Calabrese at the Cleveland Clinic held onto the memory of these patients.

There's just so many people that have these indefatigable attitudes to the point . . . where you just come out of there and go, How does he do this? I had a guy just die a month ago; he ran a college bookstore . . . and he had the worst Kaposi's sarcoma. His face was hideous; it looked like a tomato. He had to get up in the morning and sit up for like a couple of hours so his eyes would open up because he had so much swelling. His eyes were like little slits; his face was all contorted. And he was on the national board of trustees of college bookstores, and was a lecturer, and until a month before he died this terrible, terrible death, he was working. He used to come up here and say, "Do you think I should go part time?" We would just look at him, Whoa, I can't believe it. He wanted more treatment, and he was tolerating his treatment because it kept him breathing. And this is something that I would have stopped treating a year ago. I think I probably would have thought, Just make me comfortable. Let me out of this. You see these little glimpses into people that just come along, and they're just there, and you just take them for what they're worth and cherish it.

The Limits of Commitment

Despite the profound impact made by the emergence of AIDS and the sense of mission it evoked in the doctors who took care of those who became ill, there were limits to the sense of commitment. Given the tendency toward identification with those they cared for, most doctors found it difficult to talk directly about their darker feelings. Some only hinted at their difficulties in empathizing with some patients. Nevertheless, a few confessed that when patients' behavior crossed the boundary of the socially acceptable, they found it exceedingly difficult to provide care. In some instances it was the disregard for the welfare of sexual partners that evoked such responses from physicians who were otherwise steadfast. Alvin Friedman-Kien had such an encounter with Gaetan Dugas, the French-Canadian flight attendant made famous as "patient zero" in Randy Shilts's *And the Band Played On.*

While he was in New York, he would go to gay bathhouses and have unprotected sex with a variety of people despite the fact that we warned him against it. I once caught him coming out of a gay bathhouse, and I stopped the car and said, "What are you doing there?" And he said, "In the dark nobody sees my spots." He was a real sociopath. At which point I told a colleague the story. She was enchanted with him, as most people were. I stopped seeing him. I refused to see him, I was just so angry.

Such explicit refusals to treat gay or heterosexual men who endangered others were not common. More typical was a less than enthusiastic response to such patients, especially drug users. Richard Chaisson was in training at San Francisco General Hospital when he noted that some physicians were more favorably disposed to middle-class gay men than they were to intravenous drug users.

The reaction was, "Oh, geez, I didn't get into this to take care of shooters. I'm happy to take care of gay men—I like gay men—but I don't like drug users." And I had people come up to me and say, "I've got this patient, and he's a shooter, and he's a real pain in the ass. He doesn't do what I say. He's always asking me for drugs. And I'm not going to see him anymore. Would you see him?"

Chaisson did see such patients. He, like Gerald Friedland and Peter Selwyn at Montefiore Hospital in New York, were almost drawn to drug users because of how some responded to them. But for many others, the strength of their commitment was tried. These were not the patients who, in sometimes romanticized retellings, are transformed by their illness, and they did not transform their doctors, at least not in an enriching way. While he was resident at Kings County Hospital, Howard Grossman found that these patients tested the limits of his tolerance.

At the County everybody was on Medicaid, and all of the people with HIV . . . were drug addicts, virtually all drug addicts, or they had alcohol problems. Nobody went to Kings County who could go anywhere else. It was really people at the very bottom of the social barrel, and a lot of them were really difficult. I was spit on and had things thrown at me, and had people try to attack me. You were constantly tying people down.

This was not, for him, an ennobling experience, and he did not like what this encounter had done to him. After three years,

> it had turned me into a monster. I hated patients. I hated everybody. All of us. Every house staff person. Every patient was a dirt bag, a piece of shit—the worst attitudes you could possibly imagine. And why not? We had been left basically alone. We had little supervision. . . . We were thrown into this place, roaches crawling on patients . . . with all the worst excesses of city bureaucracy.

Working at the same hospital, Sheldon Landesman noted how difficult it was to call on his professional commitments to care for AIDS patients whose behavior so offended him.

> Sometimes it's really tough to identify with my patients. . . . I really need to consciously push myself, to make sure I'm not sloppy. I had a patient I saw in clinic the other day; he was a 41-year-old drug addict, recently got out of Riker's Island [prison]. He comes in to clinic drunk; he had tuberculosis which was probably untreated; he lived in a men's shelter. And what do you say about an IV drug user/former prisoner/alcoholic with active TB, who signs out of the hospital, living in a men's shelter, showing up drunk to clinic?

Nevertheless, Landesman struggled to overcome his antipathy, relying on his sense of professional duty. "You sort of have to call upon all of the ethical imperatives of your profession to say, I've got to treat him like a human being as best I can. But the identification was zero."

Just as the early shape of the epidemic fundamentally affected the experience of AIDS doctors, shifting patterns of HIV infections would, in the next years, alter the world within which the most committed of physicians worked. As of 1985, 65 percent of the cumulative number of AIDS cases were linked to homosexual behavior, 17 percent to intravenous drug use.[13] By 1990, of newly reported cases, 34 percent were Black, 17 percent were Latino, the vast majority of whom were poor. Of the cases reported in that year, 24 percent were attributed to intravenous drug use.[14]

The problems first encountered by doctors at hospitals like Kings County in Brooklyn and Cook County in Chicago would become more common, challenging the ways in which physicians caring for AIDS patients would come to view their work.

2
THE DARK YEARS
Fear, Impotence, and Rejection

The first years of the AIDS epidemic were characterized by palpable dread. Donna Mildvan called the period "medieval." The etiological agent responsible for the collapse of the immune system in those who had fallen ill was unknown. No one knew how far the disease would spread, whether it would remain confined to gay and bisexual men, drug users, and recipients of blood and blood products or would extend to the broader population. In the face of much uncertainty, public attention moved from an utter lack of interest to great anxiety. Fear of contagion and disdain for those who had fallen ill produced widespread discrimination in the workplace, in schools, and even in medical facilities. In some cases, acts of violence were directed at the sick and their families. To confront these challenges, gay organizations began to mobilize for the rights of the infected at a time when the politics of the conservative Reagan era was transforming Washington and the national political climate.[1]

For medicine, AIDS represented an extraordinary reversal. After years of therapeutic progress, physicians were confronted with a disease that rendered their interventions all but futile. There were, of course, other untreatable conditions—diseases in which, despite the most intense, costly, and sometimes heroic efforts, patients succumbed. There were also irreversible, progressively debilitating chronic illnesses that afflicted an aging population. But AIDS was different. It was an infectious threat, the kind of condition that advanced industrial societies had come to think of as primarily an affliction of the Third World. It was also a disease of the relatively young, mocking assumptions about longevity, inverting the natural order of things. As if in wartime, the old began to bury the young.

Thus AIDS posed a central question for physicians tutored in the era of therapeutic advances and optimism. If I cannot cure, what am I? What can I do for my patients? What is my role as a doctor? These were questions that would have seemed strange to an older generation of doctors. They, after all, could often do little more than diagnose, palliate, and provide succor and support while nature took its course—either healing or killing. As AIDS doctors sought to define their roles, they would have to grope their way back to the answers of an earlier era. And they would have to do so surrounded by the kind of suffering for which few had been prepared. Physicians would have to learn how important it was to listen to their patients and, however unsettling it was, to admit to them their own uncertainties.

They would have to do so at a time when many feared that they themselves would succumb to their patients' illness. Like the issue of relative therapeutic impotence, that of the vulnerability of doctors to their patients' infections was not new. In previous centuries and into the 20th, doctors had routinely fallen victim to contagion. But in the post–World War II period, the threat had been contained by antibiotics. Physicians were, of course, not immune. The threat of hepatitis B made that clear. But unlike hepatitis, which typically took years to exact its toll, AIDS was rapidly fatal. A generation of physicians had been shielded from the experiences of their predecessors. And so they had never confronted a central moral question: What is my duty to patients who pose a risk to me? Must I provide care when the risk involves the possibility of my death?—an old question, but one now posed to doctors who had not considered such a prospect when they decided to enter medicine.

The fear of infection and the limits of therapy were not the only burdens on those who had cared for patients with AIDS. They also faced institutional, professional, and social hostility. Thus embattled, the new AIDS doctors came to forge their identities.

A Disease Out of Control

Death came quickly in the first years. Dan William, who had a large practice treating gay men on Manhattan's West Side, recalled:

> In the early days of the epidemic, people had short incubating disease—aggressive, rapidly progressive disease. These people probably had extraordinarily high viral loads, rapidly declining T-cells, very, very virulent infections, and they got sick, and they died in six months to 12 months with one thing after another thing after another thing.

Victoria Sharp worked as a resident in the emergency room at Roosevelt Hospital in Manhattan in 1984. She remembered the most frequently heard complaint from arriving patients:

"I got a little short of breath when I came up the stairs from the subway." Two weeks later they were dead. Not one patient that we sent to the [Intensive Care Unit] on a respirator ever came out.

Their swift deaths distinguished AIDS patients from those with cancer, some of whom, immunosuppressed, also died of infectious complications. Deborah Cotton, who had cared for patients as an infectious disease specialist at the National Cancer Institute in Bethesda, Maryland, noted the striking difference between AIDS and the then more commonly encountered cancer:

I would see cancer patients who'd gotten very intensive chemotherapy and would get very weird infections. And so an infectious death was not an unheard of thing. What was so uncanny about [AIDS deaths] was just the speed with which they happened. The fact that they were all gay men. And that basically there was no hope; there was no presumption that any of them would live. Whereas, when you took care of cancer patients, even the worst kinds of cancer, you were going for the goal with the chemo. The idea was to try to save people, and you did believe that some of them would live, at least for a while. These guys died really fast.

Contributing to the sense of therapeutic impotence was the fact that AIDS seemed to thwart the physicians' need to assert a modicum of control. "In the earliest years," said Dan William, "the part that upset doctors was that [the patients'] illnesses were out of control."

[There] was always something going on. If they got over the pneumonia, then they developed some dread neurological problem. If maybe they were getting over that, then they had some terrible gastrointestinal thing. And we often felt we were juggling with patients in terms of dealing with all of their illnesses and symptoms.

In that way, AIDS mocked medical science's Promethean vision. "We're very puny," said a humbled Gerald Friedland. "We've only been here for a little while; we don't control nature." For Wafaa El-Sadr, an Egyptian-born infectious disease physician working at the Veterans' Hospital in Manhattan, AIDS was "a wily adversary. You were outsmarted by a disease that always surprised you. It was like being outsmarted every day."

Before they died, these patients presented doctors with a rich complex of diseases rarely encountered in clinical practice. Ronald Grossman, who had a well-established gay practice on the East Side of Manhattan by the 1970s, recalled an early patient who, like Donna Mildvan's German chef, suffered a cascade of clinical tragedies:

> [He was] a young Hispanic fellow who was clearly very ill the moment we met him. He had lost a tremendous amount of weight. He had fevers for many weeks. He had tremendously painful anal sores, and he had peculiar purple spots all over his feet and ankles. [Four months later] he was short of breath and barely made it through a bout of *Pneumocystis*. I describe him in detail because I didn't know anything. None of this made any sense to me. I'd never seen Kaposi's. I'd never seen *Pneumocystis*. As much herpes as I had treated in 10 years, I'd never seen anything that came close to this man's lesions—the size, the severity. As to wasting, well except for terminal cancer patients, we just didn't see patients waste. . . . He had no money, so we got him into Bellevue. They didn't know any more than we did. He died a dreadful death—[in] pain, demented, incontinent.

At Jackson Memorial Hospital in Miami, Margaret Fischl's caseload of acutely sick Haitians was battered by illnesses. But nothing made clinical sense.

> We recognized very quickly we were seeing illnesses that we should not be seeing. We would see *Pneumocystis* so rarely here and only in cancer patients. It was not something we saw. Disseminated cytomegalovirus was almost unheard of.

This pattern of esoteric diseases or of recognized diseases in unexpected hosts made AIDS a diagnostic nightmare, even to the most skilled and experienced clinicians.

It was all the more difficult because there were so few tests available that a physician might use to identify the underlying pathology. The causative virus was not identified until 1983; a test for the existence of antibodies to the virus was not generally available until March of 1985. Just a few physicians, like UCLA's Michael Gottlieb, with appointments at major medical centers, had access to the new technologies that allowed them to measure the levels of the immune system's CD4 and CD8 T-cells. What these counts meant, in any case, was still unclear. William Valenti, a physician from Rochester, New York, succinctly summed up the doctors' plight: "It wasn't until 1985 that we really learned that T-cells were in any way predictive of illness, so we were shooting in the dark."

Richard Chaisson, when still an intern at the University of California in San Francisco, turned to Don Abrams for advice on his first patient with AIDS. His memory of the meeting deftly underscored how dark the times were.

Donald Abrams was a fellow in the fall of '82, and we consulted him as the gay-related immune deficiency guru. And he came and told us everything there was to know at the time. It took about five minutes.

Quickly, however, doctors learned to diagnose the conditions that heralded AIDS. Ronald Grossman recalled that "the learning curve was incredible" in the early years. It was almost like going through "a simultaneous residency in all the major subspecialties at the same time. Of necessity, we interfaced with our infectious disease specialists, our oncologists, our dermatologists, our pathologists."

As they struggled with the limits of their own diagnostic and therapeutic capacities, doctors were confronted with the anxieties of their patients, both those who sought reassurance and those who believed that they had contracted AIDS. In the gay community, fear of AIDS was palpable. In New York in 1981, gay friends of Jeffrey Laurence showed him spots on their skin, concerned about the possibility of Kaposi's sarcoma. On the West Coast, William Owen recalled that his patients started coming in for every kind of mole, wondering if it could possibly be "one of these new lesions." Any flu or fever might portend the dread disease. Individuals with nonspecific symptoms visited doctors, looking for a reassuring diagnosis. These patients left physicians like James Campbell, also a gay doctor in private practice in San Francisco, feeling inordinately uneasy—and at a loss.

1983 and 1984 were very, very scary years for gay [people who] were sick with anything, because no one ever knew any day that you got a fever what the problem might be. Was it *the* disease? . . . Most of the time I felt very, very uneasy. The people who ran the fevers and were tired all the time and nothing grew out of their blood and nothing grew out of their sputum, these were the most difficult patients. You just knew that one of these days they would be sicker, and you would be able to declare they had one of those AIDS-defining illnesses. But in the meanwhile, it was just a never land of just nonspecific illness in which there was very, very little we could do.

Faced with patients' fears and clinical uncertainty, some doctors avoided disclosing their darkest suspicions. William Owen offered an ethical basis for such silence.

When people were coming in with lymphadenopathy, a lot of times we would do tests for CMV [cytomegalovirus] because it was the only thing we had. There really wasn't a whole lot that you could do about it, regardless of what you believed. So sometimes in medicine, one of our dictums is, "At first, do no harm," and so do not worry people about what later turned out to be HIV disease, when there was really nothing they could do.

When confronted by anxious patients, James Campbell confessed that he was often at a loss, ill-equipped to respond well to uncertainty.

I was just as scared as they were, and much of the time didn't really know what to say to reassure them. I said, "Everything will be okay." They would look at me and say, "Are you sure?" And I would think, No I'm not sure.

Suspecting the worst, but without a firm diagnostic footing, he was reluctant to say to patients, "Well, I think you have the Big Disease."

Many doctors may have muddied their reading of ambiguous signs and symptoms by unconsciously refusing to read them honestly, what Dan William called "doctor denial." How could physicians admit to patients what they refused to admit to themselves?

Doctor denial is having your favorite patient come to see you in the office—this is 1981 or 1982—and he says, "I'm not feeling well; I've had this terrible flu for a week and a half. I have this cough, this fever." And you weigh him, and his weight is down five pounds, and his temperature is 101, his respiratory rate is a little high. You say, "Hum, probably you have bronchitis," even though in the back of my mind I'm saying, I wonder if this guy has that funny pneumonia, PCP? I don't want to believe that. And by saying he has bronchitis and giving him erythromycin, I was in denial myself. And by not allowing the possibility of this patient having this dreadful disease, I was actually performing a disservice to him by postponing the ultimate diagnosis. In the early years, people died of PCP, not because we didn't have therapy, but because their diagnosis was delayed. . . . And this was a common problem with physicians; even physicians who should have known would often delay picking it up.

Responding to the denial exhibited by patients posed a different set of issues. Faced with a grim prognosis, some patients chose to live their lives in a way that utterly ignored the realities with which they were burdened, and sometimes their physicians marveled at their patients' capacities to live for the moment. It was, of course, from any perspective, a tragic escape, but to those who were impotent to intervene, it was an escape that provided some relief. Not infrequently, Alvin Friedman-Kien had patients with advanced disease who came into his office saying

they just bought a house on Fire Island, or they're going to Europe, or thinking about buying a new apartment, and they have absolutely no sense of reality, which I think is absolutely thrilling. Just amazing. And what could be more wonderful than somebody saying, "I've just bought a house in East Hampton," and they're terminal. They're not going to live to see the end of it, and they know it. They're just not dealing with it. It's great. Who cares?

"If I Cannot Cure, What Am I?"

However they sought to respond to their patients' needs, there was one thing doctors could not do: They could not create therapeutic options where none existed. Peter Wolfe, an infectious disease specialist in Los Angeles accustomed to curing patients, experienced himself as "impotent." Abigail Zuger referred to what treatment there was as

finger in the dam kind of medicine. When [patients] developed infections, what would now be called late-stage infections, they were treated for them, usually not successfully. Usually that was the last bongo drum because most people didn't live very long after.

Their deaths were horrifying. Donald Abrams remembers, "We didn't have anything to offer them. [They] died, and the deaths they died, I recall, were very terrible deaths; they were deformed and disfigured and wasted away, Kaposi's sarcoma lesions all over their bodies." Confronted by their own limits, their powerlessness, doctors also had to contend with the frustration and anger of their patients; San Francisco General's Constance Wofsy recalled the many times they turned on her with the remark, "You call yourself an expert?"

With a sense of urgency, doctors sought new ways to minister to their patients and to stem the growing epidemic. Their summons, according to Wofsy, "was always try harder, do more, be better, get this new drug; it was the imperative of working beyond limits, of just keeping going." But sheer will and effort were only partial responses to a disease that seemed to elude the best attempts to capture and domesticate it. AIDS treaters were also compelled to reevaluate and modify the assumptions of a medicine that taught them that a physician's claim to authority rested on the ability to treat and cure disease successfully. Painfully aware of the limits of medicine, they struggled to find creative responses to those limitations.

Some responded by adopting a posture of therapeutic skepticism. For Donald Kotler, one of the few gastroenterologists who embraced the new epidemic, AIDS was an epiphany, a discovery that curing was only a part of doctoring. With bleak humor he noted:

> I realized that physicians were suckered. After all, how long have we been curers? How long has there been disease? How long have there been physicians? Physicians have been around for 5,000 years. There have been cures for a hundred. What did they do for the other 4,900? I did get self-righteous enough to go and look at the Hippocratic oath, and, just as I'd thought, the word "cure" is not in the Hippocratic oath.

To focus on cure, Kotler came to believe, had a distorting effect on the physician's identity and behavior and a deleterious effect on patient care itself.

> I wasn't there to cure people, and, in fact, what I realized was that that was the sickening excuse of many people who didn't want to deal with patients with AIDS. If I cannot cure, why should I bother?

If I cannot cure, what am I? Gerald Friedland found his answer to Kotler's question through a cultural perspective, informed by his years as a Peace Corps doctor in Nigeria. Schooled in the optimism of infectious disease medicine, he was, nevertheless, able to call on his experience with a medicine of constraints.

> I had lived in Nigeria for two years. It really helped me a lot to know what the limits of medicine are. So I never had the delusion that we were going to conquer this thing, and I still don't. It's the wrong thing to talk about. [I think that as long as] we have the wrong paradigm, as long as we keep talking about cure, we'll always feel like failures. We're not failures; we've done great things, but people [have] the wrong expectations. What do we cure? So I think Nigeria was very helpful to me, because even the people who you could take care of with their schistosomiasis, they go back to the stream, they get it again. So we're limited. I've always felt limited as a physician.

Robert Cohen did not begin treating people with AIDS until 1988. Before that he had served as medical director of a municipal prison, Riker's Island, and as a vice president in the Health and Hospitals Corporation, both in New York City. He brought to medical treatment a hard-nosed, minimalist view that many doctors who had been treating AIDS cases for years had embraced as a protective shield.

> I never thought that curing people was what doctors did. . . . I thought they made people as comfortable as possible; if they had a very serious illness, they ameliorated, they reduced pain, simple things. They sometimes cured [diseases], although most of those were self-limiting anyway. But people who developed congestive heart failure died within five to ten years after their diagnosis. Cancer, except in a few cases, was not responsive to treatment; the sequelae of diabetes have been pretty much out of control. . . . I think that the most intense clinical experiences I had, even as an intern or resident, were hand-holding. But hand-holding is a very difficult part of medicine. I do it a lot, and I try to do it right, and it is a very satisfying as well as wrenching part of the experience.

Without the possibility of curative interventions, many doctors, like Cohen, worked their way back to an older tradition in medicine, one focused on care. "Hand-holding," in both metaphorical and literal senses, provided a means of giving comfort, psychological solace, and social support. In the last stages of the disease, doctors could reduce pain and suffering and promise not to abandon their patients. For some, like Joseph O'Neill, this laying on of hands constituted a return to real or "old-fashioned" medicine. "Taking care of, being there for somebody, not abandoning them, paying attention; I mean, what do you do when you can't cure somebody? Really being a doctor, to me, begins at that point."

Strikingly, many physicians went beyond hand-holding. They physically embraced their patients in a way that crossed the conventional clinical boundary. Charles van der Horst, who treated both gay middle-class men from the sophisticated community surrounding Chapel Hill, North Carolina, and the poorest drug-involved individuals from the eastern reaches of the state, learned to hug his patients and to touch them. Born in Holland, the child of Holocaust survivors, he had a deep-seated need to bring peace to his immediate surroundings—in Hebrew, *Shalom Bayet*. It was that need and his desire to stop the suffering of his patients that made him so apparently anomalous—a manager of large clinical trials who embraced his patients. He insisted the best thing he could do for his patients was to hold their hands from the beginning of their illness to its end. "A good plumber" could perform the technical tasks of medicine. But he, as an AIDS doctor, knew how to listen and talk to patients. It was as if the act of holding involved a kind of therapeutic touch. To illustrate, he recalled, if somewhat imperfectly, a story by Kafka, "The Country Doctor," that had had a great impact on him.

> I read it years ago in German in high school, and I've never read it since. But what I do remember—and all that's important—is that this doctor goes out on this horse and buggy to visit some guy who's bedridden, and the upshot is that they reverse positions. The doctor stays there and the guy drives off. It was a powerful image of the physician healing by touching a patient and reversing the roles. Now I have no desire to become sick, yet [I do] heal and hold.

John Mazzullo, a gay physician in Boston, also learned to hug his patients during the AIDS epidemic, an action contrary to the traditional clinical distance taught him at Columbia University's College of Physicians and Surgeons. But being close was very important to many of the patients he treated.

> In medical school, I remember we asked a teacher what would happen if our patient started to cry, and you know what he told us? Hand them some Kleenex. And it became obvious in the eighties that that was not the right thing to do. So, I hug my patients a lot.

Part of it is for me, to feel close to them. Part of it is for them, to feel close to me. But part of it is that they're going to die, and I have to have that feeling of having touched them. I don't do it with all of them; some of them would find it abhorrent. [But] I have some people that are just really suffering and are really hurting. And I can tell it, that they never get touched except by someone sticking them or poking them. So I want to touch them sometimes without a needle, to balance it out.

Such touching was also crucial for Neil Schram, a gay physician at a Kaiser Permanente clinic in Los Angeles. He talked of a night when an AIDS patient called out his name and told him he was his favorite physician because "You hug me; none of the others do." To Schram, hugging patients was terribly important.

So many of them won't be touched by anybody. . . . What people wanted most of all was a physician who treated them, in spite of their HIV infection, like a human being; and it's sad to say, but too many people had seen other physicians who didn't. The most hideous one was a patient who had gotten a phone call from a physician, being informed he was HIV positive. And he says to the physician, "What do I do now?" And the physician says, "Go home and wait to die."

Not all AIDS doctors could or even wanted to breach convention by hugging their patients, but all had to confront the limits of what they had come to expect of themselves as physicians before AIDS. There were, of course, lessons to be drawn from their earlier professional work. Oncologists, who were among the most aggressive treaters—"floggers" to their critics—brought to AIDS the experience of treating chronically ill patients, many of whom died. Jerome Groopman, at the Deaconess Hospital in Boston, described himself as primed for treating a disease like AIDS: "I was used to dealing with fatal illness, as used as you can get to it." But Alexandra Levine, a cancer specialist at the University of Southern California, found that while cancer treatment informed her AIDS work, it was through the latter that she formed an approach that allowed her to comfortably care for a patient when cure was not possible.

Number one, I had to learn to accept the fact that the patient had that illness, and that took me a little while to do. At the beginning, I would spend a lot of time thinking, Why, why? It's not fair! And

I came to somehow train myself to begin by accepting it; there's nothing you can do. The second part of the rationalization was to know I had provided the best medical care. I had to be extremely comfortable that the medical care was meticulous, that I wasn't going to [feel] guilty because I omitted something. The third part of the equation was that I will have given the patient something that few people could have given. In the area of oncology, especially solid tumors, patients are going to die, and the issue is not whether or not I'll be able to cure . . . but if I can allow the patient to live that time well and comfortably, as opposed to scared to death, I feel that I really accomplished something.

Infectious disease doctors and other physicians whose patient populations in the past suffered infrequent deaths discovered that AIDS required a paradigmatic shift in how they practiced medicine. In 1995, Constance Wofsy looked back on the evolution of her work.

I'm trying to think how many years it took before it eventually became clear that we have to accept death in young people as something that did happen, and that we were moving from "how are we going to resolve this?" to "how can we make this the least painful, relieve suffering and [achieve] the longest, best life span possible?" . . . I learned some important things: Always offer something. In a subtle way, it's sort of smoke and mirrors, but the patient has to live with something, and it doesn't have to be much. Offer a change in dose if it's within the reasonable dose change limits. If there's nothing to offer, offer time. "I think that the medications we've tried haven't been very effective. Why don't we see how things go without any treatment right now, and then report to me in a month how that's been for you." All those are offering something. It's not much, but it's something. I haven't given up, you haven't given up, you're still hanging in there.

Lisa Capaldini learned in her San Francisco practice that caring meant offering whatever was appropriate for her patient. Like Wofsy, her experience taught her the primary importance of offering something, if only, paradoxically, nothing. Recalling a patient, Capaldini remembered

looking at him and saying, "Robert, I wish there was more I could do for you. I just can't think of any other treatments we might try for your neuropathy. And the same with your diarrhea. This must be difficult for you." And he looked at me and said, "Yes. So what happens now?" And I said, "Well, I think over time you'll get weaker, and these problems will be more bothersome. I will do whatever I can to make you as comfortable and independent as possible, and no matter what, I'll be with you in this." And he looked at me and said, "That's all I needed to hear."

And it was a moment of clarity for me, that rather than react to the limits of my technical skills in what you might call a frustrated way, I realized what I still could do, that I could promise him that I would still try to palliate his symptoms, the ones that weren't fixable, and it really was a paradigm change for me. And the paradigm is to always focus on what's best for the patient at any time; and at some point in my work with them, what's best is doing a test and trying a zillion different antiretrovirals. Sometimes, what's best is spending the whole visit talking about how they're going to tell their parents they have AIDS. And sometimes what's best is helping them die with as much peace and dignity as possible. So long as I focus on what's best at that time for that person, there's always something I can do. And that has sort of let me off the hook in terms of the traditional expectations of Western medicine, which is, You should go in there and find out what's wrong and cure it. And if you don't do either, you're a failure or the patient's a failure. And in this new paradigm, there are no failures; every problem is an opportunity to help someone.

Gay physicians, for whom the boundary between clinical and private worlds was blurred, learned important lessons in "being there" and "offering something" as they cared for dying friends and lovers, lessons which they could apply to their AIDS patients. Donald Abrams, who lost four lovers to AIDS, described caring for Mark, with whom he was living at the time of his illness:

Living with Mark, I remember that we had to live every day as if this might be his last. And I found that by giving him little things to look forward to in the future I felt like I was prolonging his survival. We took a cruise together, and on that cruise he was demented and having dysentery, and it was really a traumatic experience; but I think having things to look forward to and being loved are very important. . . . I believe that, perhaps second to *Pneumocystis* prophylaxis, love and expectations into the future are things that are helpful to keep people alive.

"Being there" meant something much broader and more demanding in impoverished populations. Physicians committed to serving these communities had to focus not only on AIDS but also on fragmented lives and heavy drug use. They had to become social workers as well as primary care doctors. In Newark, New Jersey, Anita Vaughn found that despite the absence of curative or healing therapies, she could provide her patients with something valuable; she could stabilize their lives and engage them in reaching out to others.

> It's very frustrating. The patients feel you've betrayed them at times, but I'm very honest with patients and families. If people are shooting up, I make them understand that I don't [approve of such] behaviors, but I [still] love them. "You can change your life." And a lot of patients have become drug free. [We ask patients] to write [an essay and] define what quality of life was to them. Getting back in touch with God was number one, and two was to help others; they thought that if they could get that, then they had a better quality of life. So, even if we can't offer a cure, we've done a lot. A lot of patients have become educated [about] HIV, so that they are working now as peer counselors. Some of these individuals have been on welfare all of their adult life, and now they are working. You know, that's quite an accomplishment.

In the Bronx, at Albert Einstein College of Medicine, Arye Rubinstein, the quintessential scientist-clinician, responded to his poverty-stricken pediatric patients by organizing a multifaceted program.

> I realized that I was dealing with a totally different segment of the population. You cannot just see these patients for an hour in your clinic and say good-bye and assume that something is going to happen, that there will be compliance and follow-up of your instructions. It was clear from the beginning that you have to go much more into the socioeconomic situation of those families. It was an extension of [clinical] care. And that's why I started this social medicine program here very quickly. At this point we have social workers. We have outreach workers that go to the houses. You cannot treat these children without having this kind of outreach. It's a futile exercise.

Rubinstein also created a day care center for the children, which both offered them clinical and psychological services and potentially protected them from the public hysteria over HIV-infected children in the public schools. His greatest personal commitment, because both his time and his family were involved, was to create a summer camp for HIV-positive children.

> We raised funds and started a camp in the mountains—very se-cretly, because we [realized] that if anyone knew these kids with AIDS were there, they would throw us out. We took volunteers, but we came also. I came there with my twins, my twin girls. They were babies at the time. And we stayed with these kids and lived with these families. We went horseback riding with them. We went rowing with them. We went bowling with them. . . . We wanted to have the family unit there. My philosophy from the beginning was that we have to create an AIDS family center. They were very touching, mothers who knew they were dying soon, with their kids, and they were looking for another mother who had AIDS to take care of their children when they died. There were sessions on dying there, with psychologists. So my nurses went there, my social workers went there, the fellows went there. We really became an extended family with those patients.

A number of physicians found in their own religion, or that of their patients, a source of strength during the epidemic. For some, spirituality or a religious sense of mission informed their clinical work. Believing that "prayer and religion [are] a part of healing," Anita Vaughn prayed with her patients when it felt appropriate. Joseph O'Neill was inspired to use his patients' religion, even though he himself was not religious, to sustain them during the difficult course of their disease and to allow them to make wrenching personal decisions.

> I would always ask patients at some point, "Well, how were you raised, were you raised in any particular spiritual or religious be-lief?" And most would say, "Yes." And I would say, "Well, what does it mean to you now?" or just a general question about how are you integrating the fact that you're going to die into your life? It's been probably the most important intervention that I've made for a great number of patients. Now, I've not pushed anything on anybody; I don't have those beliefs. Probably my whole life will be a struggle to find something that makes some sense to me. But [I want] to bring this into the medical health care setting. One guy I took care of was a well-known professional [who] grew up in a

very prominent family, came out relatively late in life, got HIV infected. He was very bitter at [his] church because he felt he was forced into marriage. But, I said, "What was good about [your] church?" And he talked about the strength that he got from his family and [its] meaning. I suggested to him that he begin to reexplore what was positive about that experience as he prepared for death, to look at the spiritual elements of these things. I took care of him for a couple of years; and [he was getting sicker and] moved back home. And when he left, he said, "Joe, I want you to know something. Of all the things you do, the most important thing you or anyone has ever said to me was that day you raised the question about my religion and what it meant to me. I can't tell you how healing it was for me." He [was] coming to some kind of peace, coming full circle to that little boy [who] was growing up [in the West].

James Oleske's commitment to working in Newark's inner city, a mission he took on as a medical student, found its spiritual source in his Catholic, working-class background and education. If he had a calling, Oleske believed, it was "to stay in Newark to deal with [AIDS]." Oleske spoke often of his patients and their families, who offered him the reinforcement he required to remain. On a memorable occasion, he was asked to visit the church of Cynthia, a child whom he had treated and who had just died.

I knew this was a bad area—I've been here my whole career, I started in '66—and I couldn't see a children's church. So I'm driving up and down the block. [Finally, with some help, I get there.] It wasn't a church. It was a lean-to against an abandoned building. And I could see sort of flames coming from the door. So I opened the door, and here's this kerosene heater, open-flame heater, and about 15 children in a choir singing, and about eight or nine parents. Ahead of me was Sister Evelyn and her pastor and a little sort of makeshift altar with a white cloth over a stand. And they see me, and they wave me in. . . . And they had this big old stuffed chair, and when I sat down in it I realized it only had three legs, and it lurched forward so I had to lean back.

The children finish their song, and then Sister Evelyn introduced me and said that I was there to talk about Cynthia. It was around 7:30, and I'm saying to myself, "I got to get out of here now." Well, it was such an experience for me, because those kids were aged eight to maybe 14, and their parents asked some great questions. And I looked at Sister Evelyn when I first started, and I said, "Can I talk about sex and drugs and all that?" . . . Some of the men that were there asked questions about the army inventing this virus to kill minorities and [that] this was genocide, and I talked about it as honestly as I could. "Why are you saying the virus comes from Africa?" [they asked]. "Why are you blaming Black people?" And, you know, I just answered as best I could. The next thing I knew it's about two and a half hours later. It was a very positive experience.

But the best thing that happened was the minister says, "Well, you got to go Dr. Oleske, and I'm sorry that we can't give you anything, but we can give you our blessing." And with that one of the eight-year-olds from the choir came up and reached behind this makeshift altar, and there was a bottle with oil in it—obviously an old La Choy soy sauce bottle with the label off—and she puts a little oil on her finger, and then she puts her hands on my head and made the sign of the cross. And while she was holding my head, the choir sang a song of praise. And it's funny; I was really blessed.

Fears of Contagion

The first reports of AIDS that appeared in the CDC's *Morbidity and Mortality Weekly Report* suggested that the new disease might be sexually transmitted. But no one knew for certain, and certainly no one knew whether there might be other routes of transmission. For physicians whose daily work brought them in contact with patients whose symptoms were often gruesome and whose clinical course was almost always catastrophic, fear began to mount.

For gay physicians, who were typically no different in age from their gay patients, and whose sexual lives often mirrored the lives of those for whom they now cared, AIDS represented a special threat. In their patients they saw a grim omen of what could indeed happen to them. In his mid-30s during the first years of the epidemic, William Owen, long active in gay medical circles in San Francisco, recalled:

I wasn't afraid of getting it from my patients directly. I never used gloves, for instance, to examine, do a standard physical examination on my patients. But certainly seeing patients with this disease . . . made me, as a gay man, aware of the fact that this disease was probably one of the worst possible things that could happen to people who were still very young, and made me aware of my own vulnerability in terms of risk of transmission of disease via sexual transmission. I thought [back to] the period when I was more sexually active in the '70s. It was certainly a possibility that I could have been exposed.

"We were all going to die. There was no reason why we shouldn't have died," an anguished John Mazzullo said years after he knew that he had been spared. Ronald Grossman, a generation older than most of the gay physicians who came to care for AIDS patients, inspected his own body for signs of the disease he now saw so frequently in his large New York practice.

I remember the time when I caught myself examining my own lymph nodes with such vigor that I made my neck sore, and validated that I must have swollen lymph nodes. . . . I think we were all terrified.

But for some gay doctors, the story would be different. By 1985, of the physicians who had been diagnosed with AIDS, all but one had been infected through sexual intercourse. Stosh Ostrow "knew" he was carrying the etiological agent responsible for AIDS even before the virus was discovered. He came to understand the significance of his own medical situation by hearing about AIDS in California and New York at the very start of the epidemic. And so when he encountered his first patients in Atlanta, it was clear that they shared a common fate.

I developed lymphadenopathy at the end of '78. I was very sick with viral illness for about two weeks, 17 pounds weight loss, really quite ill. I got over that. And then [I] was in a seminar, sitting there, and [I] crossed my arms and felt these huge nodes and thought I had lymphoma. [I] got evaluated and that was the end of it. It wasn't lymphoma. But I very quickly realized that what was going on inside of me was what we were hearing about happening in California and in New York.

Jerry Cade did not discover that he was infected until 1987. Tested when he learned that a close friend, the deputy commissioner of health in New Jersey, had been diagnosed with Kaposi's sarcoma, he was not surprised to learn he was positive.

I had spent the last years of med school and my first internship in LA making up for lost time. Those were the years of "let's party and see how many times we can get laid." So I was worried about that. [At that] point we thought the incubation period was about two years. I started counting. I left LA in '81, here we are in '83–84, I'm still healthy, so I must be safe. . . . I think that I first tested positive in January or February of 1987. . . . I even remember part of the reason for doing so was that [by 1987] we knew the incubation period was longer. . . . And I went and tested because I almost knew it was going to be positive, and I thought, well, this will be my way of giving support, because [my friend] had been diagnosed with AIDS. And I was, and I called him, and I said, "It is." And I flew out to New York to be with him shortly thereafter, and we talked a bit about HIV disease. He, of course, was much sicker at that point in time and died not too long thereafter.

For heterosexual physicians, the fears were of a different kind. Could they acquire the new fatal illness from their patients? This was especially so for those whose practices involved invasive procedures. For Donald Kotler the anxiety took hold almost immediately.

After my first patient, or perhaps second patient, I was talking to [an infectious disease specialist], and he just used a sort of off-handed comment, "You know, this thing is probably transmissible, but we don't know what it is." Jesus, my wife was pregnant with my second child at the time. It's transmissible but we don't know how or by what? Or what to do? Well, I'm a gastroenterologist. We do invasive things, you know, sexually transmitted things through rectal mucosa. It's my job to go in and inspect rectal mucosa. I had learned when I was a fellow to orient small intestinal biopsies on my finger. I had already gotten myself stuck with a needle and cut myself with a scalpel on my first patient. And with that kind of background, then somebody comes along and tells me that there's a transmissible disease? . . . It was quite unpleasant wondering how close to be with my wife, how close to be with my kids. I buried it.

But it was not only those whose work required such probing who feared that they might contract their patients' illness. Indeed, the fears began to escalate as the understanding of how AIDS might be transmitted began to advance. Cases in hemophiliacs, first reported in July 1982, and in blood transfusion recipients in December 1982, provided evidence that the as-yet-to-be-discovered causative agent was blood-borne. That, in turn, enhanced the argument that hepatitis B, a significant threat to health care workers, represented an appropriate model of contagion. In November 1982, the CDC urged clinicians and laboratory workers to adopt barrier precautions recommended for the prevention of hepatitis B when treating patients with AIDS or when handling their specimens.[2]

"My recollection," said San Francisco's Paul Volberding, "is that my anxiety really skyrocketed when a pediatric transfusion case [was reported] in 1982. It provided compelling evidence of transmissibility."

> You see how bad the disease is, and you begin to appreciate that it's probably caused by an infection, and probably a virus because of the blood transmission. There was a period where I was more or less convinced that I had it, whatever *it* was. I had a test done of my helper T-cells [and found them dangerously low]. And I didn't tell a soul. I didn't tell [my wife] Molly; I didn't tell anybody because it was a confirmation to me that I was infected. And Molly and I had already had Alex by then; she was pregnant. So, I mean, here we are, living together, having sex, having kids, and not knowing whether or not we're carrying and transmitting this disease, and the nightmare was really transmitting it to the children. I had nightmares all the time, and it was always transmitting it to the kids. It was that sense of How could you do this to somebody else?

In fact, his wife, Molly Cooke, also a physician involved in the care of AIDS patients at San Francisco General Hospital, was concerned as well.

> I was quite visibly pregnant, and I was walking into the [intensive care unit to visit an AIDS patient] when one of the residents, a male resident, said, "Are you really sure you want to go in that room?" And I said, "What do you mean?" I had to stop and think before I understood what he was saying, and then I said, "Of course I do." But that marks when I first began to think, Gee, could we get this? It had not occurred to me before that this was something that doctors would get.
>
> Paul at this point was convinced this was a viral infection. I was cooking dinner—we were in the kitchen—and he said that the transmission looks a lot like hepatitis B and that you can account

for almost everything if you imagine a virus that's transmitted like hepatitis B. Hepatitis B was at the time the big occupational hazard for health care workers, and, you know, I thought, Shit, if this is transmitted like hepatitis B we could all get this! You didn't have to be having anal intercourse with gay men. There were other kinds of inoculation that presumably would be equally effective, and that scared me.

And then we began to hear rumors about health care workers who had gotten this. The rumors were horrible. I remember 1982 as being the really bad year for rumors. We were seeing more and more of this disease, and because we were not making the diagnosis until very late in the disease, you didn't have to wait a long time for people to die. All the initial excitement really began to be replaced by anxiety about the agent. We didn't fight about this—it was a very close time—but it was difficult.

At the end of '82 we had several discussions about if we were going to have another baby because—and it sounds so melodramatic now—but it was not clear how safe what we were doing was. And I didn't want to go ahead and have another baby and then discover that one or both of us was not going to live to see the baby grow up. So there was a very real sense of danger, that the work was potentially dangerous, and you just didn't know exactly how dangerous it was.

I had spent probably a full year feeling, at least intermittently, very scared and then on a second level very confused about my responses to my own patients—what does it mean to be frightened of your patients and your patients' disease?—before I realized that this was not an idiosyncratic, psychological aberration. . . . I can remember sitting in my office at San Francisco General reflecting on a conversation that I'd just had with a completely reasonable person and thinking about how frightened she was [and] suddenly it was, If she's that frightened it must be normal to be this frightened.

Although Volberding had received what he thought was bad diagnostic news, neither he, himself, nor his wife had yet experienced the terror of discovering a symptom suggestive of transmission. Terrible anxiety did take hold of Cooke, though, when she discovered a pink spot on her baby's ear that turned out to be nothing. It was such spots that made Donald Abrams, Volberding's future colleague, fear that he had been exposed.

One morning I woke up, and I had these red spots on the palm of my hand. I had been seeing patients in the Kaposi's sarcoma clinic, and I knew that if I pushed it and it blanched then it wasn't likely to be KS. So I pushed it, and it didn't blanch; *it didn't blanch*. I went to a Christmas party and a woman came up and she was talking to me telling me that she had melanoma, and she was getting a lot of assistance from dealing with this group called the Center for Attitudinal Healing, learning how to accept her death. And I said, "Well, you have melanoma; look at me." And I showed her the palm of my hand, and she said, "What's that?" And I said, "I don't know, but I'm afraid that it might be Kaposi's sarcoma." I was really quite petrified. And the next day was a Sunday and I called Marcus Conant, and I said, "Marcus, I don't know what's on the palm of my hand but I really, you know, I need somebody to have a look at it." I went home, and I told my lover, "We need to go. Marcus is going to see me." . . . My lover, who was this Israeli ballet dancer, who [was] very sort of pragmatic and practical said, "Think about it. Did you spill anything on your hand yesterday?" And I said, "Probably, as I was walking with this container of liquid nitrogen, some of it might have come out, and I might have burnt myself in these little splotches." So we went to Marcus, and he put my hand down on a piece of velvet, and he took pictures of it, and he looked at it, and he put on his glasses, and he said, "Well, I don't know what it is." And I said, "Well, could it be liquid nitrogen burns?" And he said, "Well, I guess it could be." He said, "But, if it doesn't go away by next week, come in and we'll do a biopsy." And two days later they were gone.

For those who experienced unexplained bouts of illness that mimicked the symptoms of their very sick patients, it was only natural to assume that transmission of the as-yet-to-be-discovered etiological agent had occurred. Jerome Groopman had such an encounter in 1983 in Los Angeles. "It was February or so of '83," said Groopman, who was only 31 years old at that time, and contracted what was a severe mycoplasma infection.

I developed prolonged fevers, pulmonary infiltrate hepatitis, and I was hospitalized at UCLA. I was really sick. And no one could figure out what I had. And I was truly frightened that I was going to be the first medical case of AIDS. I saw myself in the *New England*

Journal, not as an author but as an autopsy. . . . It turned out I had very severe mycoplasma infection.

For Michael Gottlieb, the fright was intensified by the fact that his wife had also become ill.

I had an illness that in retrospect seemed very much like the acute retroviral syndrome. And both my wife at the time and I had this, and we were sick at home in the dark because of light sensitivity, with lymphadenopathy, fever, and the feeling that you'd just fought 15 rounds with Mike Tyson. You felt like you'd been whacked.

When they felt threatened, some physicians quite naturally turned to their families for support. But others, like Kotler, kept their fears to themselves, sharing them only with colleagues, if anyone. Renslow Sherer, who was co-director of the AIDS service at Chicago's Cook County Hospital, protected his wife from the fear he felt, keeping it "in one secret place," knowing that his public reassurances regarding the transmissibility of AIDS could be wrong. "No, no, no," he said. He could not talk to his wife about the risks.

I was also a reassurer with her, and in our family, actually, and that ultimately proved to be very difficult, because I think that the way physicians cope in general is to do a lot of compartmentalizing. What happens in clinic is located in clinic, and it's there when you come back to it. But you really leave it there. . . . I was lucky enough to have family and home to return to as a buffer, not idyllic, but a place to go where they really didn't know very much about AIDS or what was happening to me. . . . There was some private fear there that I never did share with her.

How difficult the discussion of such fears could be is poignantly conveyed by Paul Volberding and Molly Cooke, both of whom understood the risks to which they had chosen to expose themselves. "I'm the kind," said Volberding, "that if I'm sick I complain about it."

If I have a sore throat I go, "Oh, I'm gonna throw [up]." That's just me. Molly is really the opposite. In her family and for her it's a sign of absolute moral weakness to complain about your health. You could be dying and you shouldn't complain about it. You shouldn't even mention it. [Also] there was so much anxiety that Molly didn't really allow me to complain or to express my fears. I understood it, I understood it very much. We were both so anxious that we couldn't talk about it, because where do you go with that? We both knew that we wanted to keep doing this; we'd made that decision, so let's just get on and do it. But it was horrible. . . . And then during that time I developed a big lymph node in my right groin, a low sort of femoral node. It was not subtle; it was kind of a robin-egg-sized lymph node, inflamed, tender. And I went, Jesus, you know, it was obviously lymphoma. I showed it to Molly, and she just froze, because she was obviously convinced it was as well, that this was it.

Molly Cooke acknowledged how unsettling she found her husband's fears.

We read *The Plague*. I'm probably as much an existentialist as I am anything else, so the stoicism of the book was quite comforting to me, and the moral strength. Paul coped completely well at work and publicly, [but] he would come home and express uncertainty about whether he should be doing this. That was intolerable to me. It's not how I deal with hard decisions psychologically myself. . . . I do as much reflection as I can tolerate, and then I decide, and then I say, "I've made this decision, and I'm going to do it." And so when he would come home and, perfectly justifiably, express his uneasiness and ambivalence to me, I finally said, "I can't provide verbal reassurance to you, because watching you work is reassuring to me." We both have a very strong sense of duty, and I said, "I think we both need to do this, but I can't right now produce what I need to do to do my work, tolerate your doing what you're doing and reassure you. I don't have enough left to reassure you." I was really asking him to make his decisions the way I made my decision, and I recognized that it wasn't really fair.

Despite Cooke's effort to "normalize" her fear, not all doctors recall the same level of anxiety. Richard Chaisson was at San Francisco General as a resident when Volberding and Cooke were so frightened. It was, he believed, his "naïveté" that protected him. "By the time I was well informed enough to be worried about it, I was obviously assured [by the research] that I didn't need to be." Others avoided fear because they worked in clinical settings where possible exposure to contagion was limited. Carol Brosgart practiced at a public health clinic in Oakland, California. "I wasn't in a house staff setting where I was putting IVs in or doing more invasive things. . . . There were very few things that one did in an outpatient setting where there was going to be transmission." But even within hospital settings where AIDS was regularly encountered, there were those who were able to treat patients with little trepidation. Janet Mitchell, an African-American perinatalogist who had committed herself to working with drug-abusing women, had done her residency at Harlem Hospital in New York before going to Boston City Hospital. She had returned to Harlem in 1988 to the Department of Obstetrics and Gynecology.

> There's no question that I waded through more HIV as a resident here than I have any place else, and if I were going to be infected by doing what I do, [I would already have been infected]. . . . So I said to myself, It's too late for me to be afraid, because I was just as macho as my fellow men were when it came to cut, cut, cut, you know, cut, slash. . . . You know, you weren't a real obstetrician unless you had blood all over you.

Blood-soaked as a resident at Bellevue, Abigail Zuger also seemed inured to the anxiety experienced by others.

> You're in this atmosphere of cowboy medicine anyway. We were all running around with blood all over us. It's kind of hard to imagine now; we were running around drenched in blood. We did all our own blood work more or less at that point. We didn't use gloves ever. We used gloves for sterile procedures but not for just [drawing blood]. I had tubes of blood in my pockets; I would come home and there they'd be. I'd throw them out in the garbage. No, I was not concerned, but I would ascribe that to a lack of intelligence on my part rather than to any kind of heroic nature.

For those who had committed themselves to the care of AIDS patients, it was crucial to adopt anxiety-reducing postures. The tension experienced by Cooke and Volberding was, for most, incompatible with sustained effort. Sometimes a leap of faith was entailed. Lisa Capaldini, who had just returned to San Francisco General Hospital after working in a nonmedical context in New York City, had to decide how to deal with her fears as she faced her first patient with AIDS.

I remember when I first went to meet him in his room, sitting down next to him on his bed and getting ready to put my hand on his to just say hello and introduce myself, and having this pause of Boy, is it okay to touch this guy? I mean, at that point we really weren't sure how AIDS was transmitted. And I'm glad I had that moment, because it's helped me be less judgmental and reactive with regard to people who have those same emotions. I was lucky enough to see all these nurses running around the AIDS ward, 5A, hugging people and touching them, and it became clear that it seemed to be a safe thing to do. That modeling helped me very much.

Constance Wofsy, whose background in infectious disease should have made her more careful, had also thrown caution to the wind.

[No, I wasn't afraid.] I was too gripped. . . . We were people with a cause, and like any cause you become overzealous, I think. The people early on who worked on the AIDS ward almost flaunted safety precautions. Our original infection control measures were written as "You do not need to wear gloves to examine the patient except for . . ." We became patient advocates to the exclusion of our own anxieties or rational observation of the data that was in front of us.

Some sought to demonstrate the irrationality of what they took to be exaggerated fears and their outrage at refusals to provide appropriate care by casting aside even minimal precautions. While at Yale–New Haven Hospital, Elizabeth Kass and some of her colleagues chose to be incautious as an act of solidarity with patients they thought were ill-treated.

There were some people there who wouldn't put an IV in or draw cultures on AIDS patients. So I think several of us found that so appalling that, if anything, we probably went the other direction. We probably did things without gloves that were stupid.

Many of the new AIDS doctors felt disdain toward their colleagues, who responded to the unknown dimensions of risk by recourse to protective gear that sometimes resembled spacesuits or the garb of the plague doctors of the late Middle Ages and that made contact between the patient and caregiver all but impossible. Howard Grossman was a resident at Kings County Hospital in Brooklyn when careful studies had already made it clear that AIDS was not casually transmitted. He was appalled by the attire worn by some of his colleagues.

> I started this with a pretty clear understanding that this was tough to transmit, and it used to drive me crazy, the masks and the gowns and everything else. I just wouldn't do that stuff. I learned very early to wear gloves, but the rest of that stuff used to just make me nuts.

For those who worked with children, the prospect of being placed at risk by their patients seemed almost unimaginable. Small and vulnerable, how could they threaten? Just as the broader society viewed children with AIDS as innocents, these physicians ignored the significance of AIDS as a blood-borne disease and of the discovery of the viral agent, HIV, in 1983. Perhaps equally important, they understood that to wear gloves, gowns, and masks would make it all the more difficult to win the confidence of their young—sometimes very young—patients. James Oleske's clinical practice in Newark was typical of pediatricians working with AIDS in ghetto communities ravaged by intravenous drug use and crack cocaine.

> Maybe I was too naive, or too dumb. I might be both, but I was not afraid. That may have been wrong on my part. I guess maybe I was never afraid of children, and I couldn't believe I could get sick from a child. . . . I can't tell you how many times I drew blood without gloves. I washed my hands; I mean I always believed in hygiene, believed in the germ theory.

Ironically, it was in an editorial commenting on Oleske's own work, published in the *Journal of the American Medical Association* in 1983, that Anthony Fauci, director of the National Institute of Allergies and Infectious Disease, speculated on the possibility of the communicability of AIDS. "If non-sexual, non-blood-borne transmission is possible, the scope of the syndrome may be enormous."[3]

It was clear that only careful epidemiological studies could respond to the growing questions posed by such speculation,[4] the lingering private fears of doctors and the dread expressed in the acts of discrimination that had begun to take place in public settings from the classroom to the workplace.[5] Such investigations were pursued in both New York and Miami. In the Bronx, Gerald Friedland, with support from the CDC, undertook a study of the households of patients with AIDS, examining blood samples of those who were sexual partners and those who merely shared a common living space.

> Because we wanted to do it in a proper, scientific way, we interspersed specimens from patients' families with specimens from patients. We wanted the lab to be blinded to whether people had AIDS or were just family members. And I had a study nurse, her name was Pat Kall, and everything was coded for reasons of confidentiality. And we're deciphering the code and determining which are the positives and which are the negatives. It was late one afternoon, and basically Pat and I are sitting in an office look[ing] at what we had. And all the positives were the AIDS patients, and all the negatives were the household members. And we went, "Thank God." And you know, that was one of those special moments. I mean, it's not a discovery, because basically we were just documenting something; but it was a revelation, and thank God it was the right answer.

Looking back on that study, Friedland noted, "I think [it was] the most important thing I've done in the AIDS epidemic—that demonstrated that HIV was not transmitted by close interpersonal contact." Margaret Fischl, who, with Gwendolyn Scott, had completed another household transmission study at Jackson Memorial, underscored the critical biomedical and public policy implications:

> We had grandmothers living in the household who were not infected that were taking care of children who were. We had older siblings who were not infected with HIV that were playing in the household, sharing bathroom privileges, kitchen utensils, fighting with each other, and it was not transmitted in that setting. . . . I think it helped bring into view how the disease was or was not transmitted. I think it also helped the public, the health care professional, that this was [a] blood-borne [virus], that this was not as easily transmitted as people were afraid it might be. This was not the equivalent to hepatitis B [which was highly contagious]. So I think it quelled some of the panic—panic is what I would call it—in the health care professionals, in the media, in the public at large.

By 1984, a broad scientific consensus had thus taken hold regarding the ways in which HIV was transmitted. The Centers for Disease Control played a central role in confronting popular anxieties.[6] The story with regard to health care workers who did come into contact with blood and body fluids that could carry HIV was different. While the basis for social discrimination was vanishing, the foundation for more legitimate concern about needle stick wounds and blood splashes had been established. But though real, the risk appeared minimal. In February 1985, the CDC reported in *Morbidity and Mortality Weekly Report* that "to date there are no reported cases of AIDS among [health care workers] in the United States that can be linked to a specific occupational exposure. . . . [Investigations of exposed workers] suggest the risk of transmission of [HIV] infection from AIDS patients to [health care workers] may be very small."[7]

To confront those small risks, the CDC and a host of public and private professional bodies promulgated safety recommendations that called for the adoption of universally applicable precautions designed to reduce the threat of transmitting all blood-borne diseases in the health care setting. Those recommendations would, in fact, dramatically enhance the safety of doctors, nurses, and other health care workers. They would not, however, eliminate all risk of HIV transmission, and that small but ineluctable burden would provide the context of work with AIDS patients. Indeed, only a month after the CDC published its recommendations on universal precautions, the British medical journal *Lancet* reported that a nurse who had stuck herself with a needle on a syringe that contained blood from a patient with AIDS, had had a positive antibody test for HIV.[8] That same week, the *New York Times* reported that the CDC had undertaken an investigation of a case involving a laboratory worker in Boston who was critically ill with AIDS. Not a member of any at-risk group, he did recall sustaining a needle stick wound.[9]

Jeffrey Laurence had been warned about such risks early on in the epidemic by Henry Kunkel, his eminent laboratory chief at Rockefeller University.

Dr. Kunkel [and those of us who worked in his laboratory] used to have lunches every day. We'd wait for him. You'd sit down at a table; if he didn't say anything, you'd say nothing for an hour; you'd just sit there for an hour looking at each other. If he said something, you started talking. [At one lunch] he said to me, "Did you know there was a registry of people who have died working in laboratories with infectious diseases?" I said, "No." And he said, "Yes, and I actually pulled it out. [There are] a couple of thousand people, some of whom have died from named viruses like Marbourg and Ebola and smallpox, and others who have died from [viruses yet to be named]."

With that warning as a backdrop, Laurence sustained an exposure to HIV some years later in his own laboratory at New York Hospital.

I was rushing. It was about 10 at night, and I get a phone call. It's a friend of mine who had breast cancer, and she's dying, and she had to talk to me. And I had to finish this experiment, so I said I will talk and work. It was a dilute culture. Concentrated cultures we do at our P3 facility, which purposely has no windows and no phones in it, and you're not allowed to have a window or a phone, just to prevent something stupid. I was taking off my gloves to put down the phone, and I spilled the virus culture on my hand. I immediately dropped the phone and poured water over it, and then poured alcohol over it, knowing that it can't go through intact skin. But how intact is skin? I was very worried about it, and I had myself tested many times. The Los Alamos person who was holding the U238 over the canister with the graphite rods with a pencil and a scissors or something stupid like that and drops it immediately knows that he's dead. He died 34 days later. And I figured, could this have been it? Did I do something like that?

More common for physicians were the almost inevitable needle stick injuries. Early in the epidemic, in 1982, before HIV was discovered, Barbara Starrett suffered such an injury while caring for a patient in her medical practice in Greenwich Village.

I had taken 40 cc of blood from a patient. I went to put a rubber stopper on the needle, and it went through my thumb. And my finger became totally black and blue, and I became hysterical. I started yelling at the patient. I gave myself 20 cc of gammaglobulin. I was scared. [I was] hysterical [that day], but then after that—I mean you can't be hysterical forever.

Four years later, in 1986, when so much more was understood about AIDS, Peter Selwyn stuck himself while performing a tuberculosis skin test on one of his methadone patients in the Bronx.

It wasn't a major needle stick; it wasn't a blood-filled syringe, and it wasn't very deep. But I panicked; I mean, I was just devastated.

I was going through the same process which I've seen since in house staff and medical students and health care workers who've come to me after they've stuck themselves or had an accident. Your first reaction is that this is overwhelming; you're gonna die tomorrow. And then just sort of free-floating anxiety, panic, feeling like, God, could this really have happened? Can't I just rewind the tape? It was so trivial and silly. Couldn't I just pretend it didn't happen? And then going through the process of first panic, and then denial, and then, you know, the same way that the stages of dealing with dying or a life-threatening illness have been described—bargaining, you know? If I just dedicate my life to only good things, then I'll be spared. My wife and I [already had] one child when this happened, but my first reaction was, my God, we have to quickly have a second child now, before it's too late. And in fact we decided, well, maybe we really should do this now. Believe it or not—it seems silly—I don't consider myself maladjusted, but this was something that I actually did—I went to a sperm bank in New York and provided a couple of sperm samples, thinking that this is it, this is my last chance. I'm soon going to be overcome with viremia from HIV, and I want to maintain my purity. I mean, really, that was totally irrational, but that was what went through my mind.

For those who had taken on a public role of reassuring colleagues about how best to reduce the threat of HIV transmission while working with patients, and for whom the doctrine of universal precautions provided a public bedrock of security and an argument against the invidious treatment of infected or thought-to-be-infected patients, the realities of clinical work sometimes provided a corrective that was not reassuring. As an obstetrician working in the heart of Brooklyn, delivering the babies of women with HIV infection, Howard Minkoff recognized the limits of his public preachments.

On the one hand, I would be going out and telling all the clinicians, "Don't worry about a thing; just use universal precautions, everything that's required." And then three in the morning you find yourself in an operating room about to do surgery knowing that the odds are that needles will pierce your glove about 15 percent of the time. . . . I remember distinctly from the earliest of times when we operated on somebody we knew was infected, that was worrisome. We used masks, goggles, but goggles in those days made surgery much more difficult. No matter what you did, they fogged up after a certain amount of time. You just hoped to get through the bloodiest part of the procedures before you were blind, and then you could take the goggles off and do the best you can thereafter. I realize this flies in the face of everything [I was] telling people, that you should be uniformly careful because the next person may be HIV positive—you just don't know it—but somehow knowing it makes you find another level. There is a certain degree to which you cannot consistently give your attention. You can do it for a certain numbers of hours, but not on and on and on.

Rejection and Isolation

Those who had committed themselves to care for AIDS patients had to confront their personal fears in an institutional climate that often mirrored the fear and hostility characterizing so much of the social response to AIDS in the early and mid-1980s. Indeed, their own identities as AIDS doctors were shaped by the way in which they came to understand the gulf that separated them from those who turned their backs on these desperately ill patients. Some came to believe that nothing more than a capacity to tolerate risk explained the difference. To others, it seemed that it was not only the risk but also the kind of patient who posed that risk that made some doctors unwilling to provide the needed care and some institutions less than enthusiastic about welcoming AIDS patients.

Some doctors could look back on institutional responses that met their needs and expectations, responses that were shaped by leaders whom they viewed as principled and compassionate. "You are doing a great job," administrators told Leonard Calabrese at the prestigious Cleveland Clinic. "We want you to keep doing this." At Boston's Beth Israel Hospital, Deborah Cotton recalled, the president would tolerate no refusals to treat AIDS patients. Those who could not or would not take on such responsibilities were told to leave. At the Deaconess Hospital, also in Boston, Jerome Groopman recalled that prejudice against gay men quickly yielded to a "Yankee tradition of service to the sick." But in many hospitals across the country, both private and public, both in institutions world famous for research and path-breaking treatments and in those with little involvement in the world of academic medicine, the story was very different.

Jeffrey Laurence experienced resistance to his AIDS work at both the prestigious Rockefeller University and then at New York Hospital. At Rockefeller, Laurence had been protected by Henry Kunkel: "Whatever he wanted to do, happened." When others, alarmed, expressed fears of contagion, Kunkel supported Laurence and his search for a viral cause of AIDS. He also stubbornly shielded him from administrators appalled by the patients Laurence enrolled in his study.

I was seeing all these patients at Rockefeller Hospital, in their clinic. Up until then, the typical patients to come in would be rheumatoid arthritis, systemic lupus, multiple sclerosis, and some of the children with genetic immune deficiencies. With AIDS, I was following a cohort of maybe 60 people. Some of them would come in their short leather pants, with the staples through their ears. Some of them would come dressed in business suits, and the nurses would have them undress and they'd have safety pins through their nipples. And they would sit there in the waiting room, and they would not look like the other people sitting there. And Dr. Kunkel told me, "People are complaining about your patients. Someone told me that they're going to drive away fund-raisers. So I said, "What are you going to do?" He said, "Nothing, I want you to keep seeing patients there!"

When Kunkel died in 1984, Laurence became vulnerable. That year he received a major grant from the New York State AIDS Institute and was chagrined to find that Rockefeller University would neither accept the award nor allow it to be transferred elsewhere. Why?

This was a large grant at the time. This was $150,000 a year. This was a lot of money. And nobody wanted it. I asked [the] head of the clinical center, [who] had taken over Dr. Kunkel's place in the interim, "Why did this happen? Tell me why. I don't care, why did this happen?" And he said, "Let's just say it's a very unattractive disease."

Laurence was not without resources of his own. Through personal contacts, he found wealthy patrons to pledge money for an AIDS research lab just city blocks from Rockefeller. He was then approached by an official in the development office, who said:

"You know, this is really very nice." He'd been in development forever; he's an Old Boy. "And the thing I like about you is you've been keeping it really quiet. So why don't you *just keep it really quiet?*"

Elsewhere, powerful shapers of hospital policy clearly articulated their desire to distance their facilities from AIDS, from the fear it engendered, from the stigma that might tarnish their institutions. Alvin Friedman-Kien noted that New York University Medical Center restricted AIDS patients to private isolation rooms. Since few such rooms were available, that policy effectively reduced the number of AIDS admissions. For Friedman-Kien such efforts reflected the fears and concerns of the institution's leadership.

> A lot of people were very proud of what we were doing. On the other hand, we had a dean at this medical school who, when I presented this stuff at grand rounds, about the tip of the iceberg and the fact that we now had this epidemic that was going to become a plague that would go on for many, many years, he got up afterwards and said, "Thank you for this very nice lecture, Dr. Friedman-Kien, but why does N.Y.U. have to be the Titanic?" Which he thought was terribly witty. But he's appalled because he realized that within two to three years, everybody saw this place as an epicenter, all the patients with AIDS were coming here, people were too frightened to come to the hospital. Patients of mine used to call up and say, "We know how involved and dedicated you are to AIDS. Would you refer us to a doctor who's less busy with those problems, so we don't have to interfere with your function?"

A policy that, in effect, limited the number of AIDS admissions obtained also at Lenox Hill, a large community and teaching hospital on Park Avenue in Manhattan. Peter Seitzman, a gay internal medicine specialist in private practice, became incensed when a gay patient of his died while waiting several days for a room. Seitzman sent the president of the hospital an angry, catechism-like letter which sought to expose the underlying ethos that had produced such an awful outcome.

> Dear Mr. Anderson: Some questions and my own answers. Question: The AIDS epidemic is the most serious health problem our society has confronted in our lifetime. Lenox Hill sits right in the center of the population most afflicted. Hospitals in smaller cities with fewer patients have opened AIDS units, both inpatient and outpatient. . . . Why hasn't Lenox Hill? Answer: Lenox Hill does not want to become known as an AIDS hospital. AIDS patients are gay men and not as worthy of the care that would be extended if the AIDS epidemic affected primarily heterosexuals. Question: Why are

AIDS patients isolated, contrary to all medical evidence of trans-missibility? Answer: Lenox Hill prefers to acquiesce to the public's irrational fears rather than help to lead the way in quelling them through education and example.

But if the great private hospitals and famous cancer centers, with their sometimes privileged clientele, resisted becoming identified with AIDS, what of the public hospitals whose clinics and wards had always provided care to the poor, and to drug users and their children? They also often avoided a too-close identification with AIDS. Prejudice was part of the story, but there was more. Underfunded public hospitals were also re-luctant to take on a new problem that would demand resources. It did not help that the resources would be expended on an "unattractive dis-ease." At Cook County, Chicago's vast but lone public hospital, two phy-sicians—Renslow Sherer, an internal medicine specialist with a history of political engagement, and Ron Sobel, an activist in the gay commu-nity—joined to form an AIDS clinic. Trying to establish it was a struggle, testing Sherer's commitment.

A new disease is not welcome here. There's not space enough for the ones we've already got, and there are too few resources. When we were trying to get an additional nurse, the head of Medicine said, "Why should I be concerned about AIDS? It's just this little fraction of all our admissions."

Ultimately, Sobel and Sherer set up a clinic, receiving permission to take two rooms on Thursday mornings. Remarkably, their labor there had to be voluntary, an addition to their workload. "Unfortunately, that meant, within the hospital infrastructure, that we started as outsiders," recalled Sherer. "We never really had the imprimatur of the administration."

In other cities along the East Coast, medical and lay administrators clearly expressed their distaste for AIDS. James Oleske was startled by the response to his initiatives on behalf of babies. First laboring in rela-tively obscure local hospitals in Newark, he moved to a more prestigious institution, the New Jersey College of Medicine and Dentistry, in 1985. During his initial year

there was a meeting in the board room. The chairman of Medicine and the chairman of this and the chairman of that, the president of the university, the dean, board of trustees were sitting around the table. The chairman of Medicine stands up and says, "Before we start, I think it should be perfectly clear that we should be deflecting AIDS money away from the school. No one should be writing grants. We shouldn't be taking money, because if we do, we're going to get sucked into this disease which will destroy my liver transplant program; it will destroy my ability to train residents. We're going to be known as a poor, inner city AIDS hospital. We've got to avoid all that." I couldn't believe what I was hearing, because I'm trying just the opposite. I'm trying to get money. Then it dawned on me that I work for a university whose public policy is "We take care of all colors; we're committed," but whose inner circle's commitment is "Don't work for this disease."

At Jackson Memorial Hospital in Miami, Margaret Fischl, unlike her colleague, pediatrician Gwendolyn Scott, contended with a hostile department and department chief. She established the adult AIDS clinic at Jackson Memorial in 1981 and became well known subsequently for conducting clinical trials of potential AIDS chemotherapies. But during the early years of the epidemic, she confronted efforts to make her feel small and isolated.

They wanted to ostracize HIV; they wanted us to have our own wards, to manage our own clinics, to not have the house staff involved. If we didn't see every AIDS patient in the hospital, even though we were working twenty hours a day, we weren't doing a very good job. And we would have our boss yell at us when, in essence, we were drowning. That was very difficult, and a lot of the physician staff I'd hired felt unappreciated and said "The hell with it" and left.

AIDS doctors on the West Coast told similar tales of tension between themselves and the institutions in which they worked or with which they were affiliated. During the early 1980s, Michael Gottlieb both treated a growing number of patients with AIDS and performed clinical research at UCLA. He described the environment there as hostile to both AIDS and to the gay community.

They had aspirations for cardiac and liver transplant programs, and they feared that if we were too well known for AIDS, that transplant patients might fear they would get AIDS getting their care at the hospital. They were phobic about payer mix. They foresaw quite rightly that ultimately a lot of patients with AIDS wouldn't have good health care coverage. And they were afraid that their house staff would rebel or that good house officers wouldn't come to UCLA to train if there was too much of one disease, particularly one that was spooky. They weren't particularly gay-friendly, either. Southern California is a conservative place. UCLA is a very conservative institution. UCLA is a state school, but the medical school has a huge private donor base in the entertainment industry and corporate culture. And I don't think it would have been perceived very well in those communities if we were seen to be catering to the gay community. And the dean of the medical school did in fact say something to me about "we're not going to let the gay community tell us what to do." But I hoped that ultimately my seniors would see the benefit to the university of having the reputation that AIDS was discovered here; I just hoped that ultimately they would recognize the worth of the program and recognize my worth.

Institutional resistance was also palpable and agonizing to Alexandra Levine, who struggled against the studied indifference of her institution. She was an oncologist, initially drawn to medicine by her experiences as a volunteer in high school at the Los Angeles County Hospital, the facility in which she later provided AIDS care.

At the beginning I had a very difficult time with administrators. My biggest frustration related to the fact that I saw what I thought was the truth, right in front of me, and no one else saw it. I had no place to see the patients. I started asking for an AIDS clinic. That would have been perhaps 1984. Under no circumstances was anyone willing to listen to me. At this point I started delivering hands-on care. No interns, no residents, no nurses, nothing. As the months went on and the years went on, it became more and more frustrating to me, because I felt all alone. I insisted upon meetings with the administrators at the county hospital, and no one supported what I wanted to do. The other issues related to homophobia, and they were real. So I was just tied up in knots. There was nowhere I could go; no one could see what was so clear to me.

Not only did those who had committed themselves to caring for AIDS patients confront institutional hostility; they also encountered the antipathy of professional colleagues as well. And such responses often affected their ability to provide care to their patients. As specialists rejected their referrals, the stigma suffered by their patients became a burden with which they too had to contend.

In 1987, Carol Brosgart resigned from her position in the Oakland Department of Health, where she had worked closely with impoverished AIDS patients, to become director of the AIDS program at Alta Bates, a community hospital in Berkeley. The medical staff at Alta Bates was divided over the need for such a program. Some saw it as responding to the community the hospital served. Others vehemently rejected it, finding it pointless. For them, AIDS was a gay disease; why not send the afflicted across the bay to San Francisco? A newcomer to Alta Bates, director of a controversial program, Brosgart often felt unwelcome.

> I was sort of a pariah because the disease I cared for was basically a pariah. I remember within a few days of coming, being in the elevator, and someone said, "Hi, are you a new doctor?" "Yes, I am, my name's Carol Brosgart. I run the new AIDS program." And just as we were about to shake hands and I said, "I run the AIDS program," he took his hand away from me. And then he said, "Oh, I'm sorry; I guess you can't get AIDS that way." . . . Well, it was incredibly distasteful to be treated as if you were a leper, just because you cared for people others saw as lepers.

At St. Luke's–Roosevelt Hospital Center in Manhattan, Donald Kotler found himself exiled by his departmental colleagues, shunted to the attic.

> The GI unit didn't let me use their equipment for fear of maybe transmitting AIDS to somebody else. For the first several years, I was stuck in this old, tiny room off the surgical suite, doing 1930s techniques, 1950s techniques. . . . I used to have to go up to the seventh floor. St. Luke's has this old mansard roof type of stuff, so I was in a room trying to do a sygmoidoscopy with my head to the side. I'd hit the wall, because the ceiling comes down at an angle. I still don't do my AIDS in the GI unit. They've established a separate room for me, because they still don't want those people there.

Such responses were embedded in striking profession-wide efforts to hold AIDS at arm's length. This was true especially with regard to dermatology and infectious disease, the two fields most directly implicated in the emerging epidemic. Marcus Conant witnessed such rejection as he sought to mobilize interest among his colleagues six months after the first cases of AIDS had been reported.

The American Academy of Dermatology was meeting [here in San Francisco] the fifth of December of 1981. We printed up a little handout and tried to hand it to doctors to tell them about the disease, the epidemiology, that it was occurring in gay men, how to recognize it microscopically, where to refer patients for a confirmative histological diagnosis. It was astonishing how few doctors would accept one of the pamphlets—not only wouldn't pick it up, wouldn't take it if pushed in their hands. There were some five thousand dermatologists here. We would say, "This is a new disease, it's called the gay cancer, and it's being seen here and in New York," and the doctors would say, "We don't have those people where I'm from," and would hand it back.

The response of many established infectious disease specialists was, if anything, more striking. In part, the new disease represented a potential threat to established research commitments; it also mocked the triumphalism of the antibiotic era, with its assumption that infections were things to be understood and vanquished. In describing the sprawling municipal hospital network in New York City, Robert Cohen, who served as its vice president, noted, "The leaders in infectious disease in all the hospitals had no interest in HIV." At San Francisco General Hospital, which would develop a worldwide reputation for devoted care to AIDS patients, the story was the same. Molly Cooke, who had been drawn to those with AIDS because she liked caring for patients "on the brink," recalled:

ID didn't want to have anything to do with it. There was an established infectious disease division, people were already working on their stuff. . . . People said, "We already have our careers started." But there's no doubt in my mind that a lot of people were very bothered by who was getting it.

It was, in fact, the reluctance of the established physicians to assume responsibility for AIDS that created unusual opportunities for younger physicians to assume leadership positions. "So there was room for younger people to come in and take ownership of it, like no other disease." But the process did not always work so smoothly, and in some instances the result was internecine feuding as those with authority were

4

101

confronted by doctors seized by their new commitment to AIDS. That the media would come to lavish attention on these young physicians only exacerbated matters. The experience of Gerald Friedland at Montefiore Hospital was both bitter and protracted.

AIDS is an intruder . . . and everywhere it goes it creates problems. . . . I [dealt] with an ID service that was repelled by it, and it resulted in an escalating personal and professional relationship of dysfunction. I just can't convey to you how terrible it was. . . . Then I became famous, and that was the worst thing, because back when I was really accused of being a charlatan, a scam, it was really envy. I was undermined at every turn. I had all these institutional struggles, and I couldn't get what I needed because I'd be blockaded. So I'd go around [the impediments] and that would result in anger. [The head of infectious disease] didn't want his people dealing with [AIDS]. He saw it as "diluting" the infectious disease training program, diffusing the efforts, interfering with what he had built. He'd built a very credible, superb infectious disease program. . . . It was like taking care of drug users is a bad thing to do. . . . But for him it was an intruder, a different style of disease, an unpleasant disease, the type of people who get it, and then I think the fact that other people were doing it and he had lost control over it in his own section. The reason he had lost control over it was because he had not wanted to be interested in it, and the thing cried out to be done, and I was very interested in it; in fact, I was more interested in it than anything else, so I wasn't going to not do it.

While institutional hostility and resistance, professional inattention, and collegial hostility were profoundly troubling, making hard work with very sick patients even harder, nothing was more disturbing than the realization that there were doctors with urgently needed skills who would refuse to treat patients with AIDS.

Sometimes refusals wore the disguise of professionally appropriate referrals. Sometimes no effort was made to mask the act of dumping. When doctors at NYU discovered that they had an AIDS patient, recalled Alvin Friedman-Kien, "they'd walk them over to my office and say, 'This doctor will take care of you. I don't see this disease.'"

In the Bronx, at the Albert Einstein Medical Center, Arye Rubinstein found little sympathy from his colleagues in that research and training institution for either his AIDS science or his patients.

We had a lot of problems, a lot of resistance. In the beginning, everyone threw their patients at us because they were afraid of them. "You take them. You do whatever you want. We don't want to see them. We don't want to touch them." Children, adults, everything. "Throw them at Rubinstein. Throw them at his team."

Neil Schram's practice in Los Angeles benefited from similar efforts to disgorge any responsibility for the care of those with AIDS. A nephrologist, he was the only doctor out of approximately 2,000 working at Kaiser Permanente who was willing, in the epidemic's early years, to accept referrals of patients with lymphadenopathy. In 1985, with the licensing of the HIV antibody test, he became the lone physician taking referrals of people who were diagnosed with HIV infection. Many of the initial referrals came as a consequence of Schram's prominence in the gay community, but soon patients were being sent from many sources. "I was getting people from all over Los Angeles."

Encountering outright refusals to treat was, for many, a formative experience. Elizabeth Kass was a fourth-year medical student at Worcester City Hospital in Massachusetts in 1985 when she witnessed such an act involving her first and only AIDS patient during medical training.

We were called to consult on a woman who had *Pneumocystis* pneumonia, and who I think was the first patient that they'd seen with PCP. . . . I remember very vividly the director of the surgical ICU, who was either a surgeon or an anesthesiologist, wanted her out of "*his* intensive care unit" because he didn't want an AIDS patient in *his* intensive care unit. I found that infuriating. . . . The interns in the coronary care unit also said, "Gee, you know, you're getting to the end of your [rotation]. Wouldn't you like to learn some procedures? How would you like to put an arterial line on that patient?" And I said, "I've never put in an arterial line before, and I'm not sure I want to learn a procedure on somebody who's in as much evident pain as she is." I had responded entirely naively, but I later found out that, in fact, the surgical intern had been supposed to put the arterial line in and tried to pay the medical interns to put the line into the patient.

And Carol Brosgart encountered a blunt refusal in early 1988, soon after she had come to Alta Bates Hospital.

A patient of mine was in the hospital and developed a nosebleed in the middle of the night. . . . The nurses weren't able to stop it.

... The ER doc came up; they put in a balloon; they weren't able to stop it. The guy is exsanguinating. They're having to transfuse him. ... I actually got called by the ID doc who was on very early that morning saying, "Can you come in to help me? I'm trying to stop the bleeding, and I can't get anyone to come in." So I came in and I started going through the medical staff roster, and everybody had a reason why they couldn't come. "Well, I'm going to be working in the student health clinic up at UC this morning." Or, "I'm attending," or, "I have a very busy schedule." Nobody wanted to come. So finally [the ID doc] and I got into a showdown, basically, over the phone with one of the guys [and said], "Look, this is your responsibility. This is a medical emergency." And finally one of the guys came in.

In confronting the refusers and the resistant, in trying to understand their motivations, in seeking to change their behavior, doctors varied. Some interpreted the rejection as a reflection of a homophobia so intense that it overrode all sense of professional responsibility. David Wright of Austin, Texas, encountered such a colleague.

We had a guy here, and it created a lot of problems for us the first six or seven years. This guy came out and he talked to me. He said, "Look, I'm not seeing any of these patients, because I believe that homosexuality is wrong and that homosexuality is against my religion, and this is the wrath of God coming down on these people." I said, "Come on, John, you don't believe that. That's a lot of bologna. I'm a Christian guy; I don't believe any of that. I practice my religion on a daily basis. Where are you reading this stuff?" He goes, "Well, that's just the way I feel about it." I said, "Well, you got to put that aside. You took the Hippocratic oath, just like I did." But he got hung up on that, and fortunately he left.

By and large, the justifications for refusing to treat were not explicitly homophobic. Sometimes they focused on clinical suitability for a given therapy. Donald Kotler, who fiercely opposed those who would not care for AIDS patients, recalled an encounter with a "natural enemy,"

a tall, thin, southern gentleman, a nutrition consultant at a major southeastern university, who said, "Why bother?" at a meeting. And I just sort of went through with him how he takes care of his people, [with AIDS who were] malabsorbers. "Would you give TPN? [total parenteral nutrition]" "No, I wouldn't give TPN. They're going to die. It's too expensive. They don't deserve it. They shouldn't have it. It's the wrong thing to do." I said, "Well, if they developed pneumonia, would you give them antibiotics?" "Of course." "If they got dehydrated, would you give them fluid?" "Of course." "If it's the only way to get the fluid in, would you put in a central line?" "If I had to." "You're the chief of nutrition?" He said, "Yes." I said, "Well, what you're going to do is you're going to treat absolutely everything else, and because of that you're going to force the patient to starve to death, because that's the only thing that you won't treat. You'll do everything else but feed the patient, so, therefore, the patient will starve to death. You are the head of nutrition?" It was a good fight. I won, so it was a good fight.

More typically, refusal centered on fear of infection. To these fears, committed AIDS doctors responded in different ways. Some were surprisingly empathic. Others were harsh and censorious. Sheldon Landesman's hospital in Brooklyn provided care to more AIDS patients in the early years of the epidemic than had been diagnosed in most states. Some of the refusers he encountered were clearly unwilling to place themselves at risk " 'for goddamn drug addicts who [are] probably spreading the disease to others.' "

Eric Goosby, who acknowledged his own fears, felt it necessary to create a context in which his residents at San Francisco General could discuss their fears of infection.

I guess compassion was how I felt. I understood where they were coming from. I had people that I was very close to who had clinical anxiety attacks around being called down to the emergency room to pick up a patient. No particular reason to think they were infected with HIV, but just the potential was enough to set up palpitations, hyperventilation, sweating, and cramps of the stomach. My response to it was—there's no way that you can get anything out of coercion. You should commiserate with them, acknowledge that this is a legitimate thing, a real thing to be afraid of. "I am afraid of it. For me, I still need to respond to the needs in front of me. I understand why you don't feel that way, and it's okay. There's enough out there to do. You ought to gravitate towards populations that are sick with other things."

Some sought to change the behavior of the fearful by providing a model of care, hoping that in so doing they could overcome the dread of contact with the infected. That this was more common for pediatricians may, in large measure, be connected to the special claims that suffering children evoke. When Hermann Mendez, a pediatrician, encountered refusals among nurses and others at Kings County Hospital, he tried to make the care of babies and children with AIDS seem matter-of-fact.

So . . . what I did every time I could was to talk to them, lecture them, role model. I mean, I'd come to the bedside, find a patient that was soiled, that hadn't been changed. I would wash my hands, clean the patient, and put the diaper on. And without saying anything else, [I would] examine all these babies without wearing gowns, gloves. Only for drawing blood, then I would insist that we have to wear gloves. Teach, and talk about the disease as something natural, something common.

Mendez's style, so gentle, was utterly different from that of the gruff chief of pediatrics at Harlem Hospital, Margaret Heagarty, who had not provided direct care to babies or children with AIDS in the service she oversaw.

There's a sociology that I've developed here, a set of social norms. Years ago I conducted something called "intake rounds." Every morning, nine o'clock, I listened to my young doctors tell me what's gone on in the last 24 hours. . . . We had a little boy in one of the rooms who had AIDS, and we had been dealing with [him] for several years, who was dying. So I inquired about Amelik. And I remember saying to them, "Who has hugged Amelik today?" And they all looked at their shoes. And I said, "Now, we do not allow children to die alone in this department, and so everyone of you is to go in and hug Amelik once a day." I've done that with other children that didn't have AIDS. And then I would go up and down the hallway and say, "Have you hugged Amelik today?"

But when such efforts did not work, Heagarty was not loath to exercise her authority to impose appropriate conduct.

We had delivered at this hospital the first woman with active AIDS. As I recall, she had Kaposi's sarcoma. And one of my young doctors had some ruddy connection to Ted Koppel, and they were proposing that night to go on *Nightline* and talk about how fearful they were to take care of this baby. And I said, "Don't tell them I'll be mad—[tell them] I'll ruin them. They'll never work in pediatrics ever [again] if they do something so asinine as that."

No one drew the ire of those committed to the care of AIDS patients more than Lorraine Day, chief of orthopedic surgery at San Francisco General Hospital. She had, as early as 1984, expressed fear of contracting AIDS because jagged bones cut through her surgical gloves, because shards often flew through the air during operations, and because of [airborne] blood [particles].[10] What would ultimately motivate her to alert surgeons about the risks to which they could be exposed was a report of an infection by needle stick of a nurse at San Francisco General Hospital in 1987. "My whole life passed before me," she told the media.[11] She went from wearing increasingly impervious protective gear—aerosolized blood can "pass through a mask like BBs through a tennis net"—to insisting that patients be tested for HIV before surgery, to withdrawing from her position at San Francisco General, where she had become a pariah. "You don't keep people on the front lines under the threat of death indefinitely," she said. And then she uttered the ultimate challenge. "There is nothing in the Hippocratic oath that says I have to sacrifice my life for the patient." But her determination to assert a right not to treat and her decision to urge others to assert such a right was especially troubling because she could not easily be dismissed as selfish and unconcerned with the plight of the socially vulnerable.

Joseph O'Neill, who was a resident at San Francisco General Hospital in the mid-1980s, was appalled by her refusal to treat patients with HIV infection. But he acknowledged his respect for a woman who "starts out in life as a dental hygienist and ends up as chief of orthopedic surgery."

More typical was the response of Day's colleague Donald Abrams. For him, it was her ability to give respectability to a position he viewed as anathema that was so disturbing.

I was speaking at the American College of Surgeons [of] Northern California and she got out there, and she did her piece of how HIV . . . was aerosolized into the air and that nobody was safe. She had all these slides of information that came from the most obscure journals of this and that that she put together to support her case, which was so bizarre. And then I gave a presentation to counter. I remember in the question and answer period that it was the most frightening thing I've ever done, because she whipped that crowd into a frenzy. She was an attractive, blond woman who was well put together for her age and took advantage of it in this crowd of macho surgeons, to the point where she was whipping them into a frenzy of homophobia. And I remember getting up there; I said, "Ladies and gentlemen, this is not Germany in the 1930s." I mean, she [had] made some comment about the gay freedom parade and bathhouses, and here we're talking about transmission in the operating room; and it was so incongruous and just so inflammatory that, for me, it was very fearful.

Neil Schram, who, although trained as a nephrologist, was compelled to learn enough about infectious disease to care for AIDS patients, was especially offended by the failure of doctors to meet their professional obligations.

When you're dealing with this hideous virus, this hideous illness, to be rejected by your physician, to be treated callously—I can't begin to tell you the anger that that creates in me. And I have to say that I'm furious with most physicians' responses. And that's why so much of the response of the epidemic has fallen on a limited number of primarily, but not exclusively, gay physicians. Because so many of the others don't give a damn and are judgmental and antagonistic and disgraceful human beings when it comes to dealing with this epidemic. On the other hand, there have been some— and no small number any more—that have been superb. But there haven't been a lot in between. It's mostly real good or real bad.

The new AIDS doctors encountered not only institutional and professional antagonism, they were also faced with an array of social responses that tended to set them apart. While many were indeed greeted with admiration—"Sometimes," said Abigail Zuger, "people decide that I'm very noble and saintly, which I don't mind"—rejection was common. Richard Chaisson could recall that "if you brought up at a dinner party [the fact] that you worked in the AIDS clinic at San Francisco General, half the room left." Passengers on airplanes would ask what he did and then "shrink over to the other side of the seat, pick up the in-flight magazine and start doing the crossword puzzle."

On occasion, the response of neighbors, fueled by fear of the new disease and the kinds of people who had it, could make providers of care very unpopular. When she attempted to turn her Greenwich Village townhouse into a home for former prostitutes, Joyce Wallace saw herself as the target of "hysteria," a fear that "12 women were going to destroy civilization as we know it." Arye Rubinstein was already well known for his care of children with AIDS when he sought permission from a town planning board to build a small extension onto his home in a suburb of New York City.

> I didn't even go there [before the zoning board]. I just sent the architect, and he was amazed when he came there. Suddenly the whole room was filled with people, neighbors, hundreds of people coming in, people were standing there. He didn't know what was going on there. Everyone opposed a three-by-eight-foot extension. One of them said, "We think that Dr. Rubinstein wants to build a gay synagogue." And it was rejected. I got very angry, and the next time, I went in with a lawyer. . . . The second time they said no, no, no, they didn't mean it, only one of the people in the community [thought I wanted to build a synagogue]—rather that they were afraid that I wanted to build a pediatric AIDS daycare center in my home. I said, "Are you crazy? I am extending 8-by-11 feet." And one guy said, "Well, with your basement together, it's a bit more"! So it was shot down again. It took me seven years to get the approval for it. And when the lawyer asked for the tapes, it was like the Watergate affair; all of the spots where the gay synagogue or the pediatric AIDS center were mentioned were all inaudible.

In other instances, physicians found their efforts to build or even renew leases on professional offices stymied. Peter Seitzman, the founding president of the gay New York Physicians for Human Rights, found himself turned on by neighbors in the cooperative apartment building where he lived. The co-op's board thwarted his effort to purchase an office with his lover in the same building. "The people in the building voted almost unanimously against us, and that was very discouraging and humiliating." It mattered little that he ultimately prevailed legally. The legacy was bitter.

The AIDS People: Newfound Connections

Confronted with therapeutic impotence and institutional and social antagonism, physicians reached out to other active AIDS doctors for support. As engaged clinicians, they were also particularly anxious to learn about new diagnostic techniques, clues to managing sick patients, and any hint of effective treatment. Although journal articles began to appear by the end of 1981, doctors depended heavily on these informal and formal linkages to obtain information that was of-the-moment.

In San Francisco, Marcus Conant used his KS clinic at the University of California in San Francisco as a center for the rapid exchange of information in the years between 1981 and 1985. He brought together oncologists like Paul Volberding and Don Abrams, infectious disease doctors like Stephen Follansbee, all very young men, and individuals from other medical specialities.

We reached out because I saw the opportunity to exchange information between specialties long before it could get published in one of the medical journals. Early in the course of the clinic, the clinic was devoted primarily to presenting all of these new patients each week, have the young guy come in, say wrapped in a towel, show the lesions, discuss the behavior [that put people at risk] perhaps, discuss the opportunistic infections. The clinic evolved over time from a purely clinical setting where we looked at patients to a more academic setting where we discussed some of the theoretical issues.

New York City's infectious disease doctors had at hand a formal network, "inner city rounds," which offered physicians the opportunity to discuss their perplexing new cases and to exchange information regarding diagnoses, treatment, and care. In the early 1980s, the City's Department of Health held formal meetings that provided a forum for case presentations for physicians. They had an important secondary function as well. Dan William recalled, "They were as much bull sessions about what are you doing, how are you managing?" In general, he noted:

There clearly were feelings of inadequacy in everyone, but because they were universal, they were quite easily rationalized as not being a measure of you being a bad person or doctor. It was quite apparent that no one knew, and since that leveled the playing field, it made it much, much easier for any given person to psychologically deal with it.

Most often, physicians depended less on such organized efforts than on informal networks. Frequently, these consisted of colleagues in the same medical center or at institutions close by. In addition to providing a mechanism for sharing clinical information, the networks served as a context for the earliest clinical studies. At Downstate Medical Center in central Brooklyn, obstetrician Howard Minkoff found in infectious disease specialist Sheldon Landesman and pediatrician Hermann Mendez his intellectual and research support.

At Montefiore Hospital, Peter Selwyn, treating and studying AIDS in intravenous drug users, began to share research and clinical problems with Gerald Friedland and others in the Department of Infectious Disease. For Friedland, the emerging connections served to provide support in the face of the hostility from his colleagues in his department.

Gay and African-American doctors often sought support from colleagues like themselves, individuals with whom they shared common values and experiences. Janet Mitchell, a Black doctor who first worked at Boston City and then at Harlem Hospital, saw her network as mainly composed of other African-American doctors and researchers, many of them women; and James Campbell found aid and assistance from members of the Bay Area Physicians for Human Rights, established in the late 1970s by gay doctors. In New York, Peter Seitzman found a source of support and advice in the New York Physicians for Human Rights, a group he had helped to organize.

We would meet once a month, and usually the most informative part of our meeting was an informal discussion after the business meeting of "what did you see in your office this week." I remember asking Dan [William] if he'd seen a lot of shingles. Nobody had even tied shingles in with HIV at that point, but we were noticing lots and lots of shingles. Nothing was done in a scientific way, but over the years we came up with strategies of treating things that have since proven correct.

Not all networks operated smoothly; competitive professional instincts intruded. Stosh Ostrow, a gay general practitioner and AIDS activist in Atlanta, characterized the small band of AIDS treaters in his city as riven with conflict. And not all doctors found the networks they hoped for in the clinical settings within which they worked. The structure and politics of academic medicine often intruded. When Deborah Cotton moved from Washington, D.C., where she had worked at the NIH and the Institute of Medicine, to Boston's Massachusetts General Hospital, she felt excluded—both as a hands-on physician and as a woman—from the established AIDS network, composed almost entirely of male physician-researchers working within the area's prestigious academic medical centers.

First of all, I didn't work at the bench, and therefore I was immediately not of their stature. So I wasn't seeing myself in the same class as a Marty Hirsch or a Jerry Groopman, and they weren't seeing me in that way either. I was seen as a worker bee in that [AIDS] establishment. They clearly needed someone like me, who would actually see the patients and feed them into the clinical trials. . . . [And], I don't think I've ever truly had a terrific professional network, which I attribute absolutely squarely to being a woman. Academic medicine is not a terribly friendly place to women, and most of the business gets conducted very much by the old boys' network. So ultimately I have colleagues that are close, but in those years I really didn't.

However important the new professional networks were, many also found deep satisfaction and fulfilment in the close relationships they forged with their patients during the epidemic's early years. Meaningful to both doctors and to those for whom they cared, these unusually intense bonds forced physicians to reevaluate their own sense of professional boundaries. While it was "very hard to develop a relationship in crisis," said one doctor, things changed as patients lived somewhat longer. Physicians, like Eric Goosby, spoke of an emerging "nexus of ties and responsibilities."

It's one thing to be in crisis where you hit an emergency room and someone is there and deals with your problem. And it's another thing when you have known this person, developed a relationship with them, seen them over a long period of time, interacted with their family and loved ones. And I think that the psychological construct that is involved in the doctor/patient relationship in that longer setting is very different. . . . And the agreement was that I may not know all the time what is going on, but I will be there with you when you go through it. And after you establish that, and by being there for them when they're sick once or twice, the bond was more intense than with any other patient group I've ever been with.

Even those who were primary care clinicians saw themselves more intimately drawn into their patients' lives than was previously true. Jerry Cade, a family practitioner in Las Vegas, compared his experience before and during the HIV epidemic.

I've always felt like a family practice necessarily involves all of the things that I like about medicine. You are closer to your patients already. You're taking care of families for generations. And that was the case even before AIDS. Certainly with HIV disease, because of all of the psychosocial concerns that came into play, I probably am more intricately involved in the lives of my patients who are HIV infected than I would have been otherwise as a physician. With HIV patients, I necessarily became more involved in their lives, partly because I thought that's where the need was.

Jerome Groopman found that, as with his long-term cancer patients, he drew patients with HIV into his life, particularly individuals with whom he shared intellectual and spiritual values.

There's a man I'm taking care of now, he's like a part of my family. He's one of my wife's closest friends, and [so is] his lover. They come to the house. He's not Jewish; his lover's Jewish. They come for *shabbat* dinner. They came to my daughter's naming; they came to my second son's *bris*. They're going to come to my son's *bar mitzvah*. And we're really close. And he's got a T-cell number of 10. He's had full-blown AIDS for almost a decade. . . . He's one of the closest relationships I've developed. It hurts a lot, and the anticipation of his dying is extremely upsetting.

Other physicians recalled how clinical distance could vanish as intense feelings took hold, how patients became friends. Wafaa El-Sadr, for example, found that even AIDS patients at Harlem Hospital with the most impoverished and shattered lives could reach out for relationships that diminished their isolation.

I don't know if it's good or bad to be as close to patients. As a physician, you get so much more out of it. It's like a glimpse into people's lives that's very unique. And when it happens, it's amazing. There's one day when you just cross that border, and you really become much closer. I could be following someone for five years, and one day it happens. It just happens.

For many gay physicians, professional distance was even harder to maintain. Old friends and former lovers often became patients. Because of deep affinity and shared experiences, patients, once strangers, became their friends. For Marcus Conant, his gay patients and his community became a seamless continuum.

> I treat friends. As a matter of fact, many of them were friends before the AIDS epidemic and became patients and closer friends as they went through the course of their disease. Many of the friends that I developed in the '80s were first patients, and then became friends, and probably the vast majority of my friends today are patients with the disease. You can't avoid that, particularly if you're in the community. And I'm not sure that at this point in my life I would want to avoid that.

Like Conant, other gay physicians experienced deep satisfaction as traditional boundaries between their professional and personal lives eroded. For Howard Grossman, it was a matter of pride.

> I take care of just about all of my friends, all over the country. So those lines blur all over the place in my life, and there really is no discontinuity between what I do for a living and what I am and where I live. It becomes very clear during the summers on Fire Island, where I go. I imagine it's what an old country doctor used to be like, because you were always "Doc."

In fact, for a few gay physicians, the continuum between patient and community, patient and friend, professional and personal, extended into their most intimate experiences. The men who were their partners were themselves HIV infected. Treating their partners, they managed their illnesses and attempted to extend their lives. Joel Weisman, who was involved in the identification of AIDS in Los Angeles and whose lover had lymphadenopathy when they met in 1980, recalled the joys and strains of his relationship with Tim, who died in 1990.

> It was psychologically really difficult for me. . . . I was in therapy when I came out and went back in the mid-80s. I was dealing with the disease, dealing with the fact that ultimately I knew Tim would die. . . . There was no separation. . . . In retrospect, we did a lot of things that we probably would have stretched out over a longer time. We loved exploring the cities of Europe. And we took our vacations to do that. And some of those vacations were taken with [intravenous feeding], TPN. They were an escape because it wasn't Los Angeles, and you weren't practicing, and I could deal with the

one AIDS person in my life as the exception. But I found the need for therapy during that time, which I went off and on with.

Like Weisman, with whom he became friends, Donald Abrams became both lover and physician to a man who was infected with HIV when he met him.

I met Mark, who was the only person that I became involved with knowing that that person was infected with HIV. I felt that I was empathic to begin with with my patients, just because I shared their life situation and the community. But having lived with a man who had three episodes of *Pneumocystis*, cryptococcal meningitis, disseminated MAC, and ultimately progressively multifocal leukoencephalopathy before he became totally demented and died in the hospice, I think gave me the full perspective of the disease. But one never knew when he was going to get another infection or what, and [just] months before he died, we had a trip to the Mediterranean.

During the time that we were together, I was convinced that I had become infected. I just had all these physical findings and I had a little lymph node behind my ear. I had all these things that I was absolutely sure were pathognomonic for having HIV, but I never wanted to determine it while he was alive, because I knew that I had been negative before I began the relationship, and so I didn't want to blame him while he was alive if I had become infected. So after he died, once I got a grip on my grief, I was in therapy, and I finally worked it out with my therapist to draw my HIV test and have the results sent to him. I walked into the office the day [the results were available]. I sat down in the chair across from him and he said, "Well, you're fine, you're negative." And we both cried for the next 10 minutes, because it was such a release.

Unlike Weisman and Abrams, there were gay physicians who could not comfortably cross personal and professional boundaries to treat lovers. Among those was Jerry Cade. As one of the few available AIDS doctors in Las Vegas, he faced the problem of caring for an ex-lover. To resolve the dilemma, he agreed to become the physician of record, but turned to a colleague to advise him on all clinical matters.

When Glen, my first lover, [got AIDS], there was nobody else in town at the time, and there was simply no one else to take care of him. So although I admitted him and had my name on the chart, I called somebody in L.A., because I was very aware of my inability as his lover to also take care of him. So what I would do was every day call my friend at USC, and say, "These are the labs, these are the charts, what do you think I should do next?"And in that way I was just playing middle person for him to take care of him. Other lovers that have been HIV infected, they go to other doctors.

Even Weisman and Abrams, however, understood that some kind of distancing was absolutely necessary to avoid emotional exhaustion. Donald Abrams recalled a seminar on physician burnout that they had both led.

[Weisman told the group], "Good harpists must develop calluses on their fingertips; otherwise, every time they play, they will bleed." And he said, "So it is with a person caring for patients with HIV disease and AIDS, that you have to develop a little callus; otherwise, if you become totally wiped out every time a patient dies, you're not going to be very useful to your other patients."

John Stansell, like Abrams, a gay physician at San Francisco General, also attempted to create a mental barrier between himself and his patients, most of whom were gay as well. As important as that barrier was, it was fragile, providing him with only a temporary reprieve.

I intellectualize a lot. I try to reduce it to its intellectual components. What can I do? What do I know? What knowledge can I gain to improve upon the outcome? What research can I pursue? That sort of thing. That's not to say I insulate myself emotionally from it. You don't. I mean, you can draw sort of a cellophane wrap between you and the devastation that's happening to your patient only to a limited extent. It's a very flimsy border. And ultimately it comes crashing down. It does that about every two months, and you have an emotional crisis of some sort. . . . You'll just decompensate briefly. But then you'll reconstruct yourself and you'll go on.

Some gay physicians found they could create the psychological distance they desperately needed by morally differentiating themselves from the type of people who presented with AIDS. Not to do so left them vulnerable to the deepest fears that they, too, might be infected. John

Mazzullo, in Boston, clung to the belief that, having rejected the sexual exuberance of the 1970s, he was distinctly unlike those he treated. AIDS would not happen to him.

> I distanced myself because there was this thing that was starting about good gays and bad gays; and the promiscuous ones, these were the ones who got it. The gay community was buying the homophobia, as we always do, that you deserve to get this because you're a bad person. It gave me some emotional distance. I didn't like the way it worked. I didn't like the fact that I recreated a we/they, but doctors do that well.

Heterosexual physicians could go a step further. To keep their own fears of illness and death at bay, they strained to maintain a psychological space by focusing on the homosexual "otherness" of those they treated. Richard Chaisson found, "The only way I was able to dissociate myself from [the afflicted] was to say, 'Well, I'm not gay.'" But as doctors, like Paul Volberding, came to know their patients as individuals, that defense crumbled.

> The [AIDS patients] were in their mid-20s, early 30s, so they were very much exactly my age, and it is really a lot harder to maintain that professional distance when the patient is like you. You can define this person as different because he's gay and you're straight, or wherever you fit on the scales, but that distinction pretty well blurs quickly, and you realize that, Well, he may be gay, but he's from Minnesota [like me] or, He may be gay, but he listens to the Rolling Stones. . . . Seeing the person as different because of sexual orientation as an element of your own defense breaks down pretty quickly. So then you have to find other ways to say, Well, this isn't me dying of AIDS. This is somebody else. And that's hard.

When all else failed, doctors, heterosexual or otherwise, had to fall back on the most basic of biological distinctions. In a somewhat different context, Sheldon Landesman expressed it succinctly and bluntly.

> The ones with the problems are the patients; or, as somebody said in relationship to cancer when they came to visit a friend who had a head and neck tumor, they realized that no matter how much empathy they felt and how sad they were about their friend, ulti-

mately they were going home to their family. They were on the other side of the tumor. Well, we were always on the other side of the disease.

Landesman and others also could rely on the deep social and cultural divide that separated them from poor, drug-using patients. Abigail Zuger was stark as she described her work at Roosevelt Hospital in Manhattan.

I'm dealing with people who are not like me. Every day, when I go to work, I go to another country. Really. You cross Ninth Avenue, and I'm in another country.

However they dealt with the divide that, in a fundamental sense, separated them from patients, whether they drew close to colleagues or found their relationships fraught with tensions, the first generation of AIDS doctors confronted so much that was common that they began to see themselves as a class apart. Gerald Friedland captured that historical moment with a striking image.

There's something a little different with AIDS people; and we call ourselves "the AIDS people," and other people call us "the AIDS people," and in every institution I've been in, we're "the AIDS people." That helps us to some extent, because there's a commonality of purpose.

3
THERAPEUTIC STRIVINGS,
THERAPEUTIC STUMBLES

Before the discovery of HIV, physicians had no alternative but to search for a way to treat the cascade of diseases they encountered in their patients with AIDS. They called on past experience and whatever expert advice they could find. In the epidemic's first years, Wafaa El-Sadr, mystified by the disease, cared for her typically poor patients at the Veterans Hospital in New York empirically and pragmatically.

> It was really scary. We had no clue what we were doing, and in retrospect we made a lot of mistakes. . . . We used medications in the wrong doses; we used stuff that there was better treatment for. We didn't anticipate things. We were just reacting. There was nothing you could anticipate, no way in which you could see a clear path for that patient. . . . You just didn't know what the heck was going on.

To Sheldon Landesman as well, clinical care in the earliest days "was quasi-chaotic. We made a lot of mistakes in the beginning. One sort of ran by the seat of one's pants, but with a certain amount of clinical intuition." But in the end, as Dan William noted, "We were all novices."

Indicative of the state of things was the reliance on radical interventions guided more by hope than by scientific evidence. At a number of academic medical centers, physicians carried out bone marrow transplants, hoping to reconstitute their patient's immune systems through a procedure already used to treat acute leukemia. Fred Siegal, who performed such transplants on AIDS patients at New York's Mount Sinai Hospital, recalled that in the 1980s, "We tried to bring to bear all the things we knew." More caustic, Jerome Groopman remembered, "They tried to transplant some people at UCLA, and they killed them. They all died. So that was a short-lived idea."

Confronted with a dying patient for whom conventional treatment was futile, Jeffrey Laurence, a typically cautious scientist and clinician, seized on a therapy that was more experiment than treatment.

New York Hospital had some extraordinarily famous people who died of AIDS, and I've been involved in the experimental care of a number of them, getting drugs that no one had access to or trying things that didn't pan out, but just to do something. I remember one very famous person, his lover dying of AIDS. And that person also eventually died of AIDS, but he was healthy at the time. We tried taking white blood cells from the healthy person, grinding them up, inactivating them. We didn't even know what we were inactivating them for; we figured we were inactivating them for hepatitis and injecting it into the person who was dying. We would do these one- and two-person experiments just to see whether we could learn something on someone—obviously with human rights committee approval. . . . It's incredibly primitive, now that we know what the answer was.

With severely limited treatment options, those, like Laurence, who cared for patients with AIDS were impelled to take risks they almost certainly would have avoided in the past. A relatively conservative practitioner before AIDS, Gwendolyn Scott found in her pediatric work in Miami that "my attitude toward medicine and toward specific treatment changed a great deal with AIDS and HIV, because you become very frustrated when you're watching a disease that you can't do anything about, and children are dying in front of your eyes; you're compelled to really try to do something." In contrast to those who practiced a conventional, routinized medicine, Margaret Fischl, Scott's colleague at Jackson Memorial, characterized an AIDS doctor as one who had to be a risk-taker. "You had to challenge the full understanding of medicine and be willing to use it appropriately and take chances and work on limited data, and then [be] willing to reassess when more data came in."

In desperation, some doctors rushed to apply therapeutic approaches they thought appropriate in cancer; but when applied to AIDS the results were often disastrous. Quoting an old saw, one doctor wryly observed about the earliest AIDS work, "When all you have is a hammer, the whole world is a nail." Jerome Groopman recalled that in the early 1980s, AIDS was seen, particularly by hospital-based physicians, as a severe and aggressive disease. "There was no such thing as asymptomatic HIV, and no one knew what to do with lymphadenopathy." Oncology had recently triumphed over childhood leukemia and Hodgkin's disease by adopting a strategy of aggressive treatment. Applying that lesson to AIDS, Groopman noted, oncologists argued that "an aggressive approach to an aggressive disease was needed."

Those who came from other backgrounds often were harshly critical of oncological chemotherapy, which further weakened the immune system. As Joyce Wallace, who saw some of New York's first AIDS patients at St. Vincent's Hospital in Greenwich Village, sarcastically observed, "The cure was worse than the disease. . . . Oncologists were doing what they knew best." And Alvin Friedman-Kien was aghast at the results of chemotherapy. He remembered his close colleague at NYU, the cancer specialist Linda Laubenstein, who was the heroine of Larry Kramer's searing AIDS play "The Normal Heart." She worked 18-hour days, treating the earliest patients with AIDS.

> She was a remarkable person. She, first of all, had polio at the age of five and had been confined to a wheelchair. She never thought of herself as being crippled and even would say, "Let's walk home together." She took wonderful care of her patients, and we worked together. [But] we disagreed; we fought a lot about the fact that as an oncologist, everybody got chemotherapy. She bumped off more people than lived, but in those days we didn't know. When we looked at an autopsy, she looked from her wheelchair and said, "No KS." I said, "Yeah, but Linda, he's died of every opportunistic infection; we bumped him off." She'd be horrified. It was like a religion; oncology is a religion for people who practice it.

Those who did not share that "religion" had to develop other ways of coping with the reality of their clinical limits.

Initially, they could only treat opportunistic infections. "We were very aggressive about treating toxo[plasmosis], bacterial meningitis, cryptococcal meningitis," recalled Ronald Grossman, in speaking of parasitic, bacterial, and fungal infections of the brain tissue and lining. "These weren't new diseases. What was new was the aggressiveness of the diseases, how quickly they could cripple or kill."

One of the most common and prognostically grim of the opportunistic infections was *Pneumocystis carinii* pneumonia, a disease that developed in more than 50 percent of AIDS patients. In the early years of the epidemic, if patients survived the first attack of PCP, they eventually succumbed to recurring bouts of the disease. "They had," said Dan William, who dreaded making the diagnosis, "a probability of dying within 12 months, and it was very, very difficult to tell patients because they were invariably in denial. It was like taking someone and cracking their head open with a brick."

A drug for the treatment of PCP, pentamidine, existed before the epidemic but was so rarely needed that the CDC maintained a limited supply, which it shipped to physicians on demand. In fact, the burgeoning requests for pentamidine in 1981 were one of the earliest signals to the CDC that something untoward was occurring. Bactrim, a second therapy, was shown in the mid-1970s to treat PCP effectively with fewer side effects and had become the medicine of choice before AIDS. Most critically, physicians had used it prophylactically in patients at high risk of *Pneumocystis*, especially those, like cancer or organ transplant patients, with weakened immune systems.

Nevertheless, few drew the lesson for AIDS. Joseph Sonnabend, who had treated organ transplant patients for infectious diseases and who was heterodox in many ways, was an outspoken proponent of the use of Bactrim prophylaxis.

From the very beginning, [I] thought that some infections would make things worse. Whatever's causing [AIDS], people die of complications of the disease. If you want to be of some help to individuals, I think one has to focus on these complications, [I] was frowned upon. The common response would be, "There's no data." But in fact there was data. People with organ transplants who were getting *Pneumocystis* were clearly recognized as being at risk, and they were given the prophylactic regimens. When AIDS came along, now we had a new group of people at risk for PCP. So why not give them the benefit of prophylaxis that other groups [had]?

Indeed, it was not until 1988, when Margaret Fischl published in the *Journal of the American Medical Association* the results of her clinical trial demonstrating that Bactrim, used prophylactically, prevented PCP in patients with AIDS, that Sonnabend's perspective was given a scientific imprimatur.[1] For those like Fred Siegal, who viewed the earlier experience with immune compromised patients as significant, Fischl's investigation was simply unethical because it had deprived of effective treatment those in the trial randomly selected to receive a placebo. Faced with such attacks, Fischl defended herself by arguing that she was "highly suspicious that lower doses [of Bactrim] would prevent infection. . . . I mean, it was a theory back then that was subsequently borne out."

Even after Fischl's study was published, many doctors remained skeptical about using Bactrim prophylactically. Fischl recalled an international meeting of infectious disease specialists at which she combatively presented her results.

> People were not believers then. They thought Bactrim was too toxic to these patients, particularly the cohort from San Francisco. And I called the doctors wimps and told them they should just treat right through it, and they would do perfectly fine . . . which is what eventually happened.

The movement toward prophylaxis of the most common of the opportunistic infections represented a critical advance. Sheldon Landesman, whose training in infectious disease and oncology had prepared him to confront opportunistic infections, believed there was no alternative but to treat immune suppressed patients empirically.

> Mostly it was commonsense stuff. After you saw your fifth or sixth case of relapse of pneumocystis, you started empirically to put some patients on post-exposure prophylaxis. And everybody had a different dosage and a different duration; it took some time to sort them out. We treated patients with toxoplasmosis. Nobody knew how long to treat the patient. But after you saw your fifth one coming back with recurrent toxoplasmosis, you started to think about trying to fashion some regimen the patient could take for post-exposure prophylaxis.

Many of the drugs used in the first decade of the epidemic were already part of medicine's armamentarium. There were, however, a few instances early on when new interventions did prove successful. Some provided dramatic turnarounds. At Mount Sinai Hospital in New York City, Fred Siegal treated two gay men with severe cases of anal herpes. They were put on a new drug, Fiac, but subsequently died, perhaps as a reaction to the medication. When a third case was admitted to Mount Sinai in the spring of 1981, Siegal searched desperately for a new treatment.

> I got on the phone and tried to find some alternative, and I spoke to someone up in Boston. And they asked if I'd ever heard of acycloguanisine, and I'd never heard of acycloguanisine, and nobody

at Mount Sinai had ever come up with this. But acycloguanisine was [marketed as] acyclovir. It was an experimental drug that nobody had, but they told me that Burroughs [Wellcome] had it, and they might be able to give it to me on compassionate use for a bad herpes lesion. They sent me the drug. And one of the most dramatic things I've ever seen in medicine was the resolution of this tremendous herpes ulcer in five days, with acyclovir. My father used to tell me about the day he first used penicillin on a woman with post-abortion infection of the uterus who was dying. They had something like 5,000 units of penicillin in 1945, and they gave it to this young woman, who was cured. It was the biggest miracle he had ever seen. So here I was, reliving this with acyclovir.

Gancyclovir became the first drug to prove effective against cytomegalovirus (CMV). It was still an experimental drug when Donald Kotler discovered its therapeutic power in his work as a gastroenterologist.

A gay man with diarrhea came to see me. He was incredibly short of breath, and in fact he could hardly walk. He had *Pneumocystis* pneumonia, and I started to treat the pneumonia. The guy was wasted terribly. I looked, and he had CMV colitis. I had heard that there was a company that had a drug. They put me through the wringer for approval for a single patient. If I was going to use their drug, I had to provide them pharmacokenetics, 24 hours of blood sampling, after. I treated the guy, and 10 days later he was better. Two weeks later, he didn't even have diarrhea anymore. That had never happened before. I sent the guy home. He came back a month later; it had all come back again. I put him back on the drug; it went away again. And more than going away again, his weight started going up. And here was a guy who was [wasting], and yet turned and went the other way. And then another, and then another, and then another. That was in '84, '85, '86.

Managing infections in a disease that doctors had first experienced as out of control proved to have a powerful psychological effect. The dread sense of impotence could at last be consigned to the dark moments of the night. It was possible to do something. If death could not be prevented, at least suffering could be controlled. Equally important, survival time could be extended. As one New York physician noted, "[It took] away a little bit of the sense of anarchy and hopelessness that both patient and provider [felt] as the disease move[d] in a sort of unremitting fashion towards the end."

Limited as they were, the achievements provided physicians with a sense of mastery; they were becoming experts. Of course, as San Francisco's Constance Wofsy observed sardonically, "No one knew what to do. You write a few chapters and you're the expert." Richard Chaisson, who would become an AIDS specialist at Johns Hopkins University, became an authority while still in postdoctoral training.

> By the time I'd finished my residency [in 1985], I probably had more experience in pneumocystis than 99.99999 percent of physicians in America. There were probably only 50 or 60 people with more experience than me, and they were either at San Francisco General and a year ahead of me or at one or two hospitals in New York.

With some infections that few doctors had ever seen, "expertise" was relative and could be acquired inadvertently. That was the experience, at once horrible and almost whimsical, of James Oleske, when he attempted to learn more about lymphocytic interstitial pneumonia (LIP), a condition characterized by an accumulation of white blood cells in the lungs of his pediatric patients.

> I remember I had four cases of LIP. And I said, "What's this? LIP?" I couldn't find anything in the textbooks, and then I was told there was a doctor down at Louisiana State University who was the world's expert on children with LIP. So I call her up, and she's a wonderful lady. She has this wonderful southern accent. And I say, "Look, you don't know who I am, Jim Oleske of Newark, and I take care of these kids with this unusual, maybe new, syndrome, but four of them have LIP on biopsy." And I proceed to tell her about the cases, and say, "I really want to know what you think, since I understand you're the world's expert." And she said, in this great accent, "Dr. Oleske, in my whole career I had one kid with LIP. You're now the world's expert."

Confronting HIV: The Search for an Antiviral Therapy

However important were the first steps toward managing the opportunistic diseases that afflicted their patients, physicians recognized that until the underlying cause of AIDS was identified and a therapy directed against that crippling pathogen found, care would be hobbled. For Paul Volberding, whose reputation owed much to his clinical testing of anti-retrovirals, the isolation of HIV in 1983 was a turning point. "The first sense that maybe there was something that could be done happened almost as soon as we knew the cause of the disease." Feeding Volberding's expectations was his belief that infectious diseases tended to be curable afflictions. Donna Mildvan, who had become an infectious disease specialist because of those same expectations, felt hopeful that, at last, the darkest period was behind her. "That was the beginning of a very optimistic phase because we had the bug. Now we knew who the enemy was. So we felt, naively, that we really could begin targeting some real interventions that would make sense."

Mildvan's first opportunity to test a drug against HIV involved the clinical trial of suramin, an antiparasitic medication used in the treatment of African sleeping sickness. It had shown promise by inhibiting viral replication in the test tube and appeared to clear HIV from patients' blood. Feisty, aggressive on behalf of her patients, Mildvan made certain they would have access to the drug by submitting a successful application that established her hospital as a site for the NIH-sponsored suramin trial.

> There was no way our patients weren't going to have access to the drug. There was no way. By then we had buried, I don't know how many, too many patients. . . . This was the birth of antiretroviral therapy. We were the first to treat our patients with something other than snake oil.

Mildvan began enrolling subjects in 1985. A self-described optimist, she maintained that posture during the early years of the epidemic by always focusing on what she could learn or change or solve, keeping her sights on whatever glimmer of light there was. Suramin became that light. Even in retrospect, she resolutely saw the suramin trial as a moment of hope for her and her patients and as a time of small, precious victories.

> The first patient we enrolled was this skinny, sweet lady who was so sick, oh God, unbelievably so. But it was a joy to think that there was hope. Now we could start using the H word, hope. There had never been anything like it before. Everybody always decries suramin, saying, "Oh, what an awful drug," and "how toxic it is." All this is true. But you had to see our cohort of patients. They loved

it. It sounds strange now, but it was true. They were so well taken care of, our staff hovering over them all the time. They lived a median of 14 months following *Pneumocystis*, which was unheard of at the time. The median survival following PCP was at most four months. . . . The drug was doing something. But in the end it was just too toxic. I've heard people say, "Suramin was pure poison." If you talked to our patients, though, they braved it. "Give me any poison that gives me some hope."

The suramin trials provided Mildvan with the sense of mastery she had come to cherish in infectious disease. Initially Mildvan had to learn to distinguish manifestations of AIDS from the varied effects of the medication. She was forced to follow her patients closely, to observe them carefully, gaining in the process an ever deeper understanding of the disease. By the time the trial was ended, she felt, "There was really little new that we hadn't already seen. In those days there was no library; the vastness of whatever there was to know was right there in front of you at the bedside."

In Los Angeles, Alexandra Levine, who had long been interested in the lymphomas, started enrolling patients into a suramin trial at the county hospital. Like Mildvan, she experienced that first trial as a positive event, an opportunity to test a promising drug when there were no others. And like Mildvan, she drew close to her cohort and spoke of her patients with great warmth.

My memory of that trial is one of friendship. We called ourselves the "suramin for lunch bunch," because we couldn't give the drug until we had all the results of lab tests. They would come in the morning; we would do our regular clinic; we would have lunch; and finally we would get the results and give the infusion in the afternoon. We were asked to [reevaluate the progression of the disease in] the patients after six weeks of therapy. At that point, there was no major responses. There were little nuances of T4 cells; we didn't have good markers of viral burden at that time. When I [reevaluated] the first patient, who had KS and lymphoma, he had a complete remission of both. It was pretty interesting. That's why I can look back and remember it in a funny kind of way as a positive thing. He's still alive. He developed significant toxicity. We kept him on that drug a long time, because I didn't know to do otherwise. He developed significant peripheral neuropathy. He had no use of one arm at a certain point. He had adrenal insufficiency, and he came into the county hospital at a certain point in shock. Then we went back and looked at every other patient, and they all had adrenal insufficiency. There were many, many complications. We stopped the drug. It certainly was the end of that drug as an antiviral agent.

Both Mildvan and Levine were therapeutic enthusiasts, who could wrest some success from suramin's failure as an antiviral agent. Others, like Peter Wolfe, another member of the Los Angeles clinical trial team, were more definitively dismissive, finding no transcendent purpose to the trials. "Basically, the stuff didn't do squat; the patients did not get better." Donald Abrams, who would inch his way toward something like a nihilistic outlook—sharply critical of the efficacy of antiviral drugs—viewed the suramin trials through an even darker lens. He and his colleague Paul Volberding put AIDS and ARC patients on suramin only to find that "the drug wasn't good. We made people sick, and some people we made die." Abrams soberly recalled a patient of his who demanded to be placed on suramin. Abrams tried to dissuade him, pointing out that he was at the beginning of the disease and very stable. The patient chose to take his chances with the drug, and he subsequently died of it. "And so," Abrams reported, "I got a healthy respect for the agents that we were using and for the power that they had." For Volberding, who like others was looking for a cure, these early trials also marked the beginning of a series of roller coaster rides of high expectations, followed by deep disappointments. "The cycle of up and down became clear from the start."

With the experience of the first years of the epidemic providing a series of lessons, AIDS doctors had begun to adopt varying styles of patient management. Some became advocates of aggressive intervention; others felt there was little to do beyond managing those opportunistic infections that could be treated. Victoria Sharp, describing treatment during this period, recalled, "Clinically, it wasn't particularly complicated. In 1987, I could have taught my brother the architect how to do AIDS medicine. [There] was nothing to do until your CD4 count hit 200, and then Bactrim." At the other end of the spectrum were doctors like Barbara Starrett, who developed strong interventionist postures. Starrett prided herself on prescribing the newest drugs to her largely gay practice in Greenwich Village, including those that could stimulate the immune system (isoprinosine) and antivirals (ribavarin and HPA23), none of which would ultimately prove clinically significant. Those patients who wanted to be cared for by someone who was willing to try virtually anything that might work were drawn to her.

> In the very beginning, people died quickly of PCP. By the time '83 rolled around, we were doing things for patients. We were now using Pentamidine. We were getting shipments from the CDC. I was always on the cutting edge as far as new treatments. So we were trying drugs. I think people who were taking Bactrim prophylaxis were obviously living longer, and I think we were becoming aware of the fact that this was not a short-term disease, but this was a more chronic illness. . . . In '85, I was using gancyclovir. I had patients go to Paris and get HPA23. . . . My patients followed [Rock Hudson there]. So we were always doing something. And that's what always helped me along in the sense that, "We'll find the drug, we'll find the drug; it's just around the corner, it's just around the corner."

Though the suramin trial was short-lived, the search for an effective antiviral agent intensified and crystallized in the late 1980s in clinical research involving the drug AZT, which, in laboratories, appeared to inhibit the reproduction of HIV by blocking an essential enzyme. The saga of that drug—the hopes it initially inspired, the disappointment and rage it ultimately provoked—provides an insight into the desperation that surrounded the treatment of AIDS during the epidemic's first decade.

The involvement with suramin prepared Donna Mildvan for the study of AZT being undertaken by the pharmaceutical firm Burroughs-Wellcome. Beginning in February 1986, individuals with AIDS or serious symptoms associated with HIV infection were enrolled in a clinical trial that ultimately involved 282 subjects. Six months into the trial, it was halted by the monitoring board of the National Institute of Allergy and Infectious Diseases because the ethics of clinical trials prohibited the continuation of placebos when those receiving the medication under study were clearly benefiting. Nineteen of the 137 participants who had received placebo had died. Only one of the 145 receiving AZT was dead.[2] Mildvan, with the same verve and anticipation that so characterized her initial response to suramin, monitored her patients on the AZT trial.

> At every stage there's one patient who epitomizes the experience of the time. There was one patient who, when I first saw him was just so sick, so bedraggled and sad. You wouldn't believe how thin

and wasted he was. I'll never forget how he looked that first day. Then he was enrolled into the study, and within weeks he began gaining weight. In fact, the next time I saw him I couldn't believe it was the same patient. I sort of held my breath. Twelve weeks into the study, he was back at work full time. He had gained more than 15 pounds, and he was better; *he was better*. I can only tell you that I had never seen anything like that before. All the chicken soup and all the suramin and all the you-name-it, I had never seen anything like that before. So in my heart of hearts, I knew we had something. But I didn't dare let myself really rejoice until September 26—I think that was the date when they unblinded the study. They sent us the results, and there it was: the three deaths who had died had been on placebo. All the people who had experienced turnarounds were on AZT.

Mildvan's sense of anticipation during the trial was shared by others and, in some cases, provoked a sense of conflict for those who were committed to their patients' interests while recognizing how crucial it was for research to go forward. For Michael Gottlieb, who was a researcher in the UCLA trials that included his own patients, the tension was particularly acute because he believed he knew who was receiving AZT and who the placebo.

I pretty well knew who was on AZT and who wasn't. People were feeling better on AZT, and minor fungal infections were clearing up, and people were gaining weight. It became apparent pretty quickly. Of course, the trial was supposed to last six months, and as an investigator you're blinded to who's on drug and who's on placebo. But part of you, the doctor part, is saying, "I want to break the code. I want to know. They should approve this drug. I have 200 more patients who could benefit from this." And the investigator part of you is saying, "Gotta stick to the protocol." I was torn.

The dramatic findings of this first trial were so positive that some AIDS doctors found them almost too good to believe. At a scientific meeting not long after the placebo trial was ended, Margaret Fischl of Miami was asked to present the AZT findings as an unscheduled "late breaker." Donna Mildvan was sitting next to Gerald Friedland, who had not been an investigator in the AZT trial.

Margaret presented the results of the trial. It was the first time anyone, including any of us, saw the data. It was thrilling stuff, totally amazing: 19 deaths in the placebo group, and one death in the AZT group—a highly statistically significant result. Everything else, like the frequency of opportunistic infections, was also in the same direction. Then Gerry said, "You don't believe any of this stuff, do you, Donna?" He meant it. Do you know why? He had never seen it. I said, "Gerry, it's real. Believe it. It really is real." He was so skeptical; he just wasn't buying it. Nobody could accept it who hadn't seen it firsthand.

It was the very prospect that at last an effective antiviral medication had been identified that provided the occasion for the bitter controversy over whether the use of placebos in trials involving dying patients could ever be justified. Critics, especially among AIDS activists, argued that it was immoral to use placebos, that comparing those who received the potentially effective agent against historical controls—who had not been treated—would provide data of sufficient rigor. Others saw in the assault on the exacting standard of clinical trials a treacherous step borne of desperation. The debate was not waged with kid gloves. Martin Hirsch, a virologist at the Massachusetts General Hospital, was a strong advocate for placebo-controlled trials and became the target of activist ire:

I thought that this [trial] would be well received by everybody, and to my surprise it led to some of us being singled out as sort of enemies of the people for having allowed a placebo-controlled trial. People who should have known better said, "You didn't have to do a placebo-controlled trial. We knew the drug was good." And "People died needlessly." And [they] came out of this as the darlings of the activists, sort of because that's what they were saying, "Why should anyone have to take a placebo?" And I came out as the villain, saying, "The only way to prove something is to have appropriate controls, and until you have something that works, you've got to have controlled trials." That led to a lot of hate mail, a lot of phone calls, vicious phone calls. . . . I didn't expect any of this, and, of course, I self-righteously saw myself doing the right thing, but the others didn't.

Others were skeptical at the outset, challenging the validity of the trial's findings and the rush to embrace what they took to be a toxic and ineffective therapy. Donald Abrams, who, as a gay physician, would lead the movement in San Francisco to engage community-based doctors in clinical trials, was an early critic of AZT.

My interpretation of that data has always been somewhat different from most everybody else's. What I was concerned about all along was that the study was very small and very short; the average duration of treatment that the patients received was four months. Even though it was to be a six-month study, only about 10 percent of the patients completed the six months of the trial before it was terminated. So I thought the study was terminated too soon. By the time they actually closed the study the next month, there were nine deaths more in the AZT-treated patients, and [with] more deaths in the placebo patients, it became 10 to 23 or something, and that was much less statistically significant than 1 to 19. So I just was concerned that we had jumped on that bandwagon a little too soon.

Joseph Sonnabend, who would, for years, remain skeptical about the centrality of HIV in the etiology of AIDS, was more scathing, raising questions not only about the trial's outcome but about whether those conducting the trial were truly unaware of who was receiving the placebo and who AZT.

I didn't believe the original AZT trials. [Furthermore] AZT does something to the blood . . . which makes red cells increase in size . . . so it's impossible, unless you are lying, to tell me you don't [know who is receiving AZT]. And I thought why did they go to the trouble of even trying to blind it? I mean it's a give-away to the doctors. . . . In my estimation, [the approval of AZT] was one of the worst things that's happened. The approval of AZT was . . . I suppose [a concession] to the pharmaceutical industry and the activists—what can I say—who were screaming for their AZT.

But such reactions were unusual in 1986 and early 1987. For doctors who had stood all but powerless during the epidemic's first years, AZT represented the first real sign of hope. Just before the AZT findings were made public, William Owen's clinical experience in San Francisco was characterized by despair.

That time was the real low point of the epidemic, because there was no hope. A person would come in, and you would see him come in with this cough, and he would have an abnormal chest X ray, and you just knew in your heart of hearts that in six months that person would be dead. So it was a very devastating kind of experience at that point. . . . Often I thought to myself, How much longer can I continue in this way, continue on like this? . . . The release of AZT showed that something could be done against the virus.

The excitement was captured by Ronald Grossman, whose largely gay practice in New York had witnessed so many deaths.

I remember going to a social meeting at Mathilde Krim's house and waving my papers in the air and having this crowd sort of gather around me—showing off my ego, right? "These are the papers that will allow me to dispense this new drug." And there was a good deal of excitement about it. I had five years of enormous frustration behind me, with no treatment at all; and already a huge list of cockamamie alternative treatments had surfaced. . . . It was very exciting to be able to get our hands on this drug, and by that time enough people had experienced that wonderful early bounce—that is, T-cells rising, appetite improving, weight going up, fevers going down. In retrospect, it was a minority of people who experienced those beneficial effects, but it was enough to get the word out, "Here's a great drug."

So dramatic was the occasion that, years later, doctors could recall what it was like to write the first prescription for AZT. Other doctors could also recall the first patient to benefit from the new therapy. For William Owen in San Francisco, that patient was someone who was so profoundly affected by AIDS that he could no longer care for himself.

He was a patient of mine back in '86. He had developed AIDS-related dementia, encephalopathy; and he had to be admitted to the skilled nursing facility over at St. Luke's Hospital because he wasn't able to care for himself. He required a nasogastric tube for feeding, constant care for shaving and washing; he was totally confused. In late '86, he qualified for the first AZT that came around. We decided to give it a go even though we had to put it down the nasogastric tube. Within just a matter of a week or two he showed definite improvement, and he ended up, within the space of a couple more weeks, being able to be discharged from the facility, and actually ended up the following year, in '87, going on his own [to] a march on Washington for lesbian and gay rights. And this was a man who looked like he was basically on death's doorstep. He was really sick. So I think, when you see an example like that, you realize that there are things that we can do.

The initial limitations on access to AZT and the stringent criteria established by Burroughs-Wellcome to guide the rationing of a drug that so many wanted forced physicians to confront the disjunction between their own patients' needs and the scarcity-imposed rules of allocation. James Campbell recalled that in the face of what appeared to be arbitrary cutoff points based on a patient's immunological status, it was not unusual for doctors to "fudge" their patient's test results. In some cases, doctors went further: In one instance, a New York-based physician permitted her patients to falsify bronchoscopy reports in order to substantiate the presence of *Pneumocystis* pneumonia, an AIDS-defining condition.

We got a typewriter that looked like the typewriter from [our hospital]. We had to document bronchoscopy, and we would sometimes . . . give the typewriter to a patient, and they brought in a confirmed bronchoscopy report. We would then send away for AZT for them. For people who were really sick, where people were getting sick in front of me, where I thought the drug would make a difference, I did something. A lot of doctors did. Because you do what you think is right for the patient.

Not only was AZT initially scarce, it was very expensive, costing upward of $10,000 per year. Those without adequate insurance or Medicaid coverage could not possibly afford it. And so some physicians devised a number of ploys to bring AZT to those who could not pay for it. In Rochester, New York, William Valenti stockpiled pills provided to him by patients who, for whatever reason, were no longer taking the medication. Others asked families to return unused portions of prescriptions of patients who had died. Finally, some manipulated the Medicaid system to get AZT to those who did not have access to the joint federal-state program that covered but a fraction of the medically needy.

A month's supply of AZT, at 10 pills per day, was easily $600–800 a month. This was ruinous for most patients, even with decent insurance; and we became great criminals to overcome this problem. . . . Medicaid didn't restrict the number of pills you could use, [so], for example, if the person was taking three a day, you prescribed

10 a day. You then had an excess of seven to literally give. And I became a broker. I dispensed vast amounts of free pills, "free" being paid for by all of us out of our taxpayers' money. And the patients, who were my conduits, were incredibly eager to do this. They knew exactly what they were doing and often continued doing it even when we took them off AZT. I was very proud of being able to cushion the dreadful financial blow of this. I said to myself, and then I began saying to patients, "Nothing will stand in the way of your getting this drug if we decide you need it."

While many of the most impoverished remained beyond such inventive efforts to create a Robin Hood-like safety net, those with resources and connections scrambled to get the promising new drug. In New York, with so disproportionate a number of AIDS cases, Dan William recalled, "You'd go to a theater, and you'd hear beeps, and it wasn't beepers; it was patients with their AZT, to remind them to pop their every-four-hour pill."

But all too soon it became clear that the initial enthusiasm had "deluded many doctors and patients into thinking that this was truly the answer." "It was," said Peter Selwyn, "desperation and relief [at having a drug] that led to unrealistic hopes." "Within six months to a year," said Dan William,

the disappointments were becoming pretty obvious. A lot of patients got dreadfully anemic very quickly because they were on too high a dose. And, yes, it helped some people, but it didn't help everyone, and even those people that it helped, the benefits were short-lived. Some people had a very, very high incidence of headaches, and queasiness, and nausea, and vomiting; and later on people developed myositis or muscle inflammation; and what seemed like a panacea became more like an albatross.

The disappointments were greatest for those who had been most enthusiastic. Donna Mildvan, who had described herself as a "believer," had to confront a profound turnaround in the very patient who had symbolized to her the effectiveness of AZT.

He started to lose weight again, to go blind in one eye. It was one thing after another. I just couldn't believe it. I was so upset. We thought we were doing something. Then it turns out we were not.

I just remember walking away. I think that was the absolutely lowest point I can remember, walking away from that bedside knowing we had lost the battle again.

The obvious limitations of AZT led some physicians to discount any potential role for a drug that had been greeted with such enthusiasm; others, chastened by experience, maintained that, however short-lived the benefits, they were better than the alternative—no antiretroviral treatment. At Boston's Beth Israel Hospital, Harvey Makadon reacted in a way typical of those for whom modest achievements were worth the effort.

I worked in a hospital where the infectious disease people were very, very cynical about AZT, and so I felt like I was the lone optimist. And I felt, even though it wasn't proven to prolong life, I didn't really give a shit. I felt like it helps people in terms of fewer symptoms, and I thought that was good. And so I just started using it.

So, too, did Hermann Mendez, who had been caring for babies and children of impoverished African-Americans and Haitians in Brooklyn with little effective treatment at his disposal. It was two years from the time the FDA had given its approval to AZT in adults that it extended its approval, in December 1989, for use in children. In that period, the limitations of AZT in adults with AIDS had become clear, and yet those who worked with children pressed for access to the drug. When the FDA gave its approval, they rushed to make the drug available to their young patients.

It was clear that this was only going to be of temporary help. That's what was being said for the adult patients. . . . But it felt like finally there was something we could do about this disease. I felt empowered, that I could offer something to the patients [to] improve the quality of their lives. The first week of January 1990, I got a nurse clinician, and I said, "No more of this waiting for the administration or the department to help us with this and to organize something. You and I are going to work in one clinic every Monday and every Thursday of every week, and we are going to see these patients, period. No more of this." [We] went into an empty clinic and opened shop, and began offering AZT to the children, the sickest children that met the criteria for treatment.

Despite the limits of AZT in patients with advanced illness, research persisted into the role it might play in slowing the progression of disease. A trial to determine the impact of AZT on individuals infected with HIV but still asymptomatic—clinical trial 019—formally began in July 1987 under the leadership of Paul Volberding. Two years later, the trial was stopped when a monitoring board determined that there was sufficient evidence of an effect to make the continuation of the study unethical.[3] For Volberding, the trial's apparent success marked a professional and scientific achievement of enormous magnitude.

> 019 was remarkable because it caused a paradigm shift in how we thought about this as a disease process. . . . Community organizations used it as a reason to encourage people to be tested [for HIV]: *"Be here for the cure."* It brought lots of people into medical care for the first time, so it was remarkable; it changed everything, and it really put me in the forefront of a lot of this.

The new study was greeted with enormous enthusiasm. Gerald Friedland wrote an editorial in the *New England Journal of Medicine*, "Early Treatment for HIV: The Time Has Come,"[4] that reflected the hopes of the moment. Looking back on that editorial from the vantage point of additional years of clinical experience, Friedland noted:

> I realize now I was much too optimistic. I wanted something, and so I was a little bit carried away by my own optimism, even though I wrote in the editorial the caveats about how long the effects will last—maybe there'll be resistance—all the things that we now know.

But for those who had been skeptical of the initial AZT findings, the new study offered little reason to revise their perspective. Indeed, Donald Abrams, Volberding's close colleague at San Francisco General Hospital, was sharply critical of the design of his associate's trial, discounting the findings.

> I felt that [the study] was too short. We've actually only benefited four people [for every] hundred people with the drug. And it seemed that the drug was not really that nontoxic; nor did I believe this was going to be a constant benefit.

The most cynical viewed the willingness to embrace such suspect findings as driven by an institutional need to achieve success. Sheldon Landesman, often an outsider, assumed that it was

> the desperate need by NIAID [National Institute of Allergy and Infectious Diseases] and those in the AIDS community who supported the research effort to show some success. Here was success. Congress doesn't fund failures repeatedly.

As doctors began to come to a realistic assessment of the role that AZT might play in the treatment of HIV infection, as patients began to deal with the failure of AZT to measure up to the promise of its most ardent advocates, a process of disenchantment set in that would, on occasion, take on a kind of fury. What at first had symbolized to many the success of science came to represent to some—the most ardent AIDS advocates among them—its utter failure. Despair fueled a reaction that for Dan William was troubling in many ways. Most important, he believed, it discouraged too many who might have derived some limited benefit from AZT from considering its utility as part of their therapy.

> There was almost like a yo-yo, this rush to and then rush away, and then the drug became politicized, which was the worst thing in the world, because drugs aren't good guys or bad guys; they're drugs. They have side effects; they have indications and contraindications; but they're not personas; they don't have a personality. But they were demonized. People didn't want to take [AZT].

Nowhere was the politicization more obvious than in the wrath of ACT-UP, the activist group that used demonstrations and the media to express outrage against the government and the corporate world because of their "torpid" response to drug development. In ACT-UP's view, resources had been misdirected into a fruitless endeavor, depriving researchers of funds that might well have met the needs of people with AIDS.[5] Perhaps most enraging to these activists, was that AZT itself caused suffering in those to whom it was prescribed. For those attacked by ACT-UP, like Martin Hirsch, the experience of being the target of protest was deeply troubling and frightening, all the more so since it was something for which he was utterly unprepared.

> I have always tried to do the right thing, tried to be a compassionate scientist; and to be called all kinds of names was very unpleasant.

ACT-UP targeted me, and they targeted Jerry [Groopman] and a few of the more visible people in the Boston area as enemies and as arrogant. One of the most awful experiences of my life was when [Jerry] and I were invited to speak at—I guess it's the National Gay and Lesbian Health Forum—at the Copley Plaza Hotel. I was scheduled to give a 20- or 30-minute review of antiviral therapy and half way through the talk a group from the back, ACT-UP people—I didn't know who they were at that point—started walking down the aisle carrying banners. And I remember some of them vividly. One of them said, "Marty Hirsch and Clinical Trials Equals Jim Jones and Jonestown." And somebody behind him had a tray of Kool-Aid, passing it out to the people. And another sign said, "The Blood of 19 Is on Your Hands," which was the 19 placebo recipients in the initial trial who died. And they interrupted the talk, and I tried to go on, and I guess I finished it. And then Jerry came on after that, and they did the same thing to him, calling him a Nazi. Given his religious background and roots, [he] was particularly— as he should have been—offended. But it was an awful time, and I hated it. And then somebody from ACT-UP coined the term—this must have been 1990—The Gang of Five because according to [them] we were controlling how clinical trials were being done in the United States, and, of course, doing it all wrong; and this became very popular. In fact, at the AIDS conference in San Francisco, this was taken up by [activist] Peter Staley who gave the keynote address. I still remember him saying, "I don't know the Gang of Five. I haven't met any of them personally, but I know they're awful people." It was a scary time. . . . And I still remember listening to PBS on the radio, and listening to [ACT-UP founder and playwright] Larry Kramer being interviewed, saying, "Nobody's listened to us. We've rallied; we've picketed; we've yelled and screamed. Nobody's listened to us. What we need is a few assassinations and maybe they'll start listening to us." I was literally afraid to go to that AIDS meeting, and it's the first time I've ever been to a meeting where I kept my tag under my coat because I didn't want anybody to see my name on the tag. We were offered police protection.

Jerome Groopman, ironically, also believed that the FDA was too slow, almost "intransigent," in evaluating therapeutic agents that might benefit people with HIV infection. But the conduct of the activists outraged Groopman and left him determined to disengage from them. He recalled the same meeting that had shaken Martin Hirsch.

> What I was most angry about was they wouldn't let people talk. They were the Brown Shirts. Basically they had decided unilaterally that we were poisoning them, that this drug was poison, and that the people in the audience would not be able to make an intelligent, considered, individual decision. They had the right to highjack the meeting and to basically prevent free speech and free dialogue. And I said that, "If you want to challenge, if you want to question, fine." And the whole meeting dissolved. They marched around the room for 20 minutes screaming, "Jim Jones, AZT is Kool-Aid." . . . At the San Francisco International AIDS Conference I was running a symposium which similarly got shut down. It was really nuts, and I thought to myself, this is really so counterproductive and so wrong. I would be damned if I were to spend my whole life investing hours in fighting them.

If the response to AZT among white AIDS activists was, in part, driven by hostility toward the research establishment, the reception of AZT among African Americans was affected by deep suspicions about the origins of AIDS and by the extent to which the new therapies were viewed as an effort to inflict further injury.[6] For African-American physicians like Janet Mitchell, these responses set the stage for moments of great frustration and even anger. Her patients at Harlem Hospital were typically women with a history of drug use.

> The hostility [to AZT] comes from the fact that there is still this unsettled feeling within the community as to where this disease came from. . . . There was this whole thing about the virus coming from Africa, somehow getting from monkeys to the Africans with some sort of connotation in one of the rumors that Africans were having sex with the monkeys. So you get this picture of, "You develop this disease to kill us off; and now you're selling us this cure that's really no good, and it's a poison."

As she sought to encourage her patients in the face of such suspicions, she tried to explain why it was necessary to use a poison to kill a deadly virus.

"You've got a virus that is very difficult to kill." And then I make analogies with roaches and what not, because you can't kill them without some side effects. You spray roach spray all over; you're not supposed to put it on food. But you have to give them analogies that put them in the context of things that they can relate to.

Such efforts worked only at times. Robert Scott, a gay, African-American physician in Oakland, California, found it striking that while 40 percent of his HIV practice was not Black, every single patient who refused to take AZT was an African American. Recognizing both the limits and benefits of AZT, Anita Vaughn would press her patients who would have nothing to do with AZT, " 'There's side effects from all medications. Not to take it means that you are allowing the virus to go completely unchecked.' " For her efforts she was, on occasion, denounced as an Uncle Tom. It was not so easy for Vaughn and other Black physicians with commitments to minority patients to adopt the take-it-or-leave-it stance of another physician, whose reaction to those who asserted that AZT represented the CIA's plot to exterminate Black people was, "Okay, don't take it."

Whatever the distortions that followed from the demonization of AZT, clinical experience and a deepening understanding of the process of viral resistance had made clear by the early 1990s that antiretroviral therapy was facing a crisis. And then on April 3, 1993, a letter in the internationally respected British medical journal *The Lancet* announced the preliminary findings from the Concorde trial, a European study that mirrored Paul Volberding's placebo-controlled study of AZT in asymptomatic individuals. Unlike the American study, which had been terminated because of what appeared to be the advantage of those receiving AZT over those receiving placebo, the European trial had been permitted to run its full course. The findings were a sharp rebuke to those who had claimed that life could be prolonged if AZT treatment was initiated in infected people before they became symptomatic.

For clinicians and researchers who had been closely identified with AZT, the study represented a grave challenge. They responded with a sharp critique of Concorde's methodological underpinnings. For Jerome Groopman, the study was "flawed."

There's almost a salacious desire for things to fail. Here's a study which is enormously flawed. So you have two choices: You can say, "Well, maybe they're right, despite all of the chaos in this study," or, "It doesn't make sense scientifically." And it didn't.

How could such an ill-conceived study[7] appear in a journal as prestigious as *The Lancet*?[8] For Groopman the answer was simple.

> *The Lancet* can be great, or it can be garbage. It's not peer reviewed. Alec Monroe, who's the editor of *The Lancet*, sits there, maybe shows it to a friend at his club over a glass of port, and then decides whether it's going to be published or not. It's not like *Science* or *The New England Journal*, although those places can make mistakes as well. I mean, everyone's fallible. But it's a crummy study.

Martin Hirsch, who had also been targeted by AIDS activists, believed the Concorde trial had been misused by the press. Rather than underscoring a finding that suggested the limits of AZT in people who had not yet developed symptoms, there was a tendency to claim that AZT was useless at all stages of AIDS. Such a picture fueled the outrage of activists who viewed the entire AZT era as the product of an unholy alliance.

> There was a very depressing period when the Concorde—Concordians, as we like to call them—were saying all the stuff about AZT being useful is wrong; it doesn't work; and people like Larry Altman [the medical writer for the *New York Times*] and others for some reason jumping on that bandwagon. He used to write front-page articles often as he could, it seemed like, saying, "AZT doesn't work, and everybody who claims AZT works is a liar," or whatever. And that was a depressing time. Altman wasn't unique. It was the feeling of a large proportion of the infectious disease community that treatment wasn't worthwhile. I think Altman and a lot of the press misinterpreted or misrepresented the results of the trial, and people went from one extreme to another and sort of discounted all the early studies and drew the conclusion AZT is no good. . . . Some of the more negative of the activists used this as ammunition that the "Gang of Five" and all the others in the American treatment establishment had been selling them a bill of goods and that AZT didn't work. And then there were all these books written about the Burroughs-Wellcome/medical/NIH/academic conspiracy to sell AZT and that we were all in the pockets of the drug companies, and that this was all a big hoax.

Two months after the initial report on the Concorde trial, the IXth International Conference on AIDS convened in Berlin. The results hung like a pall over the meeting and provided the occasion for Paul Volberding to reflect on the significance of the European study that had challenged what he took to be his most significant scientific contribution.

> I think it was a very overt decision that they were going to prove us wrong by continuing their study for the full planned duration. And they did take their trial for the full three planned years of follow-up, and the study obviously showed no effect. It will require its own history in terms of what happened. Serious methodological issues that can be raised have been raised to challenge some of the basic conclusions. What Concorde did was basically suggest to people that therapy was of no value. This is where I think I'm too close to it [but] I think that's the wrong conclusion. I think it raises questions about the optimum time to use therapy. I think, in part, it's because between the time 019 came out and Concorde came out there had been a gradual disillusionment with therapy. People had appreciated the relative ineffectiveness of therapy. The whole issue of [HIV becoming resistant to the therapeutic effects of drugs] had come out in that interval, so there was more reason to be discouraged about what therapy could do. People were prepared basically for bad news. . . . It was an ego blow to have stuff that I had done and believed in challenged, and to be perceived as no longer as relevant as it was at first.

Deborah Cotton's understanding of the canons of research often placed her at odds with clinical colleagues and the committee members with whom she shared advisory responsibility at the FDA. For her the evidence produced by Concorde underscored her belief that politics, not science, was dictating the approval of drugs and the willingness to rely on surrogate markers—changes in key components of the immune system rather than on clinical signs—as proof of therapeutic efficacy. Of an earlier trial where she had cast the lone dissenting vote she had said that the proponents of approval

> were just trying to take a sow's ear and make it into a silk purse. They wanted this to be a big effort, where we could feel good and slap each other on the back and look good, and the TV would say, "Wow, now we've got another drug for AIDS!" . . . So Concorde wasn't despair for me. I mean, it was sadness in the sense that I've said all along that I hope that all of this stuff pans out; but I didn't

think that within a year or two years of this vote there would be a clinical trial that would so clearly call into question the value of CD4 as a surrogate marker. . . . [For me, Concorde was] vindication.

Whatever the limitations of its science, Concorde was seen as a validation by many physicians, who had, as a result of clinical experience, begun to view AZT as a drug of very limited utility. Sharply critical of the tendency to confuse hope and reality, Donald Kotler was blunt:

I never had tremendous expectations and, therefore, never had tremendous disappointments. What went on in Berlin [was] that people couldn't fool themselves anymore.

The post-Concorde period was characterized by what Carol Brosgart termed a "terrible malaise." Even though he was critical of the conduct of the trial, John Mazzullo in Boston "was very blue for six months." Because she was a strong advocate of voluntary HIV testing and treatment among the Black and Latino adolescents she served in the Bronx, Donna Futterman was especially hard hit.

I think, to me, one of the hardest times was when we learned that AZT doesn't work as well in early intervention as we thought. I had really very much believed that there was a real rationale for engaging people in care. And we were starting to make a difference. But learning that we still don't know the golden moment to use AZT—how do you make that [once-in-a-lifetime] decision? Is your time more precious when you're healthy or when you're sicker? And when do you want to stop the virus? But that was really hard, to feel like we were going backwards.

Some doctors, while acknowledging the limits of AZT, saw the Concorde trial and the attendant media characterization of its meaning as having sowed confusion among patients, leading them to make choices that were very troubling. Gabriel Torres, whose clinical work was based at St. Vincent's Hospital in Greenwich Village, believed that, as a consequence, patients died too soon.

I think Concorde did a large disservice to the HIV population because there was a message sent out that treatment doesn't work, and people don't hear the specifics. They just hear treatment doesn't work, treatment is toxic, and it doesn't work. So why should you even bother going to the doctor? Why even bother getting tested? I think it may have cost the lives of many people who never sought treatment, never went to a doctor, and never came in until they had opportunistic pneumonia and died.

To limit such confusion among patients and their doctors, the Public Health Service made an effort to issue careful clinical guidelines that neither sustained unreasonable expectations about AZT nor rejected the possibility that AZT could be of some benefit to those who, though infected with HIV, had not yet developed AIDS. Such efforts were not always viewed as helpful. Indeed, they were sometimes greeted with scorn—yet another example of the gap that existed between researchers and policy makers on the one hand and doctors whose sole interest and commitment was to patients desperately seeking to stave off a life-threatening disease on the other. Working in a clinic located in a working-class community in the shadow of the powerful teaching hospitals associated with Harvard Medical School, Elizabeth Kass expressed her exasperation:

> The series of recommendations that came out after the Concorde study [essentially] said you can do this, or you can do this, or you can do this, or you can do nothing. Many of us felt like, well then why don't you just say, "Do nothing. We really have no idea." It was [almost] insulting. In the trenches, I think maybe part of what it's done is increased a sense of alienation from academics.

Kass, the "trench doctor," was not alone in her skeptical and despairing outlook. Indeed, even among those closest to centers of antiretroviral research there were doctors—Donald Abrams, for example—who were skeptical, and who believed that the search for an effective antiretroviral had been a failure.

> I'm cautious, I would say; I think I'm perceived as being very cynical. Some people think I'm very negative. I always say, "Don't shoot the messenger." . . . Whereas in the past [as someone who acknowledged that nothing available really worked] I might have been seen as anomalous, I think that there's a growing number of people who are in the same camp.

Drug Trials as Health Care

With despairing patients clamoring for therapy and equally despairing doctors struggling to provide something that might work against HIV infection or the associated opportunistic diseases, a remarkable transformation occurred in the attitude toward clinical trials of potentially effective drugs. Historically, the thrust of regulation and ethical guidelines had been to protect individuals from being coerced into medical experimentation—the specter of the Nuremberg trials and the infamous Tuskegee syphilis experiment haunted the conduct of clinical research.[9] But with AIDS, a dramatic about-face occurred. AIDS activists and their allies among physicians began to demand a right to participate in trials. "Drugs into Bodies"[10] was the demand. "A Drug Trial Is Health Care Too,"[11] was a slogan that sought to blur the distinction between care and research so central to the dominant regulatory paradigm. It was in this context that physicians, who saw themselves as caregivers, often came into conflict with those whose primary concern was the conduct of clinical trials. Even those who engaged in research found themselves torn.

Ronald Grossman was so committed to gaining access to new drugs for his patients that he found himself thwarting the conduct of investigations that involved placebo controls.

> Patients got knowledge enough to realize that their chance of getting any drug was, whatever, 50/50, one in three. I made a decision I thought I would never make—I stopped referring patients to any protocol that was placebo controlled—feeling my patients' desperation to get their hands on a drug. It sabotaged some of the protocols; they were unable to recruit. . . . I can remember two or three examples of people saying, "Please, Ron, you've got to talk your patients into understanding they'll eventually get the drug. The placebo control is only for 50 percent. You've just got to do that." And my saying, "No. I'm sorry. These patients are too desperate, however much we need that information." In retrospect I wish I had been more firm with my patients. "Look, you'll eventually get the drug. This is for science." But they weren't hearing it. They didn't want it for science; they wanted it for themselves.

It was commitment to their patients that led some physicians to view with skepticism the tightly defined criteria necessary to participate in new drug trials. Aware that acknowledging deception to gain access to a clinical investigation not only violated important ethical norms but could be the basis of professional sanctions, doctors were reluctant to describe their own efforts in this regard. Jerry Cade, who had played so central a role in organizing and providing medical care to AIDS patients in Nevada, was unusually direct.

> Cheated to make a patient [eligible]? Absolutely. I agonized for about two seconds, the first time I ever cheated. I can tell you what the first thing I ever did was. There was a white count minimum for getting AZT, and we all knew you give somebody a dose of prednisone, and that elevates their white count. And I did it several times. I have no qualms whatsoever. Science is not going to be seriously disturbed; we're not going to dramatically skew the data. I have a commitment to making sure we have good academic scientific trials, but the first job is to the human being who needs the care. It's not something I do all the time, but I'd do it again to make sure a patient got drugs.

Other physicians were troubled by the implications of cheating for their patients. Jerome Groopman, who viewed himself as both a scientist and a physician, was willing to press the limits, but he would do no more.

> I will use my Talmudic background and bend every rule and look for every loophole. I won't do anything illegal, but I'll try my damnedest to stretch the opportunity because of the humanistic aspects. And I have been in pitched battles in the past. I remember early on fighting with FDA representatives behind closed doors, people who later became transformed, so rigid, so detached, so completely out of touch with what it's like to take care of people who are in need and desperate. But I will never lie or manipulate because I think it's unfair.

How doctors' perspectives were shaped by their institutional and professional roles was cast into relief by those whose responsibilities underwent a transformation during the epidemic years. As a lesbian and AIDS activist, Donna Futterman had pressed for the needs of her impoverished adolescent patients in the Bronx. Identified with her young patients, she saw herself as an outsider. Her ethics were informed by a belief that it was incumbent upon her to succeed on behalf of her patients. But when she was given a position of national responsibility for overseeing research for adolescents, her perspective shifted.

A few years ago I would have had no question about saying I would fight for my patients—whatever I felt was best for them, [even] if that meant fudging. More and more, in research, I'm coming to appreciate a different side of it, which is that we're ultimately not going to help anyone if we muddle around, and that there were some heavy consequences when people made decisions like that. I'm head of the Adolescent Committee of the ACTG, and now [in 1995] head of the steering committee of this adolescent research study. So I [no longer] advocate "Fudge it for the patient," (a) because I think it's dangerous, and (b) I'm not sure it really will help the patient ultimately, or the study.

Gaining access to clinical trials was not, however, simply a matter of confronting the stringent inclusion and exclusion criteria that were part of research design. There were, in addition, barriers of a very different kind. Until the mid-1980s, women were, as a matter of explicit regulation and conventional practice, restricted from participation in clinical research because of concerns about potential harmful effects on the development of the fetus in the event of a pregnancy.[12] As of August 1989, less than 7 percent of those involved in federally funded trials organized by the National Institute of Allergy and Infectious Diseases were women and those figures overstated the involvement of women nationally because of the enrollment of large numbers of women in a very few centers.[13]

Alexandra Levine described the situation in the mid-1980s as "hideous." As an oncologist, an AIDS researcher, a caregiver, and a woman, Levine felt compelled to join with others to end the systematic exclusion of women from clinical trials.

A trial meant the hope of treatment because if you could not join a trial, then there was no treatment at all for the disease. And one of the things that became apparent to me was that only certain people had access to those trials. [Women] were just arbitrarily excluded. And the excuse was, "What if the woman was pregnant? What are you going to do with the unborn child?" Those were the "reasons." What that meant was that if a woman was by any chance unusual enough to actually have been diagnosed and actually brave and strong and committed enough to try to push onto a trial, she was excluded anyway. . . . The way the rules and the laws were written, the woman was mandated to die, mandated to be excluded from the opportunity to participate in something that might help her. . . . I felt it very closely. I mean, I'm a woman.

After considerable agitation on the part of AIDS activists, both gay men and women, and with support from physicians committed to the interests of their female patients, a Women's Health Committee was established within the AIDS Clinical Trials Group (ACTG), the coordinating committee that managed the huge federally funded AIDS research effort. But many activists were not mollified, and those who saw in the new committee an extraordinary opportunity to address the legacy of discrimination found themselves the target of wrath. Constance Wofsy, as chair of the committee, found the challenges disturbing.

The Women's Health Committee had been put there because it was politically correct, and everybody was laughing up their sleeves. But from the instant the Women's Health Committee was formed, which was such a success—to get a bureaucracy like the ACTG to form a committee devoted to women's research—it was the instant target of activists, of animosity. I distinctly remember that [at] the first committee meeting we had our introductions, "Hello, I'm Sarah. I do this research." And a woman activist came to the microphone and said, "This committee ain't done nothin'. You ain't done nothin' for women." . . . I didn't like it. I understood it, but I didn't like it. We couldn't get work done. It was a rite of passage. Nothing was happening to us that hadn't happened to every other person in the ACTG, [who] had to chin up and work with the activists. . . . I felt that the proportion of angry, nonconstructive activists seemed higher than I was seeing in other groups; and probably because they were earlier on in the learning curve of research, there were more obstructive activists than constructive. I found it very harrowing. I really wanted this committee to work. I could see that the leadership of the ACTG easily became confused about who the activists were and the women investigators—we were just all those noisy women.

Ironically, the most bitterly contested trial involving women raised questions of whether a study involving *only* women should be permitted to proceed. Clinical trial 076 was designed to determine whether the administration of AZT to pregnant women could reduce the rate of HIV transmission to their babies. Even as clinical trial 076 was being fashioned, AIDS activists—both men and women—denounced it because it focused on the prevention of the birth of babies with AIDS rather than on the needs of the women themselves. James Oleske, who had long established his reputation as a dedicated advocate of both the children he treated and their mothers, responded with dismay as both he and his colleagues were subjected to activist attack.

> Ed Connor was the senior [principal investigator] on that study. He was getting threatening letters; and my job was to sort of accompany him to meetings as his bodyguard. And I remember meeting with ACT-UP, having them screaming at us. There was a lot of frustration about us pediatricians only thinking [of] our women as incubators, and we didn't care. It was a hurtful thing to say because that certainly wasn't the truth. And it certainly was frustrating because the gay and lesbian community took such a strong voice; yet when you talked to a black woman in Newark, her concern was if you have something, fine. And so we were having people advocating, and I don't think they realized they weren't really advocating for the view of the moms we were taking care of.

To those sympathetic to the outrage of activists who saw the research establishment as unresponsive and arrogant, the clashes that surrounded this trial were especially painful. Charles van der Horst, whose view of the world was indelibly marked by his mother's experience as a Holocaust survivor, thought of himself as someone who could see the world from the perspective of an underdog; he was torn by the schism that emerged.

> There were leaflets put on our seats at the AIDS [research] meeting from two different groups of activists telling the other ones that they were ignorant sluts, [one leaflet] saying, "You can't do this; it's unethical to give women placebo; [the other saying] it's unethical to give women AZT." It made it a very complicated environment to work in.

As fury continued unabated, Janet Mitchell, the Harlem Hospital-based, African-American perinatologist, found herself called upon by those responsible for the national research effort on AIDS to defend the embattled trial. From her perspective, the effort to thwart the clinical trial because it might result in findings that might lead to coercive policies, like mandatory HIV testing of pregnant women, was patronizing. It betrayed white activists' assumption that African-American women and Latinas could not devise strategies for protecting themselves. Fiercely and relentlessly opposed to those who would abrogate the rights of minority women, she was the ideal occupant of the role she was called on to play.

> I get this call on a Saturday morning, pleading and begging for me to come down for this meeting, because I had been going to the [AIDS Clinical Trial Group] meetings as part of the pediatric ACTG. They knew that I had been a supporter of 076 from the very beginning. Essentially, what ACT-UP did [was] to terrorize all these nice—pardon my French—little white scientists, who were just absolutely terrified by their tactics. But somehow, when you've been attacked by raving drug addicts in Harlem Hospital and what not, they were tame to me. I could not be intimidated as easily. And so I said, "All right, you all pay my way. I'll come down." And they paid my way, and I came down. And the meeting started, and they started their usual not letting anybody talk, and I let that go on for a while. And then I finally got up, and I tried to talk. And they drowned me out and I took the microphone. And they saw me change from sort of trying to be a rational person. I took this microphone and I said, "You're all a bunch of racists. That's all you are." And I started after them—they were actually holding me back. They were truly afraid of these people, which those of us in the Black community thought was real funny. All they needed to do was be hit upside the head a couple of times. You know, I'm 4 foot 10 and at that time weighed about 96 pounds, but I was climbing over the seats. I was going to show them what intimidation really was. I had uttered a word that made everybody stop and think; because I was of color it had more impact than if [a white person] were going to call somebody a racist. I was calling them racist; and the reality was a whole row of essentially white women, not poor women of color, but basically white women. Then the women activists of color left them, and you just had this group of white women.

While the pressure to include women in trials necessitated a confrontation with a paternalistic ethos, the issue of including drug users—both men and women—raised very different questions. In 1989, a front-page *Los Angeles Times* story made it clear that drug users and, as a consequence, African-Americans and Latinos were being systematically excluded from trials.[14] "Blacks, Latinos, and intravenous drug users" said the article, "the groups increasingly afflicted with AIDS virus infections, are significantly underrepresented in federally sponsored AIDS clinical trials." Involved here was the question of whether the very factor that placed such individuals at risk for HIV made their participation in clinical trials all but impossible. Advocates on behalf of drug users saw the exclusion as a barrier to potentially effective therapy. Such restrictions, they argued, were rooted in unsubstantiated assumptions about the ability of drug users to comply with the requirements of clinical trials.[15] Like women, drug users were being "mandated to die." It is not surprising that Martin Hirsch viewed such demands with suspicion.

> You'd like to have a broad spectrum, but I think more important than having a broad spectrum is having patients who will complete their clinical trials. And it's just a fact—I wish it were otherwise— that an IV drug user is less likely to complete a clinical trial than a gay male.

However, if the issue of including subjects conventionally perceived as unreliable was to be resolved, advocates for broadened access to experimental interventions came to believe that the dominance of academic research centers in the organization of clinical trials had to be confronted. Carol Brosgart, whose community-based hospital was situated across the bay from San Francisco, expressed the exasperation and sense of isolation that many who treated AIDS began to feel in the 1980s:

> Those of us who are community physicians think that we had increasingly more and more clinical expertise than the AIDS experts because we were actually taking care of patients day in and day out and nights and weekends. We felt we were giving good care. For me, over here in Berkeley, I didn't want to have to send my patients to San Francisco every time there was a problem. I didn't want to have to send them to San Francisco to get into clinical trials. And I knew other physicians out in the community who felt the same kind of thing, How can we take all of this out to the community and not always have to come into the city to get it?

Brosgart favored a local setting: "I really wanted to have the availability of clinical trials on site, one-stop shopping; and part of my model was the cancer model of clinical trials happening in physicians' offices or large oncology clinics." At issue was how to build links between the local practitioners and the research scientists, between those close to patients and those with access to funding.

The County Community Consortium (CCC), which would meet the challenge posed by Brosgart, had its origins in an idea suggested in 1985 by Dianne Feinstein, mayor of San Francisco, to Paul Volberding to open lines of communication between San Francisco General (SFGH) and private physicians who were treating an increasing number of AIDS patients. Volberding passed the suggestion on to his colleague, Donald Abrams, since so many of the physicians who expressed interest in Feinstein's proposal were friends and colleagues of Abrams, members of the gay Bay Area Physicians for Human Rights. Together, they set the initial goals of the CCC: Community doctors would take on the responsibility of managing a portion of the hospital's AIDS patients by becoming the admitting physicians of record. In return, San Francisco General would keep the community doctors current about the newest advances in AIDS care and inform them of clinical trials available at the hospital. When physicians raised the issue of using their own practices as trial sites instead of sending patients to SFGH, Abrams acceded. He would teach them research methodology; they would supply information from the trenches.

> It became clear to me that there are some issues here. As a clinician, I was also an investigator, but many of my colleagues in the community chose to be clinicians because they didn't want to do research. But with a new disease, it seemed inherent to me that taking care of patients was essentially doing research, and why should we not capture information? It became clear that we really needed to teach people how to do research, and so that became one of the things that we also took up in the consortium.

In 1987, after several false starts, the CCC undertook a clinical trial of aerosolized pentamidine to determine its value as a prophylaxis against PCP. In New York City, a group of patients and physicians, the Community Research Initiative (CRI), organized by Joseph Sonnabend, fielded its own trial of aerosolized pentamidine, patterned on that of the CCC. The first study, published as a lead article in the *New England Journal of Medicine*, showed that aerosolized pentamidine effectively prevented *Pneumocystis* pneumonia, providing a powerful boost to community-based research. Physicians like Carol Brosgart felt vindicated and empowered.

We showed that aerosolized pentamidine worked. When everybody was being so negative and saying, "Well you can't prevent PCP," we said "You could!" And the fact that it came from community providers, private doctors' offices, little clinics like mine. . . . It was so exciting that we got a drug licensed. You know, this little podunk group of neophytes and peons. And we did it, and it gave us a sense of tremendous power or empowerment and made me feel less disconnected.

Following the success of the two community-based research initiatives, the federal government and private foundations—most notably the American Foundation for AIDS Research—underwrote community clinical trial programs in various parts of the country, spurring their spread. But these efforts, like the move to lower the barriers to underserved research subjects, had their critics. They were unwieldy and slow. Donald Kotler saw the usefulness of community trials while faulting the group process that perilously overloaded study design.

It's not been a tremendous success. I'll say it allows questions to be asked and answered which cannot be asked and answered in the laboratory. After all, AIDS has been cured over and over and over again in the laboratory. It doesn't translate so well out in the field. . . . [But community-based research suffers from] democracy. Each person adds to the protocol, making it more and more complex, sometimes altered so as to interfere with the ability to satisfy the specific aim. To reach the final committee, which has to deal with money, you will see a protocol that's much too complicated for them to do. To tear the protocol down and send it back to start over, having lost six months. A never ending series of reviews and committees and inputs. Science in many ways is really a solo effort. One person driving, the one person with the idea, the creative idea to drive.

If Kotler was ambivalent in his ultimate judgment, Joseph Sonnabend was not. Ironically, as private physicians became increasingly involved in clinical research, something Sonnabend had long championed, he began to condemn community trials for reasons that mirrored those offered by academic critics. He now found only a few instances when community-based research could be justified.

I too had the idea that anybody could do [a clinical trial]. But I've come to respect it a lot more. It has its own vocabulary, its own expertise. Physicians, when they do become [principal investigators], have no idea of what's involved or what should be involved. It has changed for me. Originally, I just thought to utilize this tremendous resource. And doctors are now doing research. They venture into lucrative deals with pharmaceuticals and do it themselves. The number of people entering clinical trials has, I suppose, certainly increased. It's the quality of the trials that is of interest to me. . . . There is no reason to have a community-based program when it comes to government-sponsored stuff or where [trials] go on at medical centers and at clinics that provide primary care. What [community research initiatives] should do is identify interventions, treatments, that are potentially useful that don't really have any sponsors and raise the money to do them. To that extent, I think we do something that can justify our existence.

Sonnabend was not alone. There were others who had been advocates of community trials who turned on them, one of whom said, "I think that universities should be doing the clinical trials. This is science. I think we've wasted a tremendous amount of money and effort and resources trying to do clinical trials in the community."

The rethinking of the role of community-based trials by some of its earliest advocates was but a more recent manifestation of the despair that had prompted some to challenge research in elite institutions. At a moment when uncertainty surrounded the future course of the treatment of HIV, devoted clinicians also began to rethink earlier propositions that had so emphasized speed in the release on new therapeutic agents, even if such speed came at the price of relatively lower levels of scientific certainty.

Particularly striking was the change of heart of Donald Abrams, who had pressed for the early release of drugs but who came to believe the costs too great to bear. He hinted darkly that the demand for early release had been backed by an alliance of needy patients and those motivated by corporate greed.

At one point I voted in favor of approving things with minimal evidence that they work because the patients wanted it, but then it became clear to me that I don't think that there is a lot of benefit to providing drugs that are not useful. I know that sometimes my paternalistic protectionism is against what my community is demanding, and that is earlier access to these drugs. But I have to rely on my training and knowledge and insight that maybe is a little more advanced than some people's who have perhaps other motives for wanting these things available sooner.

Deborah Cotton had always remained skeptical of the changes demanded by AIDS activists and their allies within the research establishment, as her "vindication" by the results of Concorde suggested. She had seen the stakes clearly when she cast the lone dissenting vote at the FDA when it approved the antiretroviral drug ddI in 1991.

I voted against ddI; I felt it was a very unwise decision. It was policy masquerading as science. It drove me absolutely crazy. If we could have said, "This is a terrible epidemic—we don't know what to do— AZT isn't working—we are all going to decide that we will make ddI available, but we actually have no idea whether it's going to hurt or help," I might have been able to vote for that. . . . I think what we're going to do is five years, six years down the road, we're going to be throwing up our hands and saying, "Okay, now we got four drugs. We still don't know which one works better than another. None of them really work too well." . . . To me it was really sacrificing people for political expediency. We knew the demographics were shifting, even though none of us wanted to say it out loud. We were really saying, "Let's save middle-class gay men, even if it means more confusion when this epidemic is all about poor Black women."

Toward a More Democratic Medicine: Sharing the Burden of Ignorance

If desperate moments led to demands for a more democratic approach to research, they also provided the context for the insistence that the clinical relationship itself undergo a fundamental change. The authoritative posture, activists asserted, based on clinical expertise, had to yield to a more collaborative approach to clinical decision making. Patients posed questions, challenged proposed therapeutic interventions, and even insisted that novel clinical approaches be considered as options. They pressed for changes that went far beyond the transformations that the critics of medical paternalism had elicited in the prior two decades. And to a remarkable degree, the pressure for change met a receptive audience. Recognizing the palpable limits of their capacities, doctors seemed ready to share their authority.

Neil Schram, whose training in nephrology had taught him what needed to be done for patients with kidney disease, recognized that AIDS posed a different challenge.

> We were taught basically that a patient comes with a problem, we diagnose the problem, we treat the problem, and we send the patient home. That's how medicine works. Well, that works great when you have a treatment, but, of course [with HIV/AIDS], for a long time, there was no treatment and so we stopped knowing the answers. Not only did we stop knowing the answers, but in many instances the patients know more than we do.

Ronald Grossman, whose large AIDS practice in New York provided ample opportunity to consider the implications of therapeutic limits on clinical style, contrasted his approach to AIDS patients with what was more typical.

> We began to use words we wouldn't otherwise use with patients with other diseases, things like "You know, this has to be a partnership." Contrasting, say, with a diabetic—this is not negotiable. I never said that, but the implication was "You start insulin tomorrow, and I'll see you in a week." And nobody ever said no to that.

AIDS doctors were confronted with desperate patients, engaged in a life-and-death struggle. Many of them were well educated, often comfortably middle class, and politically engaged, and they came to their physicians armed with the belief that those to whom they turned had no right to dominate the clinical encounter. Marcus Conant, whose San Francisco practice pioneered the development of sessions in which patients could question their caregivers about the evolving course of therapeutics, witnessed the transformation being pressed for by his gay patients.

> American medicine was moving away from this notion of the paternalistic physician writing in Latin abbreviations and saying, "Now you just take that and come back in two weeks, and I'll find out if you're better or not." We were moving away from that; this was the next logical step. But suddenly you've got something that was unique in America. We had a fatal but chronic disease amongst young, exceedingly bright people. These are angry 30-year-olds.

They were very bright people, most from middle America, who realized that they couldn't be gay and live in Kansas City, that they could become a very successful computer programmer at work in the biotech industry, move to California, make a lot of money, be sexually active; and it was incomprehensible to them that they could then be infected by a fatal disease which would change that lifestyle. They became angry; they became empowered; they developed networks; they took what was happening in terms of computer technology, in terms of exchanging information. They found out they could go to medical meetings; they wanted to be involved in making decisions about their care. And they did. I think we as physicians realized that, in the first place, you couldn't buck that type. If you had tried to, you would have been viewed, I think appropriately, as a fool. And what you do is you realize that is the way it should be, and particularly when you cannot, in fact, save their lives.

Michael Gottlieb saw it somewhat differently. His gay AIDS patients were not the first to challenge the conventional and hierarchical trappings of the clinical relationship. He had seen it before in California.

I was shocked when I came to California in 1977, coming to Stanford, and my lupus patients were that way with me. I couldn't believe it, because in upstate New York, where you had farmers coming in with advanced prostate cancer and basically having no medical care, you told them, "Okay, here's what you do," and you doctored them. You were the authority. When I came to California, I realized something was different here. You had patients quizzing you and calling you by your first name, and I couldn't believe it. Fortunately it happened during my fellowship there, and I learned to like it.

Many AIDS doctors came to admire their patients' persistence. In the face of a disease that brooked no opposition, these individuals reached for the authority to shape their treatment. With their doctors having little to offer, patients brought unproven treatments to the table as worthy of consideration. In listening to their suggestions, doctors found that the burdens of uncertainty and impotence could be less onerous. "I learned," said Dan William, "that sharing the responsibility of treatment decisions made caring for patients infinitely easier when you have less than a full deck of cards."

Alvin Friedman-Kien, whose self-confident manner conveyed precisely those characteristics that might be the target of a leveling ethos, was enthusiastic about his patients' efforts in a way that was placed into bold relief by his capacity to treat some of his colleagues dismissively.

> Every patient with HIV disease is an expert, almost any with any intelligence. They often tell me about things I haven't heard about yet. I think patients are terrific. I think their enthusiasm, their participation as partners in the disease, is very exciting and important, and I like taking care of patients who participate, who aren't just boilerplates who sit back waiting for me to give them anything I want, but who say, "What about this? What about that," who challenge you. I think that's exciting. They tell me about studies that I didn't even know existed, and sometimes they find out about things that are going on in California that I didn't even know about, because the underground is very clever. And sometimes there are drugs that I'd like my patients to get that they can't, but they say, "Oh, we can get it for you; we have an underground source for it." And that's fine. If I had HIV disease, I'd grope for straws. I'd look for the same thing.

A more open, less paternalistic style imposed a new set of burdens—ones associated with the time necessary to explore with patients their ideas and concerns. Some patients, Carol Brosgart said of her practice in Berkeley, California, came in with 25 questions on their list, and she was forced to tell them, " 'You'd better choose the top two because there's no way we're going to get through that. So choose them well.' "

To accommodate patients who sought an active involvement in tracking the clinical implications of the latest research, a number of physicians organized regularly scheduled meetings. To those who were unprepared for an assertive and inquisitive style of these sessions could be exhausting. Alexandra Levine, who met regularly with her patients with persistent generalized lymphadenopathy, recalled one such session.

> The patients always came to those PGL [persistent generalized lymphadenopathy] . . . meetings armed with big binders of papers and asking this and that. It became just second nature, "Gee, I didn't hear that; tell me about that one." . . . At the end of 1986, I had been at a conference in Japan. One of the people I met was Jean-Claude Chermann, who had been working with Montagnier and who was the person who really did find the virus. I had told them

about the PGL group and at a certain point he wanted to come and visit. . . . So I organized a PGL meeting on a Friday afternoon. . . . There was a big group of people who showed up, and Jean-Claude had gotten off the plane from France just hours before. He was tired and jet-lagged . . . and I introduced him [and] got the conversation started. . . . Jean-Claude would say something, and immediately ten people would start arguing, just like we normally did. And he was getting more and more depleted. He started sweating and so forth, and at a certain point he said, "I go sit down. You do it now."

For some physicians the more egalitarian approach was so compatible with their broader political and philosophical commitments that they were almost blind to the needs of patients who wanted their doctors to assume a more conventional role. This was true for Molly Cooke.

You know, people are really different, and even within AIDS, even among middle-class gay men with a lot of expertise there are a whole variety of styles. If anything I'm not directive enough. I've learned to overcome my queasiness about being directive. You're actually probably better off being a little too directive, because to the high-autonomy people, it'll really be obvious that you're bugging them. But if you're not directive enough, people who want to be a little dependent, especially if they're men and they've got big fancy jobs and they have staffs of thousands and are captains in industry, they will flounder, because they can't say, "Take care of me."

Inevitably, whatever their personal predilections, many doctors felt threatened initially by those who shed the passivity conventionally assigned to the patient role. Neil Schram candidly acknowledged his difficulty despite the fact that he had come to believe that greater equality was desirable.

It was initially threatening. One doesn't go from the normal medical model to the new model without a little help from one's patients; and when it first starts, it's uncomfortable. It was a lot easier when people just listened to you and did what you asked them to, or did what you told them to. . . . What I consider a liberal approach to patient autonomy came from patients basically discussing things with me. My recognition of patient autonomy only came from the patients. I certainly would not have learned that myself.

It was an especially difficult transition for those who had just recently become physicians and whose professional identities were linked to an expertise they had only recently acquired. Harry Hollander, who moved from the status of a resident to the directorship of the AIDS program at San Francisco's Moffitt Hospital, noted:

There were many occasions when people confronted me with ideas, treatment strategies about which I knew little or nothing, or non-traditional treatment strategies, again which I had no background in. . . . At first it was very hard. At the end of your training years you feel a command of a body of knowledge; you feel as if you know or should know things fairly definitively. I can recall occasions of being quite upset with patients for challenging the medical dogma that I was espousing. I think as a young practitioner you want to have more control over people than you do later on in your career; and as you practice, particularly outpatient medicine, you realize how very little you have control over in taking care of people anyway. . . . It did take some time to get used to often being bombarded with new ideas, ideas that didn't make sense from traditional medical training.

But even among some of the most ardent proponents of the new, more democratic style there was a periodic yearning for the more conventional style of medical practice, when knowledgeable doctors wrote orders based on their best clinical judgment, and appreciative patients complied. This was especially noteworthy in the case of Donald Abrams, who had devoted himself to empowering the gay community in San Francisco to play an active role in the medical management of AIDS and who was skeptical of many of the proposed interventions being proffered by mainstream AIDS doctors, including his colleague Paul Volberding.

One of the reasons that I went into medicine in the first place I think was because I liked to care for people, and I probably liked to be in control. I'm often called a control freak. I've learned to let go a little bit as I've had more life experiences. . . . About two or three years ago [in 1992] I decided, gee, it would be nice to sort of be involved again in a situation where I could experience my idealized vision of my youth of what a doctor-patient relationship should be. So I chose to go back and see more oncology patients in our cancer center here at San Francisco General, because I wanted to see people who weren't going to come in and tell me what chemotherapy to give them, and allow me to make a decision on what drugs to use, and patients who I could sometimes cure.

Much of the democratization that occurred took place in the context of the relationship between white middle-class gay men and their doctors. The picture was very different for Black and Latino intravenous drug users, their largely female sexual partners, and others who were poor and had to scramble to gain access to care when they fell ill. Donna Futterman said that her adolescent patients in the Bronx, poor minority youth, "don't really clamor" for alternative therapies. It was enough to get them to consider more conventional treatments. The same was true for the adult minority patients treated by Robert Scott in Oakland, California. "I've got people on the Internet, but the vast majority of my patients who have done all that kind of research and stuff tend to be white—even though the vast majority of my patients are Black."

But even the most impoverished could make their needs known, and in the context of a heightened sensitivity to the cultural needs of patients there was a willingness—at times mingled with discomfort—to incorporate unconventional approaches to disease. Speaking of her Haitian patients in Miami, Margaret Fischl noted,

> Particularly in the beginning, when we had less information, you would see a lot of hesitation in [their] accepting what they had, accepting how they got it, accepting what they needed to do for their illness, and the whole issue of other modes of therapy would permeate what we did. We had to deal with the voodoo religion. We had to allow voodoo doctors to come into our hospital and work with our patients. . . . They came in and they did their ceremonies, and we had patients in the next bed get better! . . . Among the Spanish and Latin culture, we had to deal with their religious beliefs; we had in the beginning more chickens killed in rooms than I want to remember.

Just how far AIDS doctors, trained in the canons of scientific medicine, could go was, not surprisingly, a source of tension. On the one hand, there was a reluctance—given the limitations of medicine as they understood them—to impose strictures; on the other hand, even the most tolerant of physicians typically had limits. Constance Wofsy believed it necessary to establish firmly the boundaries of the tolerable.

> People came with very strong opinions of what they wanted. I'm by personality a limit setter, and I think I eliminated the patient

population that was very pushy beyond where I could go, in a totally nice way. I can remember a conversation saying, "Here's what's available. Here's what I'm able to do. Here are my thoughts on the subject. I'm happy to work with you within those boundaries. I don't feel comfortable with such and such a thing that you just described to me, and I don't know that I can work the best on your behalf with that."

Barbara Starrett, on the other hand, who had been engaged in psychic healing while a resident in the Bronx in the 1970s, was among the most accepting and so attracted patients who were prone to experimentation.

> Another reason my patients would seek me out [was that] I would be willing to listen and do things. SPV 30—my feeling was from the beginning that that was not going to work; but if people wanted to be on it, that was fine; we'll just follow them. . . . If I felt it were harmful, I would not do it.

It was this latitudinarian perspective that would inform the response of many physicians to compound Q, a drug that achieved some currency in the gay community, and Kemron, an agent that some African-American patients turned to in lieu of AZT.

In the early 1990s the Kenyan government, with great fanfare, began to market Kemron, a drug that it claimed could eliminate the symptoms of AIDS and perhaps eliminate HIV infection itself.[16] First developed in the United States but tested for AIDS at a government-funded research institute in Kenya, the new therapy—a low dose of alpha interferon [an antiviral produced by the human immune system]—promised to be cheap and easily administered. From the outset, the claims were met with skepticism, adding to the allure of the drug among African-Americans. An African-American physician, Barbara Justice, who practiced in Harlem, became a strong proponent of Kemron. The Harlem-based *Amsterdam News* asserted in the fall of 1990 that the failure of Kemron to draw interest was the consequence of a racist perspective, since Blacks "could not possibly have come up with an effective therapy or cure for AIDS that has eluded white scientists and researchers."

For Anita Vaughn's African-American patients, who lived in poverty-stricken Newark, Kemron had an appeal.

> A lot of patients are so disenchanted with conventional care. I've always lived with patients who totally reject any type of Western

medicine. And so patients had been going over to New York to get Kemron.

As a self-described activist, she would have wanted so inexpensive a therapy—the projected costs were $600 per year—to work. But after trying the drug with a few patients she "wasn't really impressed with the overall effects." Janet Mitchell at Harlem Hospital was similarly unimpressed. She told her patients that she wouldn't prescribe it, but "If you want to get it, that's fine. One of the things that is pretty certain [is] that taking it orally as it's prescribed doesn't do any harm." But she never would say bluntly that Kemron was "not worth the money or time." To do so, she believed, would threaten the clinical bond she knew was so crucial.

> It's sort of like when you were a child, [and] the thing that your mother told you wasn't good was the thing you wanted. Plus then it erodes the trust they have in me, because you're then denying their right to be a partner in their care. And what they will do is, they will take it anyway. . . . I deal with a lot of patients whose roots are in the South. Eating clay, eating starch is a normal part of pregnancy for a lot of populations. Eating those kinds of things and taking your iron and vitamins chelates the iron, and the iron doesn't do any good. If I say, "Don't eat the starch," then they're going to eat it and not tell me. If I say, "Don't eat it and take your iron right behind it," or "Take your iron separately and make sure you're eating all the other things," then, even though they know I'm not a believer in it, they'll say, "Well, you know, she didn't tell me I couldn't eat it, so maybe I won't." But when people feel that they are partners and that you respect their choices, they stay in care; and the bottom line for me is keeping people in care.

By mid-1993, any remaining doubts about Kemron were put to rest as a World Health Organization study conducted by Ugandan scientists found "that treatment with low dose oral interferon alpha does not benefit HIV-infected people."[17] The announcement was made during the same International AIDS Conference in Berlin that had showcased the Concorde trial.

Kemron was a drug with virtually no reputed toxicities, but the story was very different with Compound Q, a drug derived from the root of a Chinese cucumber, which in laboratory trials appeared to selectively destroy HIV-infected cells. When these results were published in the *Proceedings of the National Academy of Sciences* in 1989, they sparked immediate interest among AIDS activists and patients anxious for treatment with greater promise than AZT.[18] Recognizing that people with AIDS were beginning to import the drug from China and furious at the torpid pace of drug development and study, the activist group Project Inform in San Francisco took the remarkable step of organizing an underground trial of Compound Q in four cities: New York, Los Angeles, San Francisco, and Fort Lauderdale. It was not approved by the FDA, nor was it submitted to a review board for an ethical evaluation—especially crucial given the potential toxic side effects. The investigation sparked a bitter dispute among AIDS activists, physicians, and researchers.

Barbara Starrett was responsible for the Compound Q trial in New York and remained a proponent of its benefits long after it receded from the consideration of even the most adventurous clinicians. Her first patient was given Compound Q even before the preliminary findings of the *Proceedings of the National Academy of Sciences* were published.

The first person I gave Compound Q to . . . was very very sick . . . and I did that in the hospital. I slept on the floor next to his bed, and his sister slept on the other side on the floor the first night. And actually it was very interesting: he woke up the next day, and he was lucid for about two days. And then he drifted off again, and then he died; and on autopsy he had aspergillosis. That was probably in '88, maybe even '87.

What drew attention to Starrett's involvement with Compound Q was the death of a patient that was reported to the *New York Times* and that led to charges that he had, in fact, died as a consequence of his treatment.

He actually did not qualify [for the trial] because everybody was supposed to have been on AZT. He wasn't going to take the AZT because it was a toxin. He had also had PCP a year and a half before. And he had an adverse reaction. He was delirious, so he was having a toxic reaction to Q. And he just needed to be supported. He needed IV fluids, maybe steroids, depending on how he went; but it was the kind of reaction that had been reported and that we knew passes. Anyway, the police came. I told them he had taken an experimental drug and that this was something that was going to last 24 hours, but he needed to be monitored. He was thrashing all over the place. He went [into the hospital] on Friday night; he was better by Saturday night. On Sunday he was discharged from the hospital. On Tuesday he came, and he wanted

more Q. I still have a video of it. He's describing what he remembers, what happened, how he blacked out, what he remembers of
the hospital. And I told him that I wouldn't give him Q again because his blood counts were low. And his last thing is, "I hope my
blood counts come up so that I can get Q." But I never gave him
Q again. [Later,] he died. There was no autopsy, so we don't know
what he really died from, but it was clearly not Q-related.

The fierceness of the reaction to Starrett was captured by Howard Grossman, who at the time of the patient's death was on the staff of St. Claire's
Hospital in New York, where the patient had been taken during his toxic
reaction.

Barbara went out on a limb. She tried really hard to do the right
thing. And they were ready to screw her to the wall. It was in the
papers. [The medical director of the Community Research Initia-
tive] was very much a part of the people who were trying to get
her. They just for some reason had it in for her. And people were
going crazy. I mean, you went to an ACT-UP meeting, and people
were saying these ridiculous things.

Joseph Sonnabend was among those who believed the trial of Compound Q was scientifically without merit and ethically flawed because of
the high risk of toxicity. As a doctor, he had cared for AIDS patients from
the outset and had been subject to discrimination because of his efforts.
Nevertheless, he was often the outsider, even within the AIDS community, given his lingering skepticism about the role of HIV in the etiology of AIDS. Here, once again, he felt compelled to confront the wrath
of some activists.

The issue of Compound Q was quite an important thing for me in
the sense that it was very painful. Compound Q was a highly poi-
sonous substance. Martin Delaney, of Project Inform, who has been
personally quite abusive towards me [sent his protocol to the Community Research Initiative]. I saw the protocol, I read it, and
thought it was ridiculous; it was a terrible protocol. And anyway,
given the potential toxicities, I didn't think we should be doing it.
[Nevertheless the protocol went forward] in an underground fashion. It was sort of heroic stuff, and the emotion was kind of fierce
and incredible. . . . There was a death on this trial that I was responsible for uncovering . . . although I didn't make a report. It put

me at odds with Barbara Starrett. That was a bad situation, because it also put me at odds with the part of the activist community [that said] "Just give it to us now. We need it now. We don't care about the quality of the science."

While other physicians around the country would provide Compound Q under conditions characterized by extraordinary stealth (in Rochester, New York, William Valenti and his colleagues hid the treatment of a patient from the administrator who had been involved in securing the state license for his clinic), others refused to provide a potentially toxic treatment. "Compound Q," said Stosh Ostrow in Atlanta, "I wouldn't go near it." Speaking to an insistent patient, he said:

"Listen, there are places in town where you can get it if you want to. If you're going to do it, please let me know. But I don't want to have anything to do with it. First of all, the toxicity is horrendous. People have died from it. And there have been absolutely no studies that show that it's effective."

For some doctors, a strategic openness to their patients' wishes masked a deep hostility to the alternative therapies. Tapping the traditions of their profession, which had long sought to impose professional controls on the unorthodox, and which, early in the century, had vanquished medical traditions viewed as unscientific, they railed against the exploitation of their desperate patients. Peter Wolfe, part of a large AIDS practice in Los Angeles, encountered much that provoked his disdain.

[What] I find most disheartening are the [patients] who have decided that orthodox medicine, whatever that means, just is not giving them the answers they feel comfortable with. And so they go to chiropractors and to herbalists and to oriental medicine doctors, and so forth and so on. I think that the scientific method does have advantages in trying to help people's lives. . . . I'm a skeptic [and] an atheist. I'm absolutely not involved in spiritual things. But I do certainly recognize that most people aren't like that and [that] they [have a] need to believe in something.

To Ronald Grossman, the purveyors of much of what passed for alternative medicine were simply charlatans. His sense of outrage was palpable.

I thought this was a horrendous, criminal, cruel rip-off of patients with this disease who were so desperate. Not the alternative therapy per se, which might or might not have had some anecdotal benefit, but rather the way it was marketed. The same old business—the people who were fraudulent promoted their cures as miraculous. And it cost a shitpot of money. It never [failed]; there was no altruistic supplier of these alternative therapies, and I hated it. I watched people deplete their resources, including very costly trips to Europe. Nothing was worse than isoprenosine and ribavarin. Literally hundreds of my patients went to Mexico to acquire these drugs where it was available, and some of it was confiscated by the customs people at the border. But in any case large amounts of money were spent.

Nevertheless, to be an effective clinician, Grossman, like Janet Mitchell, felt compelled to make his peace, hold his tongue.

It became obvious that if I did not give my blessing to patients using these drugs, they would simply go elsewhere. I attempted to integrate the use of ribavarin and isoprenosine into whatever other therapies we had; and as I did that I found that patients relaxed in my presence to talk about that and other nontraditional stuff they were using, the herbs and the potions and the lotions, let alone the massages and the acupunctures and what have you. They became more compliant patients, more relaxed patients, began to see me as someone they could trust with their tales of alternative therapies helping them.

But for some it was not simply the excesses of the alternative therapies that proved distressing. They found the move toward a more egalitarian ethos itself troubling. Such opposition did not necessarily reflect a conservative or tradition-bound outlook. Indeed, one of the most forthright articulations of concern came from Robert Cohen, whose left-wing commitments had informed his professional life. He had come to direct clinical practice with AIDS patients relatively late. Yet as a practitioner in the second decade of the epidemic, he found discomfiting the egalitarian ethos that had emerged early on when medicine had so little to offer.

A lot of people will come to me and say, "I'd like you to be my partner in treatment." I tend to have an uncomfortable reaction to that. I'm not happy with my reaction to it. I would actually like to

be more open to someone's attempt to express or maintain autonomy, which is the essential basis of ethical medical practice. I think
that it's totally reasonable for everybody with HIV infection to be
very skeptical of the whole process and want to know everything,
and know my motivations. So in some things they're absolutely
right, but there is something paternalistic about this role. There just
is. To some extent I want someone to decide to continue with me
. . . based on the fact that they want my judgment on it.

Cohen's challenge to what he took to be a misguided egalitarianism
ironically bore the imprint of his own therapeutic nihilism—a perspective
he shared with others at the close of the first decade of the AIDS
epidemic.

Yet even in that climate there were doctors like Donna Mildvan who
held fast to a vision within which science would vanquish AIDS. During
these bleak years, she struggled to remain an optimist. In describing the
basis for her hope, she referred to a movie from the 1950s, *The Man in
the White Suit*. The protagonist, a scientist-inventor, is subjected to relentless challenges to his revolutionary discovery by forces defending the
status quo. Eventually, even his discovery, a chemical formula that ren-
ders cloth indestructible, proves a failure. In the last scene of the film,
Mildvan remembers him

walking away, completely dejected, crushed, resigned and we think
it's all over. But then his pace picks up a little, then a little faster,
and then a little spring in his step. We hear the background music
start up again—the clinky clonk motif always associated with his
lab's bubbling flasks and test tubes. And off he bounds. He's got it!
He's got the answer. He knows just what he's got to do to that
formula. And that's the way it always is with us. We're crushed,
defeated, getting picked apart. And then we realize, "Oh, *that's* what
this means! Okay, I can fix that."

Such optimism, bordering on faith, was for others not easy to sustain.
There had been too many false starts, too much suffering and death.

4
TRAVEL AGENTS FOR DEATH

Death came to define AIDS in the epidemic's first years. In 1981, 120 fatalities were recorded, although in retrospect, it is clear that there were earlier losses among those for whom there was no diagnosis. In the ensuing years, the toll rose sharply; in 1986 the number of AIDS deaths had reached almost 12,000. By 1990, 100,000 had died since the epidemic's onset, almost a third of them in 1990 alone.[1] The deaths came swiftly as well; of those diagnosed before 1983, 75 percent had lost their lives by mid-1985. Equally striking was the youth of those who had fallen victim; about three-fourths were between the ages of 25 and 44. By 1992, AIDS had become the leading cause of death of men between the ages of 25 and 44, surpassing suicide, homicide, cancer, heart disease, and unintentional injuries.[2] Among young women, AIDS was the fourth leading cause of death in 1992. Among young African-American women, AIDS was the leading cause of death in at least 10 American cities in that year.

Given this toll and the burden borne by cities where the epidemic hit early, it was inevitable that death would shape the experience of the doctors who cared for patients with AIDS. At San Francisco General Hospital, where the AIDS service lost 25 to 35 patients per month, John Stansell likened his job to that of directing a MASH unit. Stansell's colleague, Constance Wofsy, who had come to AIDS work at the epidemic's onset, noted:

It will sound macabre, but I realized I was a travel agent for death and that my role was to make the process as drawn out, as comfortable, and as full of interesting things as it was possible to do. And I couldn't prevent the ultimate outcome, but I could manage it.

No training would have been sufficient to prepare physicians for the professional demands that would attend the new disease, the number of dying patients they would encounter, their patients' youth, and the suffering that would mark the path to death. Many doctors saw their medical education as having failed to provide even the most rudimentary skills for responding to the needs of those for whom they were caring and their families. Lisa Capaldini, trained at the University of California in San Francisco, would find that working with dying AIDS patients had a profound professional and spiritual impact. She recalled:

> I remember very early in med school having a sense that something was wrong, insofar as it was clear treatment wasn't working, that we didn't deal with it very up front; nor were we as doctors very good about comforting our patients and their families. There was just sort of a sense of embarrassment or anger. And there really wasn't a sense of death as part of all our lives and [that] treating someone with great care and skill is as important as when someone's in the intensive care unit and getting very technically complex treatment.

But far more was involved than learning how best to care for and comfort the dying and those who loved them. What doctors would discover—and for this there was even less preparation in medical school—was that death presented challenges to their own sense of well-being. During the bleakest years of the epidemic, when therapeutic options seemed so limited, many doctors learned that despite a professional training that emphasized the virtue of clinical distance, they could not shield themselves from the sorrow they came to know in the course of their work.

AIDS = Death

It is not surprising that death would present a special burden to physicians whose medical careers had prepared them mainly for patients who would come to them at moments that were full of promise, rather than on occasions marked by fear or pain. Howard Minkoff said of his years at Kings County, "You have a lot of ghosts in you. You watch a lot of people die. That's unusual for an obstetrician who goes into a field where you expect to almost never see anybody die." For his colleague, pediatrician Hermann Mendez, who had first encountered dying children in his native El Salvador, pediatric AIDS represented a return to something he thought he had left behind. Ruefully called the "Angel of Death" by some with whom he worked, he said,

> I became used to death [at home]—I mean, from the autopsy room to the emergency room where we would receive very, very sick children all the time—very much used to it. . . . I got reeducated in the United States. I came fresh, full of desire to practice differently, with a different population, and I allowed myself to be reeducated, so my losses were hard losses.

For physicians trained in the antibacterial era, a disease that killed almost all who were infected was beyond experience or expectation. The infectious diseases they knew and used as possible analogues of AIDS—hepatitis B, for example—led physicians like Joseph O'Neill to infer initially a significant but still limited fatality rate.

> There was a time we thought only a small percentage of people who were positive went on to have AIDS. We thought that it was like hepatitis, that only a small number of people would go on to be chronic carriers and maybe people would just have this virus.

In the Bronx, Arye Rubinstein convinced himself that his pediatric patients could survive their disease.

> There was a tremendous excitement. The first patients that we had were not so sick. [Early on,] the first patients all survived. So we didn't look at a fatal immune deficiency. This excitement somewhat abated when the first patients were dying. We were very attached to these children and to their mothers, and when the first ones started getting very sick, people got very depressed in my division. We didn't [think this was going to happen] because the kids responded very nicely to gamma globulin, stopped having infections, were growing nicely. And then the first one came up with CNS [central nervous system] symptomatology and became demented. It was a terrible picture.

By 1987, however, in the light of the epidemiological evidence and their own experiences, physicians' expectations had changed. They understood, with chilling clarity, that AIDS was almost uniformly fatal and that they would be escorting almost all their patients to their deaths. Paul Volberding, recalling the stress and grief he experienced at that time, "remember[ed] what it felt like to see a new patient, to see a strapping, attractive young man come in and feeling, shit, this person's dead; I'm looking at a healthy dead person. It's just a matter of time." That somber sense of the inevitability of death echoed in the remarks of John Mazzullo of Boston when he spoke of his own patients in the early 1990s, when the range of therapeutic options had changed the clinical management of AIDS.

> You could do everything right: not smoke, run, go to the gym, eat, take your AZT, ddI or whatever, your acyclovir; go to every doctor's appointment, be a goody two-shoes, and you still die. Everybody knows when they come in here that I'm not going to save them. That's not the point of coming to see Dr. Mazzullo. I am not going to save you. We're going to use every tool that Western and Eastern and God-knows-whatever medicine has; we're going to do it. But you're still going to die.

Revealing a positive HIV-test result to a patient became for many doctors the awful moment when a journey with grimly predictable signposts would begin. A remarkable number of physicians first learned through AIDS how to inform patients of a fatal disease; but some remained at a loss for how to proceed. Wafaa El-Sadr, who had come to America from Egypt, found herself personally and culturally at a loss.

> I have a lot of problems giving people bad news. Although people think I do it well, I don't think so at all. I just hate doing it. I've tried over the years to listen to how people do it, and mimic. It's like medicine; you learn and you mimic. Somebody, teach me how to do it! I was never taught how to do it. [And] people in Egypt, when they are ready to die, people take them home. You never told anyone they were really going to die. That was considered cruel. . . . It was not to be done, another world, and to this day I have a lot of trouble telling people.

In Oakland, Robert Scott, after 15 years as an AIDS treater, still felt that telling a patient of a positive HIV-test result was "the hardest thing I have to do; I almost think it's easier to tell someone they have cancer." James Campbell, an older, experienced gay doctor in San Francisco, acknowledged that the two most depressing moments of his work involved telling a patient that death was imminent and informing someone that he was infected with HIV.

The ordeal of bearing bad news again and again was sometimes too great. Gwendolyn Scott, initially the lone physician in the pediatric AIDS clinic at Jackson Memorial in Miami, found the cumulative stress unbearable, almost forcing her to abandon her position.

It was very, very difficult to deal with all of this information that was so negative and caused so much grief and heartache. I can honestly say that I saw the first hundred patients by myself. There was no one else. And I think that if I hadn't at that point gotten help in the sense of new faculty being added, I don't think I'd be here today. Because I really think there was a point, and it was probably a low point in my career, where I just didn't feel I could tell one more person they had HIV. I've done it so many times; it's so stressful. I had to really convince myself that this was important. I knew it was important. I knew it was something that I had to do, but it was very difficult.

As doctors experienced the escalating toll of deaths in their offices and hospitals, they frequently had difficulty coming to terms with the carnage. One of the rare office-based physicians who kept a careful count of patients who died of AIDS was Ronald Grossman.

Our cumulated total of deaths, in [a] practice in which I rarely took new patients after these early years, was just over 500 cases as of the end of 1994. And the exponential growth [of annual mortality] shows one case and one death in 1982, [then] eight [deaths], 16, 23, and quickly escalated into the 50s; [this] has drifted downward a little bit, as we prolong people's lives; but for any physician of primarily young people, to have ushered 500 to their deaths in a fairly closed practice [is] an extraordinary experience.

Others could only estimate. Joel Weisman in Los Angeles thought he had lost well over a thousand patients to AIDS by 1995, as had Barbara Starrett in Greenwich Village by 1997. Approximately 550 of Eric Goosby's patients were dead by 1996. Anita Vaughn, in Newark, estimated that over 150 of her patients had died in the 18 months between 1994 and 1996.

Some doctors needed to keep count, but most just stopped. To make such body counts was to give their losses an objectivity they could not bear. Janet Mitchell, then a Harlem Hospital obstetrician, had long ceased keeping a quantitative record.

I stopped counting. I couldn't; I couldn't. It's something you don't think about, you know. In the beginning I did, and it was just too depressing. And so you have to have a protective mechanism for your psyche. You don't want to look back and say, "You know, I've taken care of a hundred HIV-infected women and 90 of them are dead." Then you look at yourself and you say, "Why are you doing this?"

Robert Bolan, a gay physician-activist in San Francisco, simply said, "I don't know [how many have died] because I don't want to know. It's just a number. Hundreds and hundreds, maybe even thousands. I don't know."

But if they could not count the dead, doctors in private practice kept stored records, file boxes that, like cardboard memorials, bore the names of the uncounted dead. In 1996, Howard Grossman, a gay physician in Manhattan, pointed to "18 file boxes of old charts, and maybe three of them are of people who left my practice; the rest are people who have died."

With these boxes of the dead, physicians like Stosh Ostrow in Atlanta could recover traces of patients he had lost.

We have boxes and boxes and boxes of deceased files. . . . It's frightening. . . . I've been [treating AIDS] for 12–15 years now. We just went through and pulled things, and I couldn't believe— I keep saying I want to sit down and look at the names of these people, because a lot of them I don't remember.

In storerooms and closets, these boxes, monuments to the magnitude of AIDS deaths, reminded doctors like Lisa Capaldini about what they and their patients had endured as a consequence of the epidemic. "I know I have about 10 legal-sized boxes of charts of people who have died. And every once in a while, when I'm in the back room and see those, it reminds me of what I've been through."

The Hour of Death

Since cure was impossible, death inevitable, many physicians often fell back to demonstrating their prowess by organizing a "good death." They tried to counter the virulence of the disease in its last stages with all the old and newly won knowledge at their disposal. To do so required, first, that the fear and pain of dying be confronted. Ronald Grossman tried to make his patients understand

> that I will 'do everything I can to keep them from suffering. . . . [I want them to know] everybody's really afraid of the process, and that [it's] really important to me that people not have pain and suffer.

But to limit pain and suffering was not to be confused with making death pleasant, said Dan William. Death remained a trial that doctors could only help patients endure.

> [For] the majority of people who are dying, their greatest fears are concrete. I'm cold, I'm wet, I'm incontinent, I'm hungry, I'm in pain, I can't sleep, I'm shaking. It hurts. [You] have the ability to make the transition comfortable. I don't think you can ever make it pleasant.

As patients wasted away, were deformed by KS lesions, became incontinent, demented or blind, physicians did their best to protect the last remnants of their patients' dignity, symbolized for John Mazzullo by the image of a bed with "clean sheets."

> They're going to die of this fucking thing. And they're not going to do it on the subway. They're going to die in a bed with clean sheets. I have this image of how we're going to make this death into a victory. So I try to make the death a victory.

To die with dignity, a patient had to come to terms both with the imminence of death and the stigmatizing cause of the disease. Many of Gerald Friedland's patients in the Bronx had experienced the ravages of drug addiction before they contracted AIDS.

> We would preside over their cruel deaths. And in a stigmatized, unknown disease, it was quite a trip. But I got very good at organizing people's deaths in this very complicated and painful and unknown situation. . . . You've got to get [the] person to be at peace with himself or herself, and deal with issues of blame and guilt and death and dying. I learned to talk to people about it. I learned to use clergy a lot, something I'd never done in my career. And I learned to work with groups.

Dying peacefully was particularly difficult for patients unreconciled to their homosexuality. Donna Futterman, a colleague of Friedland's at Montefiore Medical Center who cared for HIV-infected adolescents, recalled her first AIDS case, a gay man filled with self-loathing. "He was a young Latino gay guy, probably in his early 20s, who just invested so much energy in hating himself for being gay. And he was lying in his hospital bed dying and basically trying to convince himself out of being gay." Guilt-filled patients could also punitively hasten their own deaths. Jerome Groopman described one of his Hasidic patients.

> He was gay, and he felt he needed to punish himself. So he, despite numerous potential interventions that would help him, decided to kill himself basically by allowing things to progress unnecessarily.

Not only did doctors need to ease their patients' suffering, but they also had a critical role to play in helping them and their families understand that further efforts would be futile. It was not a role, Howard Grossman noted, that he embraced easily.

> There's a time when I stop everything. Mutually determined, but it's usually up to me to say, "I think it's time." And people are usually waiting for me to say that. It took me a long time to accept that.

Among the many memories of the years of treating AIDS patients, these were among the most poignant for doctors. Charles van der Horst, a physician whose AIDS clinic in North Carolina treated some of the poorest rural patients in the state, recalled a meeting with a farmer and his wife in which he finally convinced them to let their son die.

> To watch a crusty North Carolina farmer, simple, uneducated, who never expresses emotion—I remember this farmer and his wife— we'd had this long discussion. Their son was now totally gone, demented, bed-ridden, huge terrible ulcers. I said, "We have to stop. We're torturing him now." The mother cried. And I say, "I know you're suffering. I know as a parent there's nothing [worse] than for me to tell a parent that you've got to say good-bye to your child." And so the farmer sits there, that wrinkled, sun-burned redneck face, and a tear sort of drips down his cheek. And that's really difficult.

It was, of course, easier when patients themselves understood that further intervention would be of little value. Stosh Ostrow in Atlanta recalled with admiration the "brilliant death" of his friend Stan who had recognized the need for leave-taking.

I have seen people who have hung on and hung on and hung on and have died miserable, horrible deaths. And I have seen some brilliant deaths. My friend Stan had a brilliant death. . . . He was on disability; he became more and more debilitated. He came to my Christmas party on a Saturday. Sunday he went in the hospital because he was so short of breath. And our commitment was to have him die comfortably. And he didn't want to die before Christmas—his partner was a Christmas freak. He died the day after Christmas. About two hours before he died, he said to his lover, "You know, I forgot to ask Stosh how to let go." And he was gone. He didn't suffer; he didn't hang on.

There was a danger that in such admiration the seeds of a new rigidity about the elements of the "good death" would be found. As with giving birth, Carol Brosgart argued, there were many right ways to die.

It used to drive me crazy when I was in pediatrics, and also when I was going through my own birth classes, about this sort of righteousness of natural childbirth, and that there somehow was only one way to have a baby, and that you'd be a failure, if for some reason or another you ended up having a C section. And there's a little bit of that in HIV too, about the right death, and that if you don't die at home surrounded by the right music and the right incense and the right friends, it's been a bad death. And not everyone can die at home and for some people there really isn't a home. What I want, I think, for all of my patients is to not die alone, to die comfortably without pain, and surrounded by people they love or things they love.

Doctors often sought to connect or reconnect their dying patients with their families. When they succeeded, that could be the occasion for great satisfaction. But such efforts could be trying and profoundly frustrating. Joyce Wallace, whose early AIDS practice was in Greenwich Village, recalled a number of instances when families adamantly refused to be reconciled with their children.

I had a boy, a man, he worked for me; he really wanted to see his father before he died. And the father said he was going on a cruise, and they were coming to New York, and he wouldn't even come to see him. He had to go out to the airport to see them. . . . And then later, when he got sicker, I called his father, and his step-mother got on the phone and she said, "Well, he has AIDS, doesn't he?" as if that took her off the hook, there was no need to visit him. "He has AIDS, doesn't he? He has this disease!" I spoke to one father in Oklahoma whose son said to me wistfully that he wished he could see his family before he died. So I called his father. Maybe it was nervy of me to do that, but I said, "You know, your son would really like to see you, and now is the time to come, because I don't know how long he will be making sense." And his father said to me, "Well, I don't want to show him that I approve of his lifestyle."

At other times, families were present, but blind. Under such circumstances doctors could feel compelled to force them to overcome denial and face the inevitable. Joseph O'Neill, for example, was still a medical student caring for an equally young AIDS patient at San Francisco General Hospital when he had to pull the patient and family sharply toward the realization that the moment of death was near.

He was very sick; he was wasted. He was paraplegic and in just awful pain. He was a gay man living in San Francisco; his parents lived in Florida. They came out in total denial of what was going on. They loved this guy, their son, passionately . . . and all they wanted to do was to fix everything. And they wanted the best doctors, the best that money could buy. "And what does Dr. Volberding say about this?" and "What does Dr. So-and-So . . . ?" I mean very kind of controlling [behavior]. "He wanted chocolate pudding, and they sent peach pudding. I'm going to call the head of the hospital." They were very hard to deal with. And here I am, this medical student, working with a resident who wasn't even paying that much attention to him because he was no longer an interesting case. And the patient was very much the same way, you know, "The room's too bright," "I asked for water, and I didn't get ice in it, and I wanted ice." . . . And meanwhile here's like this skinny dying young man who's worrying about the flavor of his pudding— you know, I mean the whole thing was wrong.

I remember this; this is where I really learned something about doctoring from him. One morning I was just talking with him and sort of listening to him, and he looked at me and said, "Am I going to die?" And I said, "Yes, you are going to die." And he said, "When?" and I said, "Very soon." And he said, "Oh. Do my parents know?" And I said, "I think they do, but have you talked with them about it?" And he said, "No, I couldn't talk with them about it. It's too hard. I couldn't talk about it." And I said, "When your parents get here today, you have the nurse page me, and I'll come." And about an hour later we were rounding, and I got paged by the nurse saying they were there.

I came back down and walked in the room, and they were just doing all this stuff. And the whole time—this had been going on for three weeks—I had never seen one of his parents touch him, lay hands on him. I mean, they did everything but. They were running around fixing the blind, I remember they were fixing the blinds in the room. And I went out and brought in chairs, these folding chairs, and I set up chairs around his bed, and I said, "Stop it." And I mean, there was just me, no nurse, no one else, just me, this little medical student, you know? And I said, "Sit down. We have something very important to discuss here." And so they sat down, and I said, "What we have to discuss is the fact that [your son] is dying." And I said, "I just want you to talk about it. So I'll leave the room if you want, but this is what's happening. There's nothing more we're going to do. Your son is dying, and you really need to spend some time with him."

And I remember his parents, they started crying. And they got up, and they held him, and in three weeks they had never touched him. And I left them, and I said, "You have to say good-bye. It doesn't matter what he's eating. It matters that you spend some time together." And I was on call that night. Maybe two hours after they left, he died.

As the hour of death approached, physicians had to make a critical personal judgment about how close to remain to their dying patients. Some dealt with impending death by retreating. Fred Siegal admitted,

There are certain things in medicine that you sort of have to inure yourself to, and one of them is people dying—I couldn't sit *shiva* over everybody—so you basically do your best and move on. I've really mourned a few patients, but I think that, generally speaking, when I see that somebody's going to die, I manage to withdraw to some extent. That doesn't mean I don't go see them, but I manage to emotionally separate myself from it. I think you have to do that or go nuts.

Others, like John Stansell, whose lover and all of whose old friends had died of AIDS, rejected Siegal's response. He believed it was crucial to draw even closer to patients who lay dying. He had long observed that when faced with life-threatening illnesses like AIDS, doctors showed a deep reluctance to remain engaged; and that, he believed, represented the ultimate failure.

We tend to separate ourselves as death approaches, and nothing could be more inappropriate, because having lived through the process of dying with someone I loved very much, I realized that's the time for the most involvement. It's the most emotionally and professionally taxing time of patient care. . . . All those viral load tests, those CD4 counts, the latest drugs, that really doesn't matter. It's the solace, the comfort that you bring just by being available to your patient, being there, letting them know that you'll go through this process with them. That's what's really important; all the rest is just icing.

To Lisa Capaldini, for whom medicine has involved a spiritual journey, confronting death work resonated with her earliest aspirations.

I think that my spiritual background has really influenced me a lot in ways that I'm sure are largely unconscious. I remember that one of the reasons I wanted to be a nun when I was a girl was that it just seemed to me that a life purely devoted to just being kind to people and prayer—that didn't have an endpoint—it just seemed very process-oriented. And I think that's kind of what my dealing with all the death I deal with is like. I try to be in the process and not view the end of that process as a purely negative thing.

When Capaldini saw patients for what she thought would be the last time, her leave-taking revealed the depths of her attachment. "The last time I see them alive, I will kiss them good-bye. And when I do that, many times tears come to my eyes. I think those tears speak the truth."

For Eric Goosby, the very moment of death produced a strikingly spiritual response.

> At that point you are not just the physician, you are a human being in the presence of another human being who's leaving the corporeal world. I had convinced myself very definitively, very clearly in my mind, that I could feel that person leave their body. If you want to call it a soul or whatever, their life being, that which makes them the personality and the person that I'd been interacting with, is gone. And it is as if someone flipped a switch. You are left with nerves, muscles, arteries, veins, et cetera. It is a body, but they are not there. I can feel them leave, and it is a very moving moment. The last gift that person gives to me is that message, right between the eyes. But I have a very physical reaction to it; I can feel it with my whole body.

The inability to forestall death in their often-young patients forced physicians to confront the question of professional failure. Jerome Groopman ruminated on the impact death had had on him.

> I had seen people die; I had seen young people die; I had seen transplant patients die. It still has an impact on me. The death is sort of yours, in a way. I mean, it's really your patient. [One has] a sense of failure, a sense of guilt, a sense of loss, and a sense of understanding sometimes that there are things in life that you can't control.

Michael Gottlieb's response was shaped by his family history.

> I wasn't in any position to help my father [when he was dying], because I was 16 years old. By the time my brother was ill, I was a doctor; and at some level I felt that despite everything I did for him—getting him to the best people, being involved in his care on a day-to-day basis, albeit from a distance—he was in New Jersey, and I was in Los Angeles—I felt that I hadn't done enough for him. And, of course, AIDS being a disease for which so little was available, I felt that I wasn't doing enough for my patients, and this led to feelings of sadness and inadequacy.

But for doctors to continue in their work, they needed to find ways to react to death that permitted them to view themselves as something other than failures. Sheldon Landesman, who had shielded himself from patient relationships that were too intimate by focusing on the social distance that separated him from the poor minority patients that came to Kings County Hospital, protected himself against a sense of failure by limiting radically his sense of responsibility for the outcomes of his interventions.

> I've always adopted a stance in medicine—and it may be related to my previous work in oncology—that I took neither credit nor blame for what happened to my patients. My job was to do the best I could, and then I'm out of the equation. I don't deserve the excessive credit that patients tend to give you nor the blame occasionally that occurs or that you inflict on yourself when the patients die. I've never viewed myself as fighting against death.

Richard Chaisson was, if anything, more direct: "I don't consider it a defeat when somebody dies. If I did, I'd have surrendered long ago."

Some went even further, seeking to characterize the end of life as a kind of triumph against the suffering that dying with AIDS often entailed. Echoing the words of Constance Wofsy about the journey to death, Marcus Conant, a central figure in the San Francisco AIDS community, came to accept death and then went on to redefine his role in a way that permitted him to preserve a sense of professional efficacy.

> I diagnosed KS [in my psychotherapist] and watched him die. He didn't die; he choked to death on Kaposi's sarcoma in his throat. I mean, a horrible death for a wonderful man. What happens early on is you begin to realize that the enemy can be AIDS, and it can even be the government, but that the patients are going to die and that you must accept that at an intellectual level. And so your role, your challenge, is to bring to the patient the best care that's available. . . . But it must go beyond that, that what your role really is is to make that process as comfortable for them, as exciting for them, as useful for them as it can be, so that when they die you actually feel good about the role you played in their life; that you don't feel you lost; you actually feel you won.

Those who came to accept the inevitability of death viewed with dismay the willingness of some doctors to pursue every last therapeutic option. From the vantage point of his large gay practice in New York's Chelsea section, Howard Grossman had reluctantly come to recognize that it was his responsibility to say to patients, "enough," and to see aggressive and single-minded attempts to prevent death in dying patients as utterly misdirected. When he could save patients from such efforts, he felt he had succeeded as a physician.

> [I] cover for one person who won't let anybody go. When somebody's dying, instead of taking things off and putting them on morphine, his response is to throw 10 new drugs at them, because maybe they'll get saved. They never do. And he won't stop [liquid nutrition,] TPN. And two of his patients, who had been through hell—they must [have been] in the hospital for four months already—died this week when I was on call. And I felt very successful when that happened.

The recognition that nothing could be done to prevent death, the effort to face the limits of medicine stoically, did not always succeed. Something deeply embedded in the socialization of doctors and the devotion of doctors to their patients all contributed to a lingering attachment to a curative role; and it was that out-of-reach goal that haunted even those who spoke with apparent serenity about the "exciting and meaningful journey." Even those doctors who sought to teach their colleagues about the futility of self-recrimination found themselves beset by doubts. Gerald Friedland, who could speak and write so movingly about the redefined role of the doctor caring for dying AIDS patients, had to admit that a sense of failure remained a specter for him.

> I think we all have these feelings, that if only I had done this, if only I had done that, maybe he wouldn't have died. And I know it's not true, but there is this sort of fantasy belief that we have the ability to stave off the Grim Reaper. It's part of why many people go into medicine. You can't not feel a little bit like a failure. It's very humbling. . . . I preach that we shouldn't feel that way, but we do.

Hospice and Its Limits

With nothing available in the epidemic's early years to delay death and with so many AIDS physicians coming to recognize the futility of aggressive interventions that did little but prolong suffering, it is not surprising that hospice care—first developed for cancer patients in the terminal stages of their illness—seemed attractive. And patients who were willing to forgo curative interventions did indeed benefit from an approach to care that stressed the management of pain and suffering, the involvement of family and loved ones, and the acceptance of death.

But the story was not always so straightforward. It was not simply that for many young patients and their caregivers giving up on the struggle for life was difficult; it was that many patients, while accepting the inevitability of death, were reluctant to give up clinical interventions that could improve the quality of their remaining months. John Mazzullo in Boston was pressed to employ the less costly hospice option for his patients by the guardians of the fiscal integrity of the health plans within which he worked. His response captured not only the limits of hospice care for AIDS patients but the way in which clinical choices and financial considerations could play themselves out in an era of managed care.

One of the vice presidents of [a managed care plan] came to discuss the use of hospice in my AIDS practice. We had used hospice very liberally in the late '80s/early '90s, but something changed it, and that was IV gancyclovir and foscarnet [two new antivirals]. And who is going to stop foscarnet or gancyclovir and go traipsing to live in a hospice with the fear that the very next moment [they] might not be able to see? So people die at home or in the hospital under intravenous therapy. And this is hard for the HMOs, because the hospice benefit is $75 a day; intravenous gancyclovir is $64,000 a year. So they have a big problem, that patients don't want to die blind. And [they would ask,] "What is it, John, in your practice? Is it you or your patients that are not doing hospice?" I say, "Probably a little of both." They didn't like that answer. "Well, your style— we have to look at your style."

The viability of the hospice option for AIDS patients was further compromised by the social-class background of many of those who were dying. Gerald Friedland's experience in the Bronx underscored the issues that would become more pertinent as increasing numbers of drug users were diagnosed with AIDS.

We had a wonderful person who joined our AIDS team. Wilma was an oncologist who had decided that chemotherapy, and all that, basically sucked, and that she was torturing all her cancer patients. And she became a director of a hospice at Beth Abraham. . . . Wilma was a big, tough woman who had a reputation of being a sort of staff sergeant type, a heart of gold. And she started coming to our AIDS rounds. And so I said, "Wilma, what's an AIDS patient going to do in your hospice?" She said, "Well, hospice is about dying. These are dying patients. We're going to take AIDS patients." . . . Wilma then started taking our AIDS patients; and we'd bring them to hospice, and they would die in hospice. And it was like they were dying in heaven, it was so beautiful. They were treated so wonderfully, and the families were so appreciative. But we always got them there too late—it's very hard with AIDS to know when to stop, because they're young people, because oftentimes they have things that you can still treat. . . . But it was easy when they became demented, and in those days a lot of patients became demented.

But it had to close. Do you know why? It turns out that the hospices are a middle-class construct for old people dying of cancer. We had drug users in the Bronx dying of AIDS. The reimbursement mechanism for hospice required that 85 percent of hospice care be in the home and 15 percent in inpatient facility. And it turned out that with the AIDS patients 85 percent were in the inpatient facility and 15 percent were at home. And why is that? No home! Drug use, afraid to give pain medicines because they're already drug using in the house, dangerous neighborhoods. All sorts of nurses wouldn't go into them. No care provider, no care partner for outpatients. They couldn't afford it, given the reimbursement. They wound up going out of business.

Even the inpatient aspects of hospice for AIDS patients presented difficulties that its advocates did not anticipate. In Jamaica Plains, Boston, Elizabeth Kass became the medical director of the first Medicaid-Medicare certified hospice designed for dying AIDS patients. There were the inevitable tensions about what kind of care was appropriate in a hospice; but more telling were the tensions between the embracing vision of those who sought to comfort people dying of AIDS and the men and women who came to the hospice.

Someone who's been living on the street, a sort of hard-bitten drug addict who's learned to lie, cheat, and steal to stay alive and function, isn't into a beautiful death. They're not into a beautiful death at all. The original people who envisioned this thing wanted lots of acupuncture and massage and meditation and all this; well, that didn't wash very well with some of the shelter people. I still remember the guy who cooks there, a fabulous cook; [he] had been a gourmet cook, did these wonderful, wonderful menus. The staff loved him. And some of the patients loved him. And then you'd get these people who'd say, "What's the matter with this guy? We have to order out because he can't cook a fuckin' burger. What's this peach soup?" . . . Some of the people who initially came with the sort of missionary zeal about bringing beautiful death to people couldn't deal with the nonbeautiful people. And the internal politics were continual. There were a lot of people with a very idealized vision of what a place would look like for HIV-infected-patients, gay men, well-off HIV infected patients, not homeless, ungrateful drug users.

Elizabeth Kass remained with the hospice for about five years—until 1995—but then resigned. A staff that included workers who were hostile to drug users and resentful of patients with behavioral problems, and an agency that could not confront the problems posed for hospice by a changing population with end-stage HIV disease, made the work to which she had committed herself unfulfilling.

Grieving

In ways that seem out of keeping with the clinical posture of contemporary medicine, many AIDS doctors experienced a level of grief and sorrow that made plain the extent to which they had been touched by the plight of their patients. While Fred Siegal, who for years had to bear the burden of providing support to his ailing wife, could say, "There's nothing that mitigates watching young people die except the realization that there's not a goddamn thing you can do about it," others could recall the tears that at least the first patients' deaths caused. Although in 1995 the pain was no longer so overwhelming for Jerry Cade, eight years earlier the story had been very different.

When the second patient died, I took off for two days. He was 23, I remember, and I just called my partner and said, "I think this is more than I can deal with." After that [I] reluctantly came back. I avoided oncology in med school because I didn't want to deal with dying patients. I mean, it's kind of a cosmic joke, I think.

After that he cried "lots and lots," but privately. "In Texas [where I was born], you don't do that in public." It was easier for women to cry in public. Carol Brosgart had indelible memories of "blubbering" with her colleagues.

However affected, some believed that their professional authority demanded a public stoicism and so had to grieve behind closed doors. Alvin Friedman-Kien recalled,

> One learns to maintain a facade, to maintain a certain kind of distraction from it. . . . My patients, I don't think, really think of me as being a warm, feely person because I've developed a facade of being very clinical and a scientist. What my inner feelings are is quite different, and I'm very much affected by it. A patient who I'd been following for 16 years died two days ago. My family and my friends and everyone recognized how depressed I was. I didn't tell them what it was. They just knew.

But even for some of the most committed there was a recognition that, however painful the loss of a patient was, it was not like the sorrow that accompanied the death of a family member or close friend. Leonard Calabrese, whose patients were drawn from ballet dancers in Cleveland as well as the most impoverished residents of that city, noted:

> It's not grief—that black despair when you lose something yourself. It's different from that. It's in a different layer. It's grief, but it's kind of something that—I don't know how to describe it—it's not like when you lose a family member or somebody that's really close, that's always been a part of your life. It's just like something that's so black that you think it's never going to go away. It's not like that anymore. It's like somebody hits me in the stomach, but I'm ready for it, like "go ahead, hit me." I know it's coming, but it's just like over and over. So it's really different. I go out of my way now not to become overly involved.

Gerald Friedland's experience treating a colleague and friend helped him to confront and deal with matters unresolved since the death of his father years earlier.

> You know . . . whenever someone dies—it's you who's dying at some level. . . . When someone's really close to you in a way that's different from a professional relationship where you're trained to have distance, then that death is closer. So I felt it more closely on

one level. [He was a physician, and his] death helped me resolve the issue of my father's death—not cure it, not cure it, but he helped me. I was able to arrange with him his death in a way that made me feel that I had really helped him die, and helped his family. And I've done that with many other people, but this was so close to me, and his children, and I felt like a good boy. I felt relieved; I felt I had learned to do it right, maybe.

For gay physicians, grief over lovers and friends not infrequently shaped the ways in which they experienced the deaths of patients; the deaths of their patients made unmistakably clear what the fate of their infected lovers and friends would be. John Stansell, who began his professional life as a nurse in Washington, D.C., before going on to head the inservice AIDS unit at San Francisco General Hospital as a physician recalled:

About 1983 my best friend became ill. . . . He was probably the first person I knew close to me who died of HIV. Virtually my entire circle of friends from Washington, D.C., has died. . . . There were about, I don't know, 16 of us that were very close. I'm the only one living at this point, the only one. It's very lonely at times. . . . The hole is always there, no matter what you do. There's no becoming accustomed to the idea. It doesn't happen.

A number of gay doctors sought to deal with their grief in ways that they would ultimately be compelled to see as self-destructive. Robert Bolan threw himself into an exercise regime that was punishing and that led him to ignore the signs that his own health was in danger. On a furious bicycle ride he began to experience signs of a hypertensive stroke.

I was so fucking stupid that when I had this flash of numbness that occurred on the left side of my face and the sharp pain in my neck I thought, Oh what the hell is that? My neck got a pinched nerve or something? Knowing full well that anything that causes numbness on the face is certainly well above any pinched nerve that can occur in your neck. It's brain stem, stupid. Stop the fucking bike! But I didn't stop the bike. I just kept on going—until I got off the bike path and started to climb the next hill, and I started feeling light-headed, and I thought, Robert, you'd better slow down. Robert, you'd better get off the bike. Robert, you'd better lay down. And then when I tried to stand up, I couldn't.

Only when he sought psychiatric help, was diagnosed with depression, and began treatment did he come to understand the degree to which grief had permeated his life. He suddenly noticed he had stopped whistling in 1985. "And the reason that I knew that is that probably four or five months into my antidepressant medication I was walking down the street, and I started to whistle!"

More commonly, efforts were made to bury the grief so that the intensity of professional commitments would not be disturbed. But the feelings stirred by the deaths of friends and patients could break through in a torrent of unexpected tears. While at a social event in San Francisco, Marcus Conant "just lost it."

> I started sobbing to the point that [my host] had to get me up and walk me out. And I look back on this, and it's almost like it didn't happen. I must have cried for two or three hours, just uncontrollable sobbing. And I was horribly embarrassed, you know; it's something a good Southern boy doesn't do, and certainly not a doctor. And that was the first time I realized you can't just keep storing it up inside and expecting that it will never come bubbling up. As a physician you cannot grieve as others in society grieve because you have to walk out of that room where this patient just died and deal with the patient in the next room. And you can't walk out crying and say, "Oh, by the way, I can't really function right now because someone just died."

For Joseph O'Neill, such tears came in 1994, more than a decade after he had first cared for AIDS patients as a medical student.

> A year ago my lover and I went on vacation to Australia for the gay Mardi Gras, which is a wonderful event. We walked out of the Sydney Opera House and I was talking with him and saying, "God, it's really great, it's wonderful to be [here]," and I really was thinking I was feeling fine. And I started crying, and I could not stop for a long time. And I sat on a curb and just sobbed, and all I could see were the faces of patients and friends, just hundreds, all of this death and suffering. And it was sort of like vomiting; and after I was done I actually felt better, and I felt better in a way that I hadn't felt in memory. I realized I had been carrying this—and do carry this—around, as a physician, as a gay man. When I started medicine, this thing all started, this death and AIDS and young people dying and suffering and Kaposi's and *Pneumocystis* and persistent

diarrhea and chronic neuropathy. And that is as much integrated into who I am now as being a doctor is. I'm not the same person I was 20 years ago; this has sort of permanently changed me.

It was not only gay physicians who could experience this level of grief. For Peter Selwyn, then at Montefiore Hospital in the Bronx, the occasion was in 1987, relatively early in the epidemic, and for him it opened a path for the exploration of a loss long buried in the depths of his soul, the suicide of his father when he was a baby.

I went to a concert at St. John the Divine in New York and was leaving the church after the concert. And they had a little display on the side of [the nave]. . . . There was no statue, just a sign on the wall that said, "In memory of those who have died of AIDS," and in front were all these candles that were lit. And I walked by, and I just stopped, and it kind of just grabbed me. And I looked at it, and I just kept staring at it, and I just started crying and realizing that I had never experienced the sort of grief for the death of all of these patients that I'd had. And I remember feeling as if I could almost see people's faces through the candles in a sort of symbolic way. And it suddenly felt like both—there was this incredible weight that I felt and also like something had been lifted at the same time. At that moment really, I realized that there was something about death and dying and grieving that was very important that I hadn't really dealt with before. And what came back to and what had unconsciously led me to that point was that my own father had died when I was a baby, when I was a year-and-a-half old. What became clear at that point was that I'd never really either experienced or grieved the loss of my father, that it was something I hadn't done; and the reason for that was that he died under very unusual circumstances. . . . And during that process I became much more aware of ways in which I could empathically be with patients and connect with them without feeling obsessive, like I had to rescue them—in fact, I couldn't—the best way to be a care provider is where you don't invest your ego in what's going to happen, even though you do everything you can to have a good outcome.

In their professional universe, within which tears and sorrow and expressions of devastation were not uncommon, some AIDS doctors questioned the depths of their own commitment because their responses were so much more restrained. Having become an advocate for prisoners with

AIDS at the start of her career in Albany, New York, and later having organized AIDS services in New York City, Victoria Sharp knew that she was devoted to AIDS patients but wondered why she did not experience death in the way she believed others did.

> I've always been able to be emotionally close to patients and yet not become devastated when they die. I don't know where that comes from. I mean, actually, I've thought of it as a weakness because I've thought, Well, maybe you're not that close if you're not devastated by their death.

Aid in Dying

The sheer suffering, the disfigurement, the loss of independence, and the wasting experienced by many AIDS patients as they approached death inevitably led many to explore the question of how they might assert a modicum of control over the way their lives would end.[3] And when they began to consider these painful questions, they inevitably turned to their doctors. Would their physicians provide direction and some form of assistance if suicide seemed the only course left? Among doctors, these questions would pose challenges that were at once psychologically wrenching and morally troubling, compelling them to confront their willingness to violate the established canons of professional conduct and the criminal law if need be.

For many doctors looking back on years of experience, what was striking was not that some patients would broach the question of physician-assisted suicide but how few actually did in a way that truly represented a request for aid in dying. Elizabeth Kass was asked by some patients, but "shockingly few, though. You'd think I'd have a lot—I don't. I think it takes a lot of guts to kill yourself actually. And it's hard. A lot of people talk about wanting to, but when push comes to shove, I don't think too many people could do it." However, Carol Brosgart asserted, it was not lack of guts but rather the desperate desire of the dying to hold on to the lingering moments.

> I've had some patients who have taken their lives, but most people really elect not to do that. And the reality is, I think most people cling tenaciously to life and want just another tomorrow and find beauty and enjoyment in an even more limited life. I think Paul Monette's book *An AIDS Memoir* is very beautiful in that way. There's one description in there where he talks about how he and

his lover went from being so [socially involved] till a good day became getting out onto the deck. One's life can change, but one can still get pleasures out of a more limited life.

Constance Wofsy suspected that her own obtuseness may have made it difficult for her to recognize her patients' tentative efforts to explore the issue of suicide, even as her colleague Donald Abrams was beginning to describe such requests as not infrequent.

I think that in retrospect people probably did indirectly approach it, and I didn't pick up the clue or the key. And it wasn't pursued. I have had people who have sniffed around at it. In the few instances I can think of that were fairly direct, it was a cry of disheartenment and not an issue that related to the stage of disease. I don't know. Somehow I have the subtle impression that I can't substantiate that there is more asking amongst gay men, and that some of the providers who at a personal level as well as a professional level are very, very, very connected to the gay community, give and read the signals about this more strongly than other providers or patients from other populations.

Indeed, many had the impression that requests for serious explorations of the possibility of physician-assisted suicide were more common among middle-class, gay men than among others. "It's really extraordinary to talk to mothers with AIDS," said Deborah Cotton.

It's very hard to get them to focus on themselves. It's all about the kids, especially if some of them are infected. But also [it's] just about staying alive for them. One of my friends pointed out to me, he said, "Have you ever had a woman ask about assisted suicide?" And I realized never. My problem has been getting women to tell their kids that they're dying. They just hold out every hope, and they ask you to do everything. Not because they have some false sense that I can make them live forever, but if they have a four-year-old they think it would be better if they could live until she's five, and if they have a six-year-old till she's seven. They just want to stay alive for another year, because it does make a tremendous difference in a child's life.

But whether very rare or relatively more frequent, the requests for assisted suicide, when they did come, pushed doctors to consider the way in which their own moral world view should shape their professional work. Raised as a Catholic and deeply concerned with the ethical dimensions of her work as a doctor, Lisa Capaldini struggled, in her Castro district office, to understand the meaning of her patients' requests and the limits of her duty to respect their claims on her.

I realized early on, through my patients teaching me, that one of their biggest fears in being HIV positive or having early AIDS was going through the same sort of dying process that they saw their friends or lover or neighbor go through, and that for many of these people—at that time they were mostly guys—it felt tremendously reassuring to know that they had the option of ending their life when and if their quality of life was unacceptable to them. Many of them never actually planned to use whatever route they had at hand, but it was enormously comforting to know it was there. It's a little bit like the psychological pain experiments where if you tell someone, "You can stop whatever is giving you the pain on a second's notice," the people who have that option can tolerate a lot more painful stimuli than people who don't feel the sense of control.

I also remember feeling very ambivalent about it. From just a medical point of view people with AIDS can get delirious or depressed, either of which could influence a person's ability to make a sensible judgment. So I didn't want a patient who was relatively well, in the midst of a delirium, to say, "That's it."

The other issue was, of course, that it was illegal and, beyond being illegal was, within my profession, by most experts, considered a violation of not only the Hippocratic Oath that I took, but just the whole basic principle of respect for life. . . . I was very honest with [my patients], because I felt they were honest with me about [ending their lives]. I made it clear that if they were ever thinking about using what I provided them with, that they had to call me at least three days beforehand so I would have the chance to see them and verify that they weren't saying, "Oh, I have a hangnail. That's it." And I said, "I get veto power in this, and if I have any concern about it I'm going to take it away." And what was interesting to me was my patients appreciated that—that I was sort of a failsafe measure.

Like Capaldini, Molly Cooke framed her struggle with this issue in terms of her ethical responsibilities as a physician and her professional obligations to her patients, as well as against a backdrop of a growing right-to-die movement. Reluctant, beset with doubts, she was in the end compelled to acknowledge that there were some patients for whom suicide was right and for whom that meant that she had to provide some help. In speaking with her patients at San Francisco General Hospital, she said:

> During the course of this illness you will have many times when you're discouraged, many times when you're uncomfortable, many times when you're in pain. And my job is to encourage you and to treat discouragement and depression if there's a treatable problem there, to manage symptoms, and to help you live for as long as you want me to do that. And when it's not time to do that anymore, then I will certainly stop things that are keeping you alive and let you die, and help you be as comfortable as possible. But my job is not to make you die." I don't think that it's what doctors ought to be doing, and I certainly don't think it ought to be medicalized and routinized.
>
> And I think you really deform medicine and the best content of the relationship between the doctor and the sick person by medicalizing this, by normalizing it, and by setting up these ridiculous procedural safeguards that the lawyers always talk about very blithely. Two doctors certifying, psychiatric consultation—all this stuff is totally beside the point. It's totally beside the point. The point is someone who's suffering, and it doesn't really matter whether their prognosis is six weeks or six months or nine months. The problem is their suffering and the way they understand their suffering, and where they look for help. And that's the problem for the doctor; and in a strange way it's kind of a paradox at the heart of medicine. We're not, in secular American medicine, trained to deal with suffering; and that's what really bothers people in the end.
>
> My experience with the vast majority of my patients is that if you're willing to sit there and listen to them tell you how they're suffering and how they're struggling to understand why this has happened to them, that's what people mostly want. If I encounter somebody for whom in the end, after I've listened for everything, suffering is meaningless, a meaningless humiliation, and it's just pure badness, I will help that person.

Donald Abrams was less beset by doubts. For him, assisted suicide was neither a perversion nor a distortion of the physician's role. Rather, it entailed a very special duty under extraordinary circumstances.

If you accept that death is part of life, and that as a physician one of your responsibilities is to help people with that transition or make that transition as comfortable and as meaningful for the person as possible, and if you know that people are truly suffering and in pain and that that's not where they want to be, then it's not that difficult.

Concern about the suffering of patients did not always—even in the most committed of physicians—lead to a willingness to provide assistance in dying. "I really do believe," said Harry Hollander,

that one of the greatest goals of doing this sort of work is that when it is apparent that somebody is going to die to give them the best sort of death possible. And I think that there is enough leeway within acceptable medical practice and legal/medical practice that that can virtually always be done. So I transmit to people my belief that I will be able to make them comfortable, that I will be able to take care of their symptoms because in the vast, vast majority of people I have been able to do so. The only symptom that I have been frustrated to the bitter end with in a handful of people is not pain but nausea. I have come to the point where I've not been able to help somebody who constantly feels miserable and nauseated. And those have been the few individuals where I have not kept my promise.

Nevertheless, he would "not write an excessive prescription for the purpose of a sedative overdose for that explicit purpose."

Although she endorsed the right to end one's life as much as she supported the right to abortion as a matter of privacy, Carol Brosgart was troubled by the impact of suicide on those who would be left to mourn.

Sometimes checking out of life, just turning out the light, ends up being very difficult for friends and family; it's a bit of a process. And [I] compare it a little bit to birth—that there's something that everybody can gain laboring through death, provided that it's comfortable.

Working primarily with poor African-American and Latino patients in New York, many of whom were drug users, Abigail Zuger had never encountered an explicit request for assisted suicide. But if she should, she said, "I don't think I would cooperate, because I don't really approve of that kind of coping. I think people can be made comfortable enough that they don't have to do drastic things."

For Renslow Sherer, the concern was of a different sort. Caring for impoverished patients at Chicago's Cook County Hospital, where he had encountered so much reluctance to expend resources on those with AIDS, he was fearful that physician-assisted suicide would undermine whatever commitment there was. "I think that [it] can induce a culture of acceptance that's not healthy for a physician and a patient. So it's a pretty fine line."

Because of the legal context within which the issue of assisted suicide took shape and the social ambiguities within which it was embedded, many doctors felt utterly alone as they confronted choices they could not avoid. Some, like Robert Bolan in San Francisco, lashed out at the way the need for secrecy seemed to cripple doctors who had come to believe that they had a duty to help their patients die.

Do you think that there's a body of literature out there that really tells us exactly what to do under all circumstances? Of course not. There is no body of literature because of all these [legal and social constraints]. In this most important area I am extremely ignorant. This is the most important part of this disease, for Christ's sake! This is the culmination; this is when things get chaotic and scary and painful, and some people say, "I've had enough. I want out of here."

An unexpected response from an audience of health care providers greeted John Stansell as he confronted the burden of silence.

I was the last speaker on the last day, so everyone was absolutely exhausted. I thought, Oh, God, this is a throwaway. I'll be lucky not to be crucified. So I presented this, and at the end presented my views of orchestrating the good death, you know, working up through hospice care and everything but then presenting this phi-losophy of the appropriateness of aid in dying in that small per-centage of the population who have unbearable [pain] at the end of life, allowing them control over their means of exit. And I didn't know how it would come across; and I presented it, and the au-dience was just absolutely quiet, just unbelievably quiet, and that's hard to do for a thousand people. And I finished the talk, and the place erupted, absolutely erupted. I got a standing ovation! Actually

I left the podium and was called back to the podium. I was absolutely stunned by this. I had no idea that people would respond in such a positive manner. But then I subsequently realized no one had talked about this in the past. This was something that went on all the time, but no one was willing to discuss it.

But that was not always the way in which advocates of physician-assisted suicide were received. Howard Grossman, who had come to believe that he had a duty to help his suffering patients end their lives and who had joined a class action suit in New York that sought to assert a constitutional right to physician-assisted suicide, was outraged by an opponent who embodied, for him, the moralistic refusal to recognize the most elemental needs of patients who could no longer be helped.

I did something at the New York County Lawyers Society that was just awful. I mean, we did fine, and the audience was clearly on our side, but there was this woman from Sloan-Kettering who's just the worst; she was such a pig. She runs their pain control center, and she was a doctor. At one point we were really getting into it, and I was pushing her a bit, but she was so condescending. I spoke before she did, and I talked about this patient, and I talked about patients of mine who have suffered and patients who were clearly rational in their decisions to commit suicide, or to end it. She was a total bitch! She actually sat there and said, "Well, I just don't understand why doctors have to do that. Why can't a patient just go into the garage, turn on their car and put the hose in their mouth?" And I'm like, "What? Why don't we just have them put their heads in the oven?" I said, "That's really beautiful, thank you." And she clearly came out of a very Catholic background. She made references to that all the time. She, with her nurse practitioner, clearly had religious objections that they were voicing. It was so scary to listen to them talk—and yet they would be very convincing to a wide range of people. They made it out that nobody could ever do this safely or in any way that was compassionate or legal or anything else.

Even among those committed to the idea of physician-assisted suicide there was sometimes a reluctance to smooth the path by writing prescriptions for drugs that could be used when their patients were ready. Peter Seitzman, a gay physician in New York, was concerned that patients were sometimes afraid to raise the issue themselves and so would actually broach the subject himself. Nevertheless, his own experience made him cautious.

> I had one episode where, early on, in the early '80s, somebody wanted to commit suicide. And I gave him a prescription after we talked about it. And he took not enough to kill himself and then decided that he didn't really want to kill himself in the first place. And I said, Oh, my God, I almost helped this person kill himself who really didn't want to. And I didn't really think it through enough. So, since then, I talk about it with people, and I tell them that I can perfectly understand that they would want to, and I want to help them if I think it's reasonable. . . . But even then I tell them that most people are ambivalent, and I don't want to be the one that's instrumental in pushing them into committing suicide. So I want them to demonstrate their commitment to it. I say, "There are ways you can find out what you need to take. There are friends who can help you get drugs if you want. You have to demonstrate to me that you are really committed to doing it. And if I think that you really are, and you tell me what you're going to do, and if you're going to do it the wrong way, then I'll tell you. And if you really can't get what you need, and I think that you've demonstrated that you're committed, then I'll help you with that too. But I won't just write a prescription for future use."

Others, however, had few such concerns. In recalling those they helped to die, they evidenced little discomfort and focused on how they had sought to protect themselves in the face of the threat of possible prosecution. Jerry Cade was dismissive of the idea that others did not share his convictions.

> I don't know very many physicians who don't [receive requests for aid in dying], and we all have pretty standard protocols. Certainly all the physicians I deal with say, "This is up to you." We write a prescription for a barbiturate, encourage our patients to take our names and labels off of it, and leave the power of that choice in the patients' hands—which is what I think doctors should be doing. It's totally absurd that our patients should not have control over the end of their lives. I've done it. Every physician I know has done it. And I'll continue to do it. And what happens, I would say, for every 10 prescriptions of Nembutal that I write, probably only one

or two patients actually end up taking it. Most of it's just an incredible need to know that I've still got some semblance of control." It's just totally ludicrous that any state or federal law would take that control away from somebody who's dying.

Robert Scott, an African-American Oakland-based physician, spoke of his willingness to share the final moments of his patients who chose to die. He would sit with them as they took their lethal medications, "sipping wine" as they fell asleep. Of attending the death of a close friend, he said:

> I remember the evening very well. At his home, we got enough Demerol and Seconal together with alcohol. And you just fall asleep—you don't wake up. It's very simple, just very simple.

Much rarer than either prescribing sedatives or the termination of life supports was the willingness to cross the boundary into active euthanasia, a step with more serious legal and moral implications and one that even the most committed advocates of physician-assisted suicide typically refused to take. Barbara Starrett, who was willing to do almost anything for the patients in her Greenwich Village practice, would not start a morphine drip with a dose designed to end life. Open to taking great risks, she was not willing to take a step that she believed required a definitive act on the part of the patient who wanted to die.

> I had one patient who wanted to die, and he was on a morphine pump. And I showed him how to use the pump and showed him what he could do. And he couldn't do it; he wanted his lover to do it. His lover said, "I'm not doing it." He'd say, "I don't want to live any longer." And I said, "Well, you're strong enough to do it yourself." And maybe in that sense I was like, I don't know, moralistic or judgmental or cruel, but to me, I didn't think it was essential for his lover to do something he didn't want to do. And I wasn't going to do it, because I felt the patient, if he really wanted to do it, would do it on his own.

One physician was able to describe having chosen to give force to moral convictions that few within medicine would publicly embrace. But even he felt compelled to seek the protective cover of anonymity in describing his effort.

I actually helped a patient die at home who was too ill to take medicines orally. And in his case he had horrible diarrhea and vomiting and had gotten sick very quickly over about a month, which was great because he was able to live a pretty functional life until then. And he and I had talked about this very early on when he started to get sick, and he was very clear that he did not want to be in bed soiling himself for the rest of his life. . . . He was getting IV treatment already, so he had an IV access in place. His sister came to town, and he felt comfortable disclosing our plan to her. And I came out, and a colleague of mine, a dear friend as well as a nurse, helped me administer a combination of phenobarbital and versad to him, followed by a big bolus of potassium, which, after he was asleep, stopped his heart. . . . He was in his beautiful bedroom; his cat was on his bed in the cradle of his arm. His sister was on one side of him; I was on the other. And I remember, when we were getting ready to start infusing, I said, "Would you like to open the line or would you like me to?" And he said, "Oh, I'd like you to." And I said, "You know, there's something missing. I want to put some music on for you. What would you like?" He was a real big opera fan, and I put on the trio from *Cosi Fan Tutte*, where Dorabella and Fiordiligi [are] saying good-bye to their two boyfriends who are going off to war. And the music has a sense of flow, imitating the water the boat's on. And they're singing about a safe journey. And I thought, I hope this experience is like that for him. I hope he feels safe. He's surrounded by three people who really love him, and we're going to do this as comfortably as possible. And it was a time when I really switched from having predominantly heebee-jeebees but wanting to do it because my patients wanted it, to feeling very deep in my heart and soul that these moments with my patients were very sacred moments. It was a very sacred moment and a great privilege to be with him when he died.

However much he believed that his act represented an expression of the doctor's duty to his suffering patients, he knew, too, that the political and legal context of his actions demanded great care.

I'm always fearful of the law, but the idea is if you do this correctly, meaning technically and procedurally, you won't get caught. We don't leave anything around that would be a clue that some medicines were administered that weren't indicated. You are careful about who knows that this was done or is happening. And, frankly, in this city, the coroner's office does not actively investigate deaths at home, in the sense that most people with AIDS who die at home—a good proportion of them, I imagine—do in fact die of so-called natural causes. It's well known—here at least—that many of us are helping our patients die, and if the coroner's office wanted to put an end to this, or try to at least, they could be pursuing these cases more. I'm very grateful that they're not.

Last Rites

Physicians inevitably had to face the question of how to bring some closure to the often intense clinical relationships that developed as they cared for their dying patients. Confronted with fear and overt discrimination in the epidemic's early years, doctors had to search for those who would bury their patients. As Gerald Friedland recalled, "You couldn't get people to bury people with AIDS." But beyond such organizational tasks, many emotionally and psychologically taxing, were the funerals themselves. Carol Brosgart, like many others, believed that she owed it to her patients and their families to make the final gesture of respect.

I have AIDS physician friends who have a policy, "I never go to funerals," and they somehow carry that like a mantra, like that's really crossing the line. I've gone to a lot of patient funerals. We have a couple of deaths a week. I can't go to everybody's—I mean I have to work! And you have a life, and sometimes you're out of town, and sometimes they're local, and sometimes they're far away. And you feel differently about different people. Sometimes I've gone to the funeral just out of tremendous love and respect for the person—they meant so much to me. I often find that when I've decided to go to a funeral, it's because of the family or the lover, the people that are still living.

Joseph O'Neill didn't go to many funerals. But those he did attend stayed with him.

One was for a Jewish, gay man I took care of. I took care of him probably five years. When he came to see me he had 16 T-cells. And he did so well for so long. I really liked him a lot. Just a sweet guy, got to know his family when he got sicker and sicker and sicker. And I really felt like I had to go to his funeral. I was a pallbearer. That was tough, carrying the body of a patient that I'd cared for. There's an intimacy that you have as a physician with a patient's body that's unlike any other; and it was so powerful to carry that coffin; and then to throw the dirt on the grave of that person—it was a Jewish ceremony—that I had cared for in every way for so long was very, very hard. It was really a powerful experience.

Different in scale but equally moving for O'Neill was the funeral of a gay African-American for whom he had cared, an event that revealed the public persona of the man he had come to know intimately as a physician.

He was the choir director of the largest Black Baptist church in town, so a very prominent person in the Black community. His family asked me to speak at his funeral . . . and, I mean, you couldn't get within six blocks of the church. It was just people pouring in and out. And this guy, I mean he was such an honorable person, very, very spiritual. He really had a peace about him and had accepted this in his life, and that God was calling him home. And he really had a clarity and a vision and a peacefulness about him that I really admired. But he never told his family until the very end that he was gay and that he had AIDS, and he'd never told his church. I didn't know the Black community part of him; I didn't know what the church [was for him]. But what none of those people knew was this part that I knew, about his struggles with his sexual identity and his love for men that he couldn't tell his family and his sisters and the church, the whole sort of homophobia that was going on in his community.

In some instances, attending funerals could require overcoming religious impediments. For Arye Rubinstein, it was his Orthodox Jewish faith that posed a barrier.

I had in the beginning a lot of reservations—you can see that I wear a *yarmulke*—of going to wakes, for example, which is a no-no for us. I had mixed feelings going to those events. On one hand, we didn't want to participate in such an event out of religious reasons. On the other hand, we were very close to the patients. But with these mixed feelings in the beginning, we went to all of these funerals to support the families. In fact, the social worker we have is also an Orthodox lady, Anita. Despite advice from her rabbi, she would go to the funerals.

For James Oleske it was the fear of entering an all-Black setting that had to be confronted.

I was scared at the first few funerals—remember these were mostly Black, inner city poor people. And I remember one of the first funerals I went to. . . . It was a crowded church, and one of the aunts, who had never come to see Cynthia when she was in the hospital, she got up screaming and saying, "The doctors killed Cynthia, the doctors killed Cynthia." Of course, I'm the only white person in the building, and of course I have, unfortunately, this premature white hair that stands out like a sore thumb. . . . But I have to say, after I went through them and got over that first nervousness, it gave me some relief too. I mean it was mutual, and I didn't feel like I was a burden on the family [by] going.

But even for Oleske, attending funerals was more common in the early years of the epidemic, when the numbers were smaller.

In the beginning I went to almost every funeral. I can't keep doing that now. I mean, we had 34 kids dying last week. What would you say if I told you that a terrorist came in, took over a classroom of children. Only it wasn't a terrorist, it was a disease. It was 34 kids in our program dying.

It was not, however, the sheer burden of busy schedules that provided the justification for staying away. Anita Vaughn, whose AIDS cases, like Oleske's, were drawn from poor African-Americans in Newark, simply asserted, "I don't do funerals." Jerry Cade felt he no longer needed the sense of finality that a funeral could provide.

I went to the first two or three. For some reason, for me it was important to be there the first two or three times, probably to assuage my cosmic guilt for not having kept somebody alive. . . . It's not a closure I need anymore. I needed it at first personally, and I need it with my friends, but with my patients I'm usually pretty comfortable that we've done all we can. And so when they die— and most patients die in the hospital—that's usually okay now.

For Marcus Conant, who presided over a huge AIDS practice in San Francisco, it was the emotional toll they could exact that made attendance at funerals impossible. "I can't go to funerals, because I really cannot indulge myself in the luxury of breaking down, because the next morning I've got to do it again. But I can grieve." Wafaa El-Sadr decided she could no longer go to the funerals of children because of how she had been affected by the last one she had attended. "I really didn't do well. It's not good. It's not even good for them to see me like this."

For some doctors, it was the recognition that funerals could not provide them with the emotional succor they offered family members and friends that led to a decision to stop attending. Harvey Makadon, who, like some other gay physicians, derived great satisfaction from the experience of serving his community in Boston, sought to avoid the feeling of isolation funerals had evoked.

I find after someone dies it often feels quite lonely. . . . My own experience has been that the physician is not necessarily the person the family wants to be around a lot after someone dies. And then all the people who sometimes avoided—sometimes didn't avoid—being with the patient are the ones who kind of take over the process and organize the memorial service and do all these things. It's with rare exception that I don't feel like I'm somehow on the periphery of things.

Eric Goosby, so moved by the moment of death, believed that doctors who attended funerals misread the needs of surviving family and friends. "There's not really a place for a physician at a funeral." Whether it was his own sense of failure or the perception of failure on the part of family and friends, it did not matter. The doctor represented an unwanted intrusion. In some instances that intrusion could elicit hostility. Howard Grossman believed that "there's a fair amount of anger from friends and family when somebody dies, and I guess I'm really afraid that some of it will turn on me; and I feel uncomfortable being there."

Oddly, for Ronald Grossman, whose large practice in New York had witnessed so many deaths, it was not hostility but the intrusion of gratitude that burdened him at funerals.

I can remember very distinctly when I decided I wouldn't go to any more. People would come up, "We didn't expect you as a doctor to show up." They either said that or implied it. I went there to have my private moment of closure with the deceased and instead had to be on a pedestal, if you will, on display for the family and the friends, an exhausting and difficult experience. And I simply stopped going.

Given the number of deaths with which AIDS doctors had to deal and the psychological and logistical problems posed by attending funerals, it became necessary to fashion an institutional response that would permit doctors, nurses, social workers, and others to share their grief. The Alta Bates clinic, which Carol Brosgart directed, was not unique in this regard.

Here in the clinic [we] try to do a memorial about every three months, and we get together after work hours. Sometimes we do it here; sometimes we do it at someone's house. We try to have nice music, and we light candles, and we keep a list of everybody that dies. And we go through the list from the time we've done the last one and talk about the person. People with AIDS are just like everybody else; I mean there's wonderful people, and there's terrible people. And there are some patients when you just go, "God, that person drove me crazy; it was so hard to take care of him, or her!" And people are very open, talking about what they liked about the person and what they didn't like. And then there are the people who we just adored. And people talk, and people cry.

Consumed by Death

As coping mechanisms failed or strained under the burden of death, dying, and intense clinical involvement, physicians felt spent. In 1995, Gerald Friedland, after almost 15 years of treating patients with AIDS, and after having made the move from the Bronx to Yale–New Haven Hospital, acknowledged his physical and emotional exhaustion.

I got depressed; I have to say that I don't think I've been particularly successful in dealing with my own burnout issues. I find this work to be very, very difficult now, much more difficult than it was earlier. I'm really tired of it. . . . I really feel it. I think the institutional battles, the loss of patients—so many—it's very wearing. It's cumulative.

And Joel Weisman painted the picture of a man transformed by his sorrow.

Taking care of people with AIDS had taken so much out of me, so much physically and emotionally out of me, that I wasn't a fun person anymore. . . . You talk about chronic grief, and you talk about not being able to heal and get over people's deaths. I've walked around for the last few years as just a very sad person. I was very happy. I had a good relationship. I have a good life. I'm healthy. But I was just sad from having to deal with people who were going to die.

In Eric Goosby's AIDS unit, the famous Ward 86 at San Francisco General Hospital, he and other veteran clinicians had shared a universe in which close colleagues were so chronically depressed or depleted that the toll was initially difficult to discern.

Toward the end of 1989–1990, it started to get kind of acutely difficult for everybody. The main bulk of the people who were seeing patients at the time in the clinic were all getting fried. They'd all been involved in just AIDS care for five, six, seven years, and were completely burned out. But we all spent so much time with each other that there wasn't a lot of contrast between us, so we didn't really appreciate it as much. But all of us in the same six-month period began to have a lot of emotional lability, where we would be unable to stop an emotional feeling. Something on the radio or TV, a commercial, would trigger something in you that would put you to tears.

At times, physicians ignored or endured their state of chronic depletion, sadness, and fatigue until an acute event forced them to acknowledge their feelings. It was an accidental fall requiring months of convalescence that had allowed Joel Weisman to realize that he finally needed to let go, to release himself from the responsibility of treating patients with AIDS.

I got hurt in June [1995] and I've been away from patient care July, August, September, and October. I've had the longest break. I still feel badly when I talk to some of my patients, but I've had a chance to heal from this period of chronic grief. I had never been away from dying patients for 15 full years. It's amazing what four months of not doing it has done.

Many physicians learned to moderate their expectations, to recognize that there were people and conditions they could not "fix." With years of experience behind him, James Campbell of San Francisco noted, "We just didn't set our expectations too high." And Dan William pointed to a hubris in some of those colleagues who burned out: "a sense of [being] more than what they were; if you think you can save the world, don't go into AIDS care." Some took refuge in a personal world removed from AIDS. Women, specifically, spoke about having children. One said, "Coming home to a new baby was the best medicine anybody could ever imagine."

Many sought to diminish the pain of AIDS work by assuming duties that provided a diversion from the demands of continuous patient care. "I believed," said Donald Abrams, "that more than [the] duration of your involvement with HIV, it's the intensity that leads to burnout; and so I think by involving yourself in other aspects of AIDS—in research, in administration, in teaching, as opposed to patient care—one loses something by not having those intense, powerful experiences with patients, but one gains, I think, longevity in the field." For Alexandra Levine, whose work in oncology prior to the AIDS epidemic had compelled her to deal with death, research involving potentially effective therapeutic agents helped to hold the sense of futility at bay. "I don't know if I could have been involved in AIDS care if I didn't do the research. The research was my hope."

Not all doctors could use their scientific work as a buffer. A number had to rethink the intimacy they had permitted to permeate their relationships to patients, to rediscover the virtues of conventional boundaries. Harry Hollander, who had been a resident at Moffitt Hospital in San Francisco in the early 1980s, recalled a patient to whom he had been drawn.

> He happened to be in San Francisco but lived in New York, was a dancer with the Joffrey Ballet. He was in terrific physical condition, and he used to, for exercise, dance up and down the halls of Moffitt Hospital. And he was a lovely man, quite a favorite, and I well remember sitting at his bedside and talking with this man who was getting over his *Pneumocystis* but had heard enough that he had reached the moment of terror for him in terms of seeing that it was quite likely that this would end his career and end his life within fairly short order.

Over time, Hollander reluctantly realized he had to pull away. He had to tamp down what he called his "emotional vulnerability" to his patients' pain, illnesses, and death. While confessing to that vulnerability, he still remained unable to express the depths of his emotional experience, finding it "very difficult to talk about." His personal need to diminish the intensity of the relationships he formed with patients was both personally necessary and a bitter end to his aspirations.

It certainly was an atrophy if not the complete death of an ideal, but I think in a sense, at least at the time, a rationalization for it might have been that these were also years in which we were beginning to have a little bit more to offer people medically. If one felt as if you could provide some more of the science of medicine, one was not so obliged to give of themselves so deeply.

Hollander was hardly unique. Many doctors discovered a need to pull back because they could not maintain the intensity of the first years of patient care. For many, among them Leonard Calabrese, distancing was not a defeat—it made possible continued exertions on behalf of their patients.

I go out of my way now not to become overly involved. I try to kind of just keep a proper balance about this. I don't think anybody's got a patent on what's the best way to do it. But [as] long as I can do it on my terms, I'll do it forever.

For some, however, there was no alternative but to withdraw completely from the intensity demanded by patient care. When he realized he could no longer engage in the close clinical relationships he felt AIDS work required, Eric Goosby stopped seeing patients. Ironically, that move was precipitated by the birth of his first child.

I think it became more and more difficult in the sixth and seventh year, when I started to feel it. Being willing to give in and engage one more time, knowing what was ahead of [that patient and me], knowing that we're going to go through all of this, and knowing that that's what they need; and wanting to give it to them, but being empty, depleted from doing it the way I thought it should be done. In 1990 I had a little boy, and that's what kicked me into a very personal introspective reaction to what I was doing. My ability to engage diminished, and it was all around the issue of the realization that each of these was somebody's kid. And that this person in front of me was connected to a mother and a father and extendeds [who] had the same intense feelings that I had for our baby. And somehow that realization tumbled for a period into an inability to want to engage; and even ducking situations that I knew I would have handled differently a year before. . . . I would hesitate consciously around not wanting people to get too intimate with me because it hurt so much when we lost you. I had gotten burned so much with it that I didn't want to put my hand back in the flame.

Paul Volberding, who had established Ward 86 and who had a world-wide reputation as a leading clinician, also withdrew. Even before Goosby, he had left primary care, focusing on the organization of clinical trials and the management of his AIDS service.

It always amazes me that people are still doing high-volume primary care more than a decade [into the epidemic]. I don't think that it's an accident that I ended up being sort of eager to be involved in research and administration. I don't think I could deal constantly with the level of grief that this epidemic carries.

Most of the doctors who, as of 1995, had left direct care believed they were doing so temporarily. Eric Goosby, who went from San Francisco to a position in the U.S. Department of Health and Human Services in 1991, took up a part-time practice in the AIDS clinic at D.C. General, the grim public hospital in Washington. Joseph O'Neill, who had moved in and out of AIDS patient care, had left again in 1995 to oversee the AIDS work of the Health Resources and Services Administration, but felt confident he would soon return.

It's a little bit of a hiatus. I realize that I'm pretty damaged by the whole thing. I've been so out there and working so hard and so emotionally present to everything, that it's kind of a nice time for me to be backed away from it a little bit. . . . And things have worked out in my life, such that I can stop for a while before I dive in again. . . . I can't imagine a time that I would completely walk away from the clinical practice of medicine. Being a doctor is very integrated into my self-concept. It's just something that is almost like breathing to me. I love practicing medicine; I love helping people in that way; I like using my mind in that way; maybe I love pushing people around; maybe I love telling people what to do. I don't know what it is, but I cannot imagine not doctoring.

Although leaving direct patient care might have been unavoidable for some doctors, the consequence for their patients was often dreadful. Very sick or chronically ill patients could feel a sense of abandonment at a moment of great vulnerability. As a gay physician in San Francisco, William Owen saw the impact on his own community. "That's been a major trauma in the community, where patients suddenly lose their physician." In New York City, Ronald Grossman, another gay physician, described patients who were left by those upon whom they had come to depend.

> A patient came in who shares his care between here and the city he currently lives in. [I asked,] "Why are you back?" "Well, you know, [my doctor] has taken a leave of absence." And he gives me a strange look, and he said, "You know what that means—it means that he has burned out. I hope he'll come back. In the meantime, I'm going to come back to you for all my care." He then gives me this kind of wistful look, like "That's not going to happen to you, is it?"

For some who worked in impoverished areas, where close relationships between physicians and patients were rare, leaving patients was viewed as simply unacceptable. In Newark, James Oleske spoke earnestly of the need to persevere, to remain committed to the community and its patients.

> You got to stay with it. You can't take the next job. I try to tell medical students once you make a commitment to a community, once you make a commitment to go out in private practice, if you're really going to be an effective person, you've got to stay there, you can't give up; that's why I don't believe in this burnout thing. Because patients can't say, "I'm poor. I don't want this disease, and I want to leave Newark." They can't take the bus and leave Newark and go some place and be well and healthy. And I don't think as a health care provider that you have the right to say, "Well, I've seen too many kids die, I've seen too many problems, I'm going to change my job." I don't think we have that privilege.

At Harlem Hospital, the chief of pediatrics, Margaret Heagarty, made it clear that burnout was an option foreclosed to physicians who served under her leadership.

I have been asked by any number of young reporters, "Oh, Dr. Heagarty, how on earth do you prevent burnout?" And I say, "I don't permit it. . . ." [Burnout's] an arrogant assumption. It's a middle-class arrogant assumption. I had for years a cleaning lady who was 70, shlepped in from Brooklyn to clean my house once a day. Nobody ever said to her, "Susie, how do you prevent burnout?"

Heagarty understood, however, as did the heads of AIDS programs like Gerald Friedland and Arye Rubinstein, that her doctors needed to be heard and supported in order to carry on: "Oh, about every third day they come in and *kvetch*, and I say, "Yes dear, now go out there." Rubinstein, who had created a mental health program for his AIDS patients in the Pediatric Immunology Clinic at the Albert Einstein College of Medicine in the Bronx, offered its personnel to his nurses and physicians, beginning in 1983. By incorporating them into support groups, Rubinstein believed he had succeeded in preventing burnout: "We had no burnout here; to date we have no burnout."

Some physicians developed their own support groups to discuss the threat of burnout. In New York City, doctors associated with Roosevelt Hospital, including Dan William, organized a group under the guidance of a psychiatrist to contend with issues like depression. At San Francisco General, grief and despair became so severe that the clinicians there established several therapeutic groups. Eric Goosby, in the months before he left, joined his colleagues in deeply emotional sessions.

There were a number of nurse practitioners in the clinic who were so burned out it was pathetic, who had been there since the beginning, since '83, '84, and needed some help in (1) realizing where they were, and (2) moving through it. And we started a discussion group, and this was fortunately about six months before I left, and the discussion groups were wonderful. Paul [Volberding] and Connie [Wofsy] and Donald [Abrams] and Michael [Clemen] and myself. The docs had their group; the nurse practitioners had their group. And then we had a big group. We met twice a week and talked this out. And it was the most amazing, cathartic time that the clinic has ever gone through. Everybody was in tears and crying. We had never had an opportunity to express grief. We had never acknowledged that we had grief. We layered it [over] hundreds of times. . . . And just the ability to say, "Yes, I hurt too. Isn't it a bitch?" went a tremendous way in allowing people to say, "I guess I'm okay" and start the self-healing process that I think all of us are still doing: to try to place it into some construct that has personal meaning and was not this futile flail.

Such encounters allowed Goosby to come to terms with the resentment he felt toward those who, for whatever reason, had stopped treating AIDS patients and to overcome the sense of abandonment he shared with patients whose doctors had left them.

Connie [Wofsy] and Paul [Volberding] went through what they had experienced. Both of them stopped seeing patients around '84, in terms of following patients. Connie came in and out of it. She'd go away a year, come back. Paul was pretty much out of the clinical area. Even though he's a gifted clinician, he never continued. . . . And those of us who were seeing patients understood why Paul saturated and pulled back, but there was an element of resentment too. Paul, in this group, verbalized his feelings and broke down in an uncontrollable outburst of sorrow and crying, as did Connie later and all of us at different points as we told our stories. And it gave me an appreciation for Paul that made me feel much better about him in terms of—he'd been there; he'd gone through it; he knew what he was dealing with. And that was important for everybody to hear.

Most doctors preferred more traditional, less tempestuous solutions to diminish the threat of burnout. Some, like Howard Grossman, who acknowledged his own struggle with behavior he came to understand as self-destructive, took an apparently stoical posture, enduring their sense of loss and grief without letting those emotions overwhelm them.

I know people who work in HIV who have turned [their pain] off. I'm not sure they last that long, frankly. And I know plenty of people who chose to have the pain who burned out. The trick is to experience the pain and not run from it and learn to live with it.

For a few physicians, spiritual or religious belief was the source of strength against the specter of burnout. James Oleske, a Catholic, employed the language of vocation when he spoke of his enduring commitment.

When I say my morning prayers, I ask for two things: [to] stay humble and to persevere. . . . I just think that [AIDS] was my problem, and I was called to deal with it. . . . Not called. I was sort of there when it happened. I was called to stay.

Those who saw in burnout a spiritual crisis that threatened their professional work sometimes found the strength to continue through a kind of reawakening. Lisa Capaldini—like Oleske, a Catholic—found in the rekindling of her spirituality an antidote to her growing sense of estrangement and depression. In the early 1990s, after almost five years of treating AIDS as a private practitioner, she had difficulty continuing.

Things were empty; things felt like chores. I would see the list of patients on my schedule and try to anticipate what their problems would be and how I could get through these things efficiently and promptly. It's like the difference between making bread when you're in a hurry to do it and it's a chore, versus loving to make bread and enjoying every step of it and savoring it. I was just out of touch. Part of it was that I wasn't feeling all the wonderful spiritual, emotional connections because what was coming in was very little and what I was putting out was so much.

At a retreat, she joined a group of clinicians similarly suffering spiritual loss. In discovering that her experiences were hardly idiosyncratic, she started what Goosby described as "a self-healing process," finding that it permitted her to integrate her sense of the "nonrational" and the sacred into her practice.

I went to this retreat. I went to this one called "Rekindling the Flame," about getting back in touch with why you went into this profession and work. It was amazing to be with health practitioners like me who were struggling with similar stuff. And the common denominator was we all deeply cared about our work, but we had lost touch with some of the spiritual dimensions of it. It was just a very overpowering thing to realize it was okay to talk about issues of meaning and loss, and that you weren't a baby if you had struggles with that. . . . [It] really helped me come out of the closet as a person who, for example, loves Byzantine or iconic Madonna and Child figures, and feels a very strong connection with that insofar as a physician dealing with AIDS, I am a little bit like Mary. You know, a regular woman who becomes the mother of God. I mean it's a task you're not ready for but when called to do it, you do it. I can both have a sort of motherly, instructive, protective function with [my patients] and, at the same time, as individual people they have a particularity and a sacredness that goes beyond anything I can do for them. Three or four years ago, I wouldn't even have given myself permission to think like that, because it sounded too "out there" and too self-indulgent or too metaphorical or too Catholic, or whatever. But it's a very powerful image for me; it helps me.

For Charles van der Horst, the horror of AIDS and the death of his patients precipitated the deepest despair. As a resident, he had been drawn to the Judaism his parents had abandoned, because it offered him *shalom bayet*—in Hebrew, literally and metaphorically, a peaceful space in his life. Sabbath services provided that peace.

Saturday morning, light streaming through the windows, no organ or anything like that, singing songs that I didn't understand, but they were wonderful melodies, great ancient melodies; and it was very [much] like doing a mantra, very relaxing, peaceful, soothing to the soul. I liked the idea of the continuity, something that was 5,000 years old. It was beyond me. It began before me and will be going on for thousands of years after me. I liked that sense.

In the late 1980s, in the midst of developing an AIDS clinic in North Carolina, van der Horst suffered a spiritual crisis. Not unlike Elie Wiesel, he, the son of a Holocaust survivor, kept asking himself, "Where is God?" in the midst of this death and dying. His deep religious sensibility deserted him, leaving him bleak and stripped of the peace he had found.

I think it was probably a small version of my mother's response to the Holocaust. "How could God let something like this go on? How could a caring, loving God allow all this suffering?" And so I would say the prayers, and I would go to the synagogue, but I had a very hard time with it. . . . I think the best example is standing up and doing the *Ameda*. It's a prayer where you do praises to God over the various aspects of what God has done. But in the crisis, I would stand up and it was all meaningless to me. The words were like dust. I would say them, and they literally had no meaning. Who was I talking to? I didn't know who I was talking to. I didn't get the shiver down my spine that I always got. It was not a good period. I didn't know what was going on—was God abandoning me, or was I abandoning God? I busied myself in my work. But my religious life was gone.

His feeling of despair lifted once he, like Lisa Capaldini, found he could "sacralize" his relations with his patients.

If I was an historian, I would look at the documents about my relationship with my patients. In 1988, I start developing these re- lationships with people, with the first and longest being Nat Blev- ens, because I'd followed him all the way back from being a fellow. Then I get this rich relationship. I experience the simultaneous pain and joy of being able to articulate and speak with Nat and hug him and kiss him and express my doubts about being his clinician—that I don't know if I'm capable of making unbiased decisions to help him. And him saying, "That's okay; that's why I want you to be my doctor." So in a sense, then, I think I was able to find God again. I think that in allowing yourself to develop a relationship with an- other human being, it is a holy thing, whether they're your patient or your spouse, your parent, your friend, your child.

Paradoxically, then, the intense, highly personal relationships with AIDS patients that could result in burnout provided some practitioners with the rewards that sustained their commitment or drew them back to AIDS work. Despite the debilitating demands of the patients and their disease, doctors were often invigorated by the chance "to make a differ- ence" and by the gratitude they received in return. Goosby, for example, spoke of the "dynamic that's set up with a patient and a physician" in terms of "energy exchange." Many spoke of the opportunity to develop a bond that sustained them during years of treatment and after the pa- tient's death. Ronald Grossman, in what might be taken as a secular restatement of van der Horst's spiritual connection, summed up what allowed him to endure.

The secret to why I haven't burned out—and I think I can speak for other colleagues who've stuck it out as long as I have—is that the humanistic side of medicine makes it tolerable. However painful it is to lose somebody that you really like, it is the process of having gotten to like them and know them during the illness that can sustain you when they head down the hill to the terminal phase and then to death. It is not the worst thing in the world, as it turns out, when we grow up, to have experienced wonderful people who then leave you. I think it's a lifetime lesson.

Nonetheless, he had to temper his remarks. "There have been times," he recalled, "when the Grim Reaper has marched through this office to the tune of a death a week for long periods; [then] I and my staff are hard pressed to sustain our enthusiasm and not show our grief."

Parting

"You won't die on me?" the patient searchingly asked the doctor he was consulting in the aftermath of his own physician's death from AIDS. This startling question was broached by anxious patients with HIV disease more frequently than ordinary medical practice might have suggested possible. By 1990, when the medical newsletter *Medical World News* published an account of doctors who had died of AIDS, the CDC had estimated that 350 physicians had fallen victim to the epidemic, approximately 100 of whom were from New York and California.[4] Not all such physicians, virtually all of whom were gay, treated patients with AIDS, but many did. An understanding of what it was to treat patients with HIV-related illnesses while struggling with AIDS oneself is largely lost to memory. John Stansell, who had remained asymptomatic despite his years of HIV infection, captured the significance of sharing an illness with his patients.

> I don't think you can get distance. It's always there. It's like you had a hump on your back. There's no defense mechanism really which can separate you from the fact that you're HIV positive. There is not a day goes by or an hour goes by that I'm not constantly reminded of that fact.

Some sense of what it is to be at once very sick *and* a doctor may be learned from Constance Wofsy—the "travel agent for death"—who through much of the time she cared for AIDS patients and assumed other epidemic-related responsibilities confronted breast cancer and then metastatic disease. She struggled with the difficulty of traversing the terrain between being a patient and being a doctor. As a woman with breast cancer, she felt turned into "a thing" by probing physicians, her dignity threatened, her cherished privacy invaded. She covered her body with a sheet as she, like any other patient, waited to be examined in a cubicle that afforded little to protect her modesty. As a doctor she felt called upon to be in charge, to engage in what she sardonically called "male-speak" with residents and interns. As a patient she felt her disease was out of control. She had to deal with the almost unbearable tension between her sense of the obligation "to be there" for her patients when she wanted more than anything to be cared for herself. She had to confront the fact that as her disease advanced she needed to have less patient contact. All of this was brought into relief as she recalled a dedication ceremony she had attended in mid-1995.

Last night we went to the dedication of a middle-school auditorium to be named for a music teacher who has very, very, very advanced AIDS. She's been teaching in the public schools for a very long time. She's an extraordinarily vital person, and she was at the ceremony last night. She was brought in by paramedics on a stretcher, on a non-rebreather mask, with four tanks of oxygen set up. And they had built a platform, and she stayed for the whole ceremony. Students had written a song about her. They had people from her church, from the Board of Education, from a corporation where she had done an award-winning educational film for children. I know her doctor, and I'd known of her infection for about a decade. And the irony, why this is such a remarkable story, is that at the time she was infected my children were both of school age. She was their teacher. I gave the first talk at that middle school. The principal realized that they had to address AIDS; they had to address it for the parents, and they had to address it for the kids. And, as many doctors did, I went one evening, and they got as many parents as were interested in coming to hear about what the realities were. And then I gave a lecture to the entire eighth grade class in the auditorium, which was a real hoot. They asked about things like anal sex, and, needless to say, there was a lot of fear and a lot of prejudice.

Last night—although it was never spoken, it's known to everybody who was present at that dedication why she is so severely ill—to a person, everyone hugged her. And the audience was oblivious, 100 percent oblivious, to the nature of her disease. It's the full circle of the doctor going out into the schools because there was absolutely no one else to do the education. Now, it would be unheard of for a doctor to go into the school, because who needs it? There are more AIDS educators around than there are librarians. But the doctor went to the school and dealt with stigma and disease and prejudice, and 10 years later one of the teachers was bid farewell with absolutely no evidence that she has anything that could possibly be fearsome or stigmatizing by the very population that had to learn it in 1986.

Constance Wofsy's tearfully and haltingly recounted story of that evening and its meaning for her was informed by the fact that, unbeknown to most of those who surrounded her in that auditorium, she who had come to that very room a decade earlier as a healer was now, like the teacher being honored on the stage, dying.

Constance Wofsy died just a year later, on June 3, 1996, a year in which 37,525 AIDS fatalities were reported. By then 375,000 had died since the epidemic's onset. Wofsy's life ended before she could fully appreciate the significance of the clinical advance that was heralded six months before her death: highly active antiretroviral therapy that would profoundly change the experience of HIV disease for both patients and their doctors.

5
THE WANING OF THE EPIDEMIC?

Turmoil and Doubt

More than a decade after the onset of the epidemic, there was a pervasive sense among many doctors that the effort to meet the clinical challenge of AIDS had stalled. Although there had been progress in the management of HIV-related opportunistic infections, attempts to identify powerful antiretroviral agents had achieved little that could add dramatically to the life expectancy of those with AIDS. For those not given to optimistic interpretations, the situation seemed bleak indeed. Drawing on her experience with patients in Boston, Elizabeth Kass had adopted a posture of profound doubt about what medicine could offer people with AIDS.

> I remember going to these conferences [with a colleague] and listening to people say with conviction, "Oh, absolutely everybody should be on drugs, and the more drugs the better." And we'd sit there and say, "How can they say that with conviction in the face of all this data?" . . . You look at your patients who are not on drugs and your patients who are on drugs, whether it's been their choice or yours, and you'd see that they're really not doing all that much differently, and you think, obviously, there are so many individual factors we don't understand. How can one be anything but humble about this disease? And how can anyone stand up and be dogmatic about what makes sense?

Even among those who had involved themselves with research, whose careers merged a commitment to clinical care and the investigation of new therapeutic options, there was deep pessimism. Donald Kotler, who had years earlier expressed exhilaration over the discovery that gancyclovir could effectively be used to treat CMV colitis, was especially bitter about the false promise of highly touted antiretroviral treatment and about those whose careers had been built on research. Referring to the antiretrovirals approved after AZT, he noted:

> After the first time, are you going to be stupid enough for the second drug? For ddI? Is that the cure? Is d4T the cure? Is 3TC the cure? It's like the same story over and over again. What it takes to not be a stupid fool is to accept the fact the first time you see the patient that the patient will die of this disease. I've helped a lot of people. I haven't cured anyone. The people who have made their careers doing phase 1 trials of one new antiretroviral after another have done very well for themselves but in some ways haven't helped anybody. What do you expect from the "inner circle," the [Gang] of Five at the ACTG?

Such a carefully circumscribed therapeutic perspective enabled many doctors to persist despite the gloom that pervaded the search for an effective antiretroviral therapy. Like practitioners in oncology, a field so many had spurned, they would continue to focus closely on their individual patients, using their growing clinical acumen to contend with pathological decline. James Oleske found solace in a parable that defined both the limits and the purpose of his efforts under these dismal conditions.

> One of my first patients that died, her mother sent me a little story that she said reminded her of how we approach patients. It was called "Courage." It talks about an old man walking the beach at dawn. As the old man walked the beach, he [saw] a young woman ahead of him, picking up starfish and throwing them back into the sea. The old man caught up to the young woman and asked what she was doing, and she stated that if the starfish were left to the morning sun they would die. And the wise old man looks down the beach and says, "There are millions of starfish. And the beach goes on for miles. How can your effort make any difference?" And the young woman looks at the starfish [and says], "It makes a difference to this one."

Not everyone could find in such a focus an antidote to the toll being taken by AIDS. To continue to function as providers of care, they needed something more: a robust faith in scientific research as the eventual source of a cure or vaccine. It was a vision that appealed to Marcus

Conant, who, despite his intense involvement with patients, was, in desperation, drawn to the image of the hard and heroic scientist untouched by what he contemptuously termed "social work values."

> I think the thing that has kept me involved is not the personal satisfaction of seeing people get better [or] the personal satisfaction of helping someone through the dying process, but the intellectual challenge of "can we finally get a vaccine and stop this disease?" . . . That becomes very hard to stay focused on. Donald Francis expresses it better than anyone I know. He was trained as a pediatrician, and he talks about walking into a camp where these children are dying; and he had to step over these dying children to go into the tent to isolate the virus, because only then would you stop the epidemic. And that's what it's really all about, having your priorities straight but also understanding that the academic challenge is sometimes even more important than the compassion of wanting to help this child who's on the ground. That stopping to help that one child may not be nearly as important as getting in that tent and isolating the virus and finding a cure.

Ironically, it fell to Jerome Groopman, an oncologist, to find grounds for optimism, even as others had all but given up hoping for dramatic changes in the prospects for effective therapy. Sardonically, he referred to his Jewish optimism—"things could always be worse"—to explain his resilience. But more pertinent was his faith in science, based on the experience of treating cancer in children.

> I believe, right? That's the basis of faith. I believe that science has the potential to improve the situation. It has the creative impulse. There's no guarantee that it will happen or that the time frame will be anything that we want, but it's done it before, and I think it has a real possibility of doing it again. Not that it will "cure" it, but I think that marked improvements in the quality and longevity of the lives of people with HIV will be achieved. I've believed that from very early on; and part of it comes from having experience. Look at leukemia. When I was in fifth grade there was a guy, Eric Gold, who I remember very well, who was a classmate. No one said what he had. He became yellow; he became bald. In a sort of lower-middle-class neighborhood in Queens, he was the first kid to ever get a ten-speed bike. Then he disappeared about two months later. I found out years later that he had childhood leukemia. He was

treated with some primitive regimen, probably in 1959 or 1960, and he died. Uniformly fatal disease. Curable now in 85 percent of kids. Okay? Three decades.

Among the factors contributing to Groopman's belief in eventual scientific success was a remarkable research finding in early 1994. In February of that year, the Data Safety and Monitoring Board of the National Institute of Allergy and Infectious Diseases recommended the interruption of clinical trial 076, designed to determine whether the administration of AZT to pregnant women infected with HIV could reduce the rate of maternal-fetal transmission.[1] Women who had received AZT in the trial had a transmission rate of 8.3 percent; among those who had received a placebo, 25.5 percent of the newborns were infected. AZT had effected a two-thirds reduction in the rate of transmission. Howard Minkoff, who, over the prior decade, had delivered babies to almost 500 infected women in the heart of Brooklyn, noted:

[This] is a most dramatic moment. It's a first cure. . . . Those children for whom it works have been cured; they've been spared a short life of pain and certain death. For the woman whose child survives, it's hard to overstate the benefits.

The turmoil that surrounded the trial, as well as the reception that greeted its successful findings, place into bold relief the ways in which distrust and social inequality framed the world of AIDS clinicians. Activists, fearful that the results would be used to justify the mandatory screening of pregnant women, challenged the scientific validity of the trial's findings.[2] Some even minimized its clinical significance. Mardge Cohen, who came to AIDS work at Chicago's Cook County Hospital through her commitment to women's health issues, was striking in this regard.

I don't see this perinatal AZT thing as a major, phenomenal, incredible victory except for Burroughs-Wellcome, [which] could then come back and actually feel better about what they've done. I mean, I think that probably for people who have never had AZT it might reduce it from 25 percent to 8 percent—that might be true—though in Chicago . . . [untreated women have an] 18 percent perinatal transmission.

Those who viewed the results of 076 as a remarkable breakthrough felt that the lingering debate only served to confuse the women who could most benefit. Judith Currier, who had worked to enroll women in the clinical trial in Boston, was appalled by the effect opposition had had on women she now cared for in Los Angeles.

> Some of the criticism has actually almost been detrimental for patients in that it suggests that you shouldn't believe the results of the study. . . . What people seem to be objecting to is what policies are made as a result of the study, [but] what's happened is that they just hear that it's bad. They say, "076 equals bad," and "I shouldn't believe this." I think that [it's] really a shame that that message has gotten across.

Although AIDS activists (some doctors among them) feared that pregnant women would be coerced into taking AZT for the benefit of their offspring, many found that once they explained the potential benefits of the new regimen, the women they cared for became ardent claimants. Carol Brosgart, who had long been an advocate for women with AIDS, noted,

> These women get very excited about the possibility of being able to reduce the risk and wanted to get on AZT *yesterday*. They didn't have the political feelings about AZT, even among pregnant women I was seeing who were Black. I have not seen a single woman who did not want to take AZT.

Such enthusiasm among patients mirrored that of clinicians who had felt ineffective for so long and who now believed they could finally offer those with HIV infection something more than palliation. Suddenly, much of the talk of how physicians should rediscover their calling to comfort in the absence of therapeutic options began to recede. For Janet Mitchell, the results of clinical trial 076 allowed her to return to her original mission as a doctor. "It was extremely important because it was bringing me back to what I was trained to do, and that is to offer some alternative to just letting the disease run its course."

But amid the surge of therapeutic enthusiasm there were those who recognized that for the women most in need, the regimen dictated by clinical trial 076—AZT three times per day during the second and third trimesters of pregnancy, intravenous AZT during delivery, and the treatment of the newborn for six weeks—assumed that women received prenatal care. For James Oleske, who, long before AIDS, had committed himself to working with the poor children of Newark, this was the ultimate and most bitter of ironies.

> When 076 came out, [it was] very gratifying that we could reduce from 24 or 25 percent to 8 percent the transmission rate. I have to say it [was] almost immediately followed by a low. My intense frustration [was] that the majority of women at this [hospital], which enrolled the first woman in that study, still would not have access to AZT.

Breaking the Therapeutic Impasse

AZT had made possible the remarkable reduction in the risk of transmitting HIV infection from pregnant women to their babies, but by 1994, it had come to symbolize the limits of therapeutic progress. Almost four years had elapsed between its approval by the FDA and the licensing of ddI, a second drug in the same class as AZT. Within the next two-and-a-half years, two additional antiretroviral drugs were licensed, ddC and d4T. At the end of 1995, 3TC was approved. It was the availability of this range of drugs that made possible a conceptual shift in the treatment of AIDS. Donna Mildvan compared this advance to the treatment of tuberculosis: one drug would inevitably fail because it would set the stage for viral resistance, rendering the therapeutic agent impotent.

> It took us a while to figure out. Too long in fact. TB can't be treated with one drug. Neither can HIV. We were all too slow in figuring that out. But early on we didn't have the drugs to put together in rational combinations.

For Michael Gottlieb, the advances in therapeutics had, by 1995, made him more hopeful about his patients' prospects but only "slightly so."

> I am using AZT, ddI, and 3TC in combination when possible. We have lovely tests for viral load; we can measure the quantity of virus and we can mix and match drugs and look at their effect on the viral load over a period of weeks. So I can start someone on AZT, 3TC, and ddI knowing their baseline viral load, and I can check it again in a month, and I can see whether I'm having an impact on curbing replication of the virus, which, after all, is the principal problem.

Deborah Cotton, ever skeptical, did not share the enthusiasm of those who had, like Mildvan, seized on combination therapy as a way out of the therapeutic impasse of 1995.

Now the virologists have sort of taken over, saying, "This is a viral disease, stupid, so any drug that lowers the amount of virus in the blood is going to work." Important people are saying, "We have some potent new drugs, and now we have these wonderful markers, and we're going to be able to not only know when the clinical trials are working by using these surrogates, but, even more, we can individualize therapy. I can give you drug A and watch how it lowers your viral load and keep you on that, but as soon as your viral load goes up I'm going to hit you with B plus C plus D." And people are coming up with these kinds of strategies; and, of course, in my view there's still no basis in fact for any of this. . . . It doesn't feel wonderful to go in there and say, "I honestly don't know if ddI is better than AZT is better than d4T in this setting." It feels much better to say, "I've just measured your virus, and it's starting to go up, [so] now we're going to switch to this therapy." And it might be right! That's the other thing.

It was not, however, the combination of drugs in the same class as AZT that was to signal a radical transformation in the therapeutic world of those confronting HIV. Rather, it was an entirely new class of drugs known as protease inhibitors that promised to reduce the blood level of HIV to undetectable levels. While research on these drugs was ongoing, word of their potential efficacy began to spread. It was not until January 1996, at a national conference in Washington, that news of the protease inhibitors was first publicly presented. Howard Grossman attended the Antiretroviral Meetings and struggled to make sense of what he heard.

I remember sitting there in the conference and thinking, Okay, well, this is a lot better than what I thought it was going to be, from the last couple of years' worth of dribbles and leaks and things like that. But there's all these questions, and, I don't know. We'll see. I'm not sure what I'm going to do. But by the end I thought, This is ridiculous. This is really exciting data. Be excited about it.

Carol Brosgart, like others who had been treating patients with AIDS for more than a decade, was also skeptical, recalling the flush of enthusiasm that had surrounded AZT.

At the retroviral meetings, as Abbott and Merck are presenting their protease data in an almost orgasmic fashion, [a senior AIDS clinician] was sitting next to me, and he said, "What does this sound like? It sounds like AZT in 1987." And that's right. "AZT saves lives." And the question is "For how long?" and "At what cost?"

Six months later, Brosgart, together with thousands of other physicians, AIDS researchers, and activists attended the XI International AIDS Conference in Vancouver, Canada. It was a meeting that was suffused with an optimism at times bordering on euphoria. Not only was it demonstrated that the protease inhibitors could radically reduce viral load and provide patients with periods during which they were symptom free, but some even suggested what, a short time earlier, would have been considered unthinkable: the possibility of eradicating HIV in those who were infected. The key, it was argued, was to treat early in the history of an individual's infection and to treat with a powerful combination of drugs, both protease inhibitors and nucleoside reverse transcriptase inhibitors.[3] "Treat Early, Treat Hard" became the clinical rallying cry. Surrounded by enthusiasts, Brosgart was troubled.

It bothers me when things are portrayed as the standard of care, when it's an evolving time of trying to sort out a standard of care. And there are still so many unanswered questions. [On the one hand,] if you take someone very early in disease and you treat them with three or four drugs—with all the toxicities and costs and ways that make them a patient when they might have had 10 years or more of being asymptomatic—is that right? . . . There's still not an answer to when to start and what do you start with, and do you need two drugs, or is it three drugs, or is it four drugs?

Beset by doubts, Brosgart was compelled to question her own motives.

I was sitting in this session being very bothered by some of my colleagues who were presenting, saying, "Absolutely. Yes. [If] somebody comes in with primary HIV infection, treat them with three or four or five drugs." And they were presenting data, and the data was compelling. But it was data on five patients, and it was over a very short period of time, showing that you could reduce viral load. And I'm sitting there wondering, But will that make a difference in five years? Or 10? I'm trying to think it out, and then, as I'm doing all of this, I'm going, Well, am I just being a naysayer? Is there something in me that would want to maintain people in a state of illness? Why am I not feeling aggressive, like I want to go out there and hit early and hit hard? Why am I not as enthusiastic? Why am I not jumping up and down? I was trying to understand it. Is it the true scientist in me that's really still questioning what do we know and what don't we know? Or is it that if, all of a sudden, we had a cure and everybody could go home, what would I do with my life? And I started thinking, Well, what is it that I would want to do in my next career. Were my motivations good and honest, or was there something self-serving in them? And I started laughing, because the reality is that's not where we're at yet, and we're a long ways from it.

In the aftermath of the Vancouver session, other physicians, relying on their own clinical experience, began to challenge what they took to be a wildly unsubstantiated view of the data at hand. Harvey Makadon, who had recalled the thrill of writing his first AZT prescription and who could be scathing in his estimation of naysaying researchers with little clinical experience, took a posture of studied sobriety.

There's no question that the new medications have, for a time, led to people feeling better. And they don't need to come in as frequently, and they haven't been in the hospital as much, and there aren't as many crises. But that was sort of true when AZT first came out too. . . . I think if you cut away the public hype, you're left with you and the patient and some medications, and the differences are not astronomical. [But] I'd be crazy if I didn't say I feel better now about seeing patients and being able to treat them.

As they considered the implications of the therapeutic regimens now being proposed for their patients, physicians were acutely aware of the burdensome side effects that could make the protease inhibitors so difficult to tolerate. Barbara Starrett—so ready to make the most novel of therapies available to her patients in New York—described the physical changes induced by the new treatments.

We still don't have the perfect drugs. Every one of my patients [on protease inhibitors] is walking around looking pregnant. The bloating is phenomenal. One patient [said], "If this is how I have to live, I'm going to stop my proteases." He was in so much pain, and I couldn't believe what his belly looked like.

This image of AIDS patients in the mid-1990s stands as an ironic counterpoint to the time when wasting was so common. Deborah Cotton captured the earlier moment when she recalled,

> [When] we started the AIDS clinical trials unit, we saw our patients on the same floor as the obstetric patients. They shared a waiting room. I'd follow my patients both on studies and regular patients, and the OB patients would be sitting there. Each week the OB patients would be getting fatter, and my patients would be getting thinner.

John Stansell was able to appreciate the discomfort of his patients because, infected himself, he had decided to embark on treatment with protease inhibitors.

> I've had a constant state of gastritis for the last two-and-a-half months due to Crixivan. I'm one of the world's most compliant patients now—they'll never get anyone as compliant as me—but I'll tell you it just tears your stomach out, just tears it out. And that has frustrated me. I've felt like stepping up to the plate and screaming at Merck.

And so, removed from the media-enhanced excitement of Vancouver, doctors and their patients had to confront once again the difficult question of how to balance hope—with its inevitable risk of disappointment—with skepticism, which could lead to a reluctance to take on the challenge of therapies, the long-term prospects of which no one could predict. "I don't think it's so important that *I* don't feel disappointed," said San Francisco's Harry Hollander. "I don't want my *patients* to feel disappointed at this point. I'm trying to be as objective a filter of information as I can for them, so they have some realistic idea of what they're in for."

> With the protease drugs, for example, it is one thing to hear about these marvelous results in viral suppression; it is another thing to figure out, How am I going to take 12 pills a day on an empty stomach when some of my other medications want me to take those pills on a full stomach after a meal? How am I going to pay for the medication? What about these so-called minor side effects, which are not so minor for me? So there is a big leap between translating scientific advances that occur in a very controlled clinical

trial setting to the realities of life as an individual living with HIV in the context of all the other problems, medical and otherwise, that they're dealing with.

Some of the most cautious evaluations of what the protease inhibitors might signify came from clinicians with a deep involvement with research, both epidemiological and viral. Richard Chaisson's hostility to those who were therapeutic enthusiasts was shaped by an ever-present reminder of death among his Baltimore patients.

It's hard to go to a [memorial] service and be deliriously happy about new therapies, because, clearly, people still die. The new therapies are nice and good developments, but they're only small steps, and ultimately we are still faced with the lethality of AIDS and the mortality of our patients. . . . So my enthusiasm about the new therapies is tempered by the realization that reality will set in soon for everybody; and we'll realize that they are good, but they're not cures, and people are still going to progress and are still going to die in spite of these drugs. The only thing that is going to be a cause for real celebration is an effective vaccine. That will be a cause for declaring victory.

Martin Hirsch was, if anything, more restrained. As a researcher closely linked to the early history of AZT, he thought it dangerously foolish to overstate the promise of the protease inhibitors and stressed, instead, the necessity of developing new classes of drugs that could challenge the inevitability of HIV resistance.

At the first International AIDS Conference in Atlanta—it was 1985—I gave the first talk there on treatment. And this was just after AZT and interferon and others had been discovered; they hadn't even been tried in patients yet. And I made a statement [to the effect that], "We're on our way," which was widely quoted, and people saw that as a voice of optimism. And then during some of these periods of pessimism they said, "You know, you led us astray," blah, blah, blah. There aren't very many penicillins that come along and eradicate something. Protease inhibitors are nice advances, but the euphoria of today will not be there two years from now when resistance starts appearing. I'm already worried. There's nothing in the pipeline. We have these reverse transcriptase inhibitors, and within a month or two three licensed protease inhibitors, and there are more protease inhibitors coming. But what's after that? So I'm already getting a little pessimistic, while everybody else is optimistic.

Yet, there were physicians fully aware of the difficulties that the new drug regimens involved and alert to the treatment failures among their patients, who saw in the protease inhibitors and in the promise of yet a newer class of non-nucleoside reverse transcriptase inhibitors—the first of which was licensed in mid-1996—the promise of a new therapeutic world within which the management of HIV would be radically transformed. Alexandra Levine, who, despite moments of grave doubt, had never yielded to nihilism, was utterly buoyant. "This is," she said, "very, very big."

Number one, because, as a class . . . they are just far more potent than any of the other drugs you have ever had before. Number two, for the first time, we can knock down virus in both uninfected cells and in already chronically infected cells. So you can hit the virus at two opposite poles of the life cycle. And the third concept is true, valid combinations. And that's [just the same as in] my life in oncology. And now that the protease inhibitors have come, the combinations that are possible and available are scientifically valid combinations. Now it's for real.

Recalling a meeting of the Presidential AIDS Advisory Committee on which she served, Levine noted,

We just started going around the room, and one of the first people to speak was David Baltimore, [the] Nobel Laureate, [who said] that for the first time in the history of the epidemic he was truly optimistic about what we were able to do, that the world had changed and this was a very, very exciting moment. All of the people sitting in that room were people who knew very, very well that you don't say things inappropriately in a public forum, and you don't give false hope. As we went around the room, everyone [supported Baltimore's optimism]; I have goose bumps now just thinking about it, because I realized it wasn't just me in my own little way realizing what was happening. This was for real, and everyone knew it was for real, and it was extremely exciting. It was one of the real high moments of my life professionally.

Levine's excitement mirrored the changes she had seen in her patients.

> I have a whole group of patients who have not wanted to be treated over the years. . . . They've said, "No, that stuff is poison. I'm not using it." Now those people are coming to me on their next regular visit saying, "When can I get Ratinivir or whatever it is?" So the naysayers are going away with this.

Dan William saw the transition as every bit as dramatic as the shift in air travel from biplanes to the era of jet planes. Permitting himself both hope and a hint of humor that would have been impossible earlier on, he said:

> I think we're entering into the disease as chronic illness rather than a terminal disease. This has yet to be shown, but that's sort of my prediction, and I think it's quite likely that AIDS wards are going to be emptying out, not unlike iron lung wards in the fifties, that people are going to be doing better, and they won't need to be in the hospital as much, and there will be fewer AIDS-associated opportunistic infections, and the end result will be that I'll have more vacation time.

Minorities, Medicaid, and Managed Care

The social world into which the powerful new therapeutic agents made their entry was very different from the one that had existed in the epidemic's first years. Drug users and their sexual partners had always represented a substantial aspect of the epidemic on the East Coast. But the picture had been different elsewhere. In many parts of America, AIDS was experienced as a disease of white middle-class gay men. Gerald Friedland could recall how different his universe was from that of his West Coast colleagues.

> I remember the first International AIDS Meeting in Atlanta [in 1985]. Paul Volberding gets up, and he gives a talk about AIDS in San Francisco, and he shows this picture of the Golden Gate Bridge and sunset over the highlands and how we love San Francisco, what a wonderful place, and this wonderful model of care, with flowers at the bedside and people coming in and holding hands and chanting mantras and all kinds of stuff like that. And I'm saying,

Oh, shit. We're in the fucking Bronx, you know? It's sort of grungy and there's nothing to advertise, and I couldn't show a picture of anything other than a burned-out building maybe. And this is the kind of AIDS that we're dealing with.

By 1995, the picture had changed. While AIDS in San Francisco was still primarily a gay disease, AIDS at San Francisco General began to take on the demographic contours of every other condition treated at the public hospital. "AIDS," said Paul Volberding, "is becoming 'County.' "

The patients that we see now are about 180 degrees different from the patients we saw early in the epidemic. A lot of the patients with HIV are people with drug histories, with thought disorders, home- less people.

Friedland wryly noted that Volberding and others remarked to him in the 1990s, "Oh boy, now we're dealing with East Coast AIDS."

As the incidence of new infection with HIV dropped dramatically among gay men, and as infections continued to spread among poor drug users and their sexual partners, the public image of the epidemic began to undergo a transformation. The face of AIDS, it was said, was changing. To Anita Vaughn, whose Newark clinic had always served the impov- erished, the fact that so much was made of this change was a source of some amusement.

I laugh because [I] was [at a] national AIDS update a couple of years ago, [and] the theme of the conference was the changing face of AIDS. And I said, "It's the same face of AIDS that I've always seen, from the very beginning, [intravenous drug users] and women."

Changes in the social class composition of the AIDS epidemic, when added to the growing number of those impoverished by illness-related loss of jobs and social benefits, dramatically affected how hospitals and physicians were paid for their services. As they lost their health insurance and exhausted their resources, men and women with AIDS increasingly came to depend on Medicaid, the joint federal-state health financing program for the eligible poor. By 1987, it paid for more than half of all AIDS hospitalizations in New York. In San Francisco, the figure was 30 percent.[4]

Given this pattern of dependence on Medicaid, it is striking how very few AIDS doctors in private practice would take new patients covered by that public program. In this they were not very different from other office-based practitioners who found the Medicaid reimbursements for care too low to be economically acceptable. What made their decisions so striking was that they were the very physicians who had so committed themselves to the care of AIDS patients, for whom such care entailed a sense of mission. The refusal to care for Medicaid patients persisted even when some states created radically enhanced reimbursement fee schedules for AIDS.

Marcus Conant, like others, justified his decision not to care for Medicaid patients by noting that public sector clinics could provide the needed services. "We would make the phone calls; we'd refer them to the appropriate physician at the university next door where they got excellent care that was reimbursed by the state. And one did not feel that you were abandoning the patient."

Lisa Capaldini, for whom AIDS care was so explicitly informed by a sense of vocation, had struggled with the issue of MediCal (California's Medicaid program) both because of the low reimbursement fees and the nature of the clientele involved. In the end, the demands of her practice compelled her to exclude the most needy.

When I first started out, I saw whoever wanted to see me. I'd kind of gotten into my Mother Teresa mode, which is to say, Well, Mother Teresa never turns anyone away. How can I justify that? And I shared this with several of my friends; and the friends I found the most helpful were my nonmedical friends, because they'd say to me, "Well, Lisa, you aren't Mother Teresa. You're a doctor. You're a human being. And you've got to pay your staff. It's okay for you to make a decent living." I feel like I've chosen to restrict how many low-income patients I take, and I don't feel great about it.

Others were less troubled. For Howard Grossman, Medicaid represented a bureaucratic nightmare. But, more starkly, he believed that it was beyond the call of his commitment to care for those who had failed to secure for themselves adequate private insurance. And while he could extend himself for a time to those who had lost their protection, he believed that they should ultimately be shifted to publicly funded clinics.

I don't take Medicaid. When I first started in practice, I decided I would try taking Medicaid, and they kicked back my first three office visits with messages [like] "We don't pay for abortions." And I tried calling about it, and I ran into the Medicaid block. And I just said, "Forget it." It was just too much bureaucracy. They didn't pay enough to justify it, and it just wasn't worth it. I've taken care of a lot of people for free. In almost every situation where I've taken care of people for free, it blows up in my face. Those people get more angry than anybody else. They expect more than anybody else. They demand more. I realized that the people who pay me appreciate what I do. The other thing I realized is people make their own beds—especially true in the gay community. There are so many gay men who come from good middle-class families. They know about insurance. They know how to do that but they decide to party instead of having insurance. Well, it's not up to me to pick up that tab, and if they end up at Bellevue because they spent all their money on drugs and parties, I feel really bad for them, and I will work to help Bellevue to have the best service that there is, but it's not my job to make up for it.

Remarkably, while many of the most committed AIDS doctors were bitterly critical of those who refused to care for AIDS patients because of fears of contagion or because of anti-gay bias, it was almost impossible to find physicians who would challenge the choices dictated by the economics of private practice medicine. Alvin Friedman-Kien noted, "I'm blessed in that I was fortunate enough not to have to worry about making a living out of my profession. I can't be critical because I'm not in that position. I'd like to be critical, and I am deep inside, but I can't do it overtly because I'm not there."

Although private practitioners could insulate themselves from the burdens associated with caring for the poorest (in 1996 only about a third of AIDS patients receiving care had private insurance, while 90 percent of children with AIDS were covered by Medicaid),[5] they could not protect themselves from the increasing demands being imposed on the health care system by managed care. And here they shared the sense of dismay born of the erosion of professional discretion experienced more broadly by American physicians. Arye Rubinstein, using a Yiddish term of derision, simply and directly referred to managed care as "managed *dreck* [shit]." And Abigail Zuger spoke with disdain of the care delivered by a pioneer in the organization of prepaid group practice. It was the inadequacy of the care previously received by patients who ultimately came to her that she found so appalling.

I think managed care is an affront. I have personal experience with AIDS patients, several of them, who were taken care of in HIP, which is the oldest managed care [organization] in New York. The mismanagement was just obscene, and it's because their access to specialty care was so limited by these managers. It really kind of makes you shudder.

For Robert Bolan, who had been caring for AIDS patients in San Francisco since the early 1980s, the need to get permission to provide the care he considered appropriate—despite the fact that he was involved in the development of a managed care plan for AIDS patients—was the source of outrage.

The biggest impact on me is that very few people have indemnity insurance. That means basically reduced fee-for-service billing, with restrictions and mother-may-I shit associated with it. Those are my biggest nightmares; those are the biggest fuckin' nightmares in the world because they each have their own formulary; and if I wrote fluconozol, they'd say, "No, we won't fill fluconozol. You've got to use Nizoral." And it's different for each one; and I can't, won't, take the time to figure out who's got what and attach a formulary to the chart of every patient. So I have a lot of yelling matches over the phone. I've channeled a lot of my anger and frustration directly toward the insurance companies and carriers, and I think that for the most part they're the scum of the earth. My favorite line when they won't authorize a treatment is "You know, I'll bet that if this were your brother or your father or your son that we're talking about we probably wouldn't be having this conversation, would we?" I've had people hang up on me with that line. I've had people burst into tears with me on that line, and I don't care.

But in the struggle to maintain a quality of care, more than the control over professional discretion was at stake. Reduced fee schedules forced physicians to make modifications in their own practices in order to preserve their earnings. Howard Grossman, who would not treat Medicaid patients because of the level of reimbursement and the intrusions it would entail, was compelled to alter his clinical style with privately insured patients.

The impact of managed care for me has been that I make less money, but I'm also trying to figure out how to spend less time with patients and how to be more efficient. I'm running a business. I have five employees to support and myself and this big new space. Somebody's got to pay those bills, and I have that responsibility, and it's as much of a responsibility as it is to the patients. So if a person . . . comes in [with] a list of 40 questions, it's like, "I'm sorry, you're not paying for that time. You're going to have to come back." Or, "Pick the 10 most important questions, or the five most important questions, because that's all we have time for." And some people get very offended by that; and at this point my attitude is if they get offended because I'm telling them that they're not paying for more service than they're getting and they leave, that's okay. I'm not the only doctor in town. . . . Lots of people think they deserve unlimited time, and I can't do that anymore. Plus the managed care stuff makes me a bit angry, mostly because I'm watching this tremendous transfer of wealth to the insurance companies; and that's hard to watch. It's hard to watch people not understand what managed care is all about.

Not all AIDS physicians were so hostile to the changes being pressed by managed care. It was not surprising that Harvey Makadon, who had administrative responsibility for a managed care plan at Boston's Beth Israel Hospital, would find the demand for efficiency justifiable.

It used to be no one cared. We saw our patients. I have three hours; if I wanted to book four 40-minute patients, that would be my whole morning. Now, no one cares about the complexity of my patients. There's a rule that we need to see an average of seven patients a session; and I guess you could say you don't have to abide by that; but at the end of the year, you're not even eligible for any incentive unless you see an average of seven patients a session. . . . Maybe it's partly because I've been in a leadership role in the practice that I feel like I can't just flout those kinds of issues. I feel like I have to set a good example. And I have to say, I like it. I actually like the fact that we're being more productive, we're seeing more patients.

There were some office-based practitioners who shared Makadon's outlook, for whom the transformations were long overdue, even salutary. Although he disliked what he termed the "Big Brother" aspect of the supervision entailed in managed care, Dan William, whose New York

AIDS practice dated from the epidemic's first days, was enthusiastic about the possibility that it would force efficiencies that had been resisted.

> I love [managed care] because I've always despised waste in medicine, and medical care in the United States has so much waste that it's outrageous. The waste is a function of both physicians and patients. For HIV care it used to infuriate me that patients would say, "I haven't been in in three weeks. Let's do some more T-cells." And you don't do T-cells every three weeks. It doesn't give you information that you can act on. Managed care allows me to say, "No, sorry. Can't do that. That's not appropriate for your care. I'm the gatekeeper, and we have to control some costs, and we'll do it as appropriate."

Whatever the limits imposed by managed care and the increasing poverty of AIDS patients, there was one element of federal policy that physicians recognized as providing a singular benefit to their patients: the AIDS Drug Assistance Program (ADAP), which subsidized the purchase of AIDS-related medications for those who were uninsured or poorly insured.[6] In generous states, the program went far to assure access to drugs that would have been out of reach except to the very wealthy and the very poor covered by Medicaid. Given the way in which income and wealth affected access to treatment and care in the United States, the program seemed all the more remarkable. For Elizabeth Kass, the result was filled with ironies.

> There's [an] HIV drug reimbursement program, and that covers HIV meds. Okay, it's a little cumbersome. . . . You can get them acyclovir, you can get them AZT. The problem is everything else. If somebody happens to be hypertensive, diabetic, you might not be able to get them blood pressure medication or insulin or any of those things.

But not all state programs were generous. Some created waiting lists; others failed to cover all the drugs from which patients could benefit. Anita Vaughn had to confront limits in her Newark clinic, which served mainly poor minority patients.

> A hard day, in this day and age, is trying to provide care for folks when there's no money to do it. And it's getting worse now. . . . If

you have Medicaid, city welfare, or insurance that'll pay for it, you get Epivir and the protease inhibitors. Right now, patients are coming in, and they want to get on a protease inhibitor, for instance. They can't if they don't have those, either Medicaid or city welfare or any insurance that'll pay for it. They can't get it. ADAP is not paying for it . . . and so patients are suffering. . . . It's very frustrating. It's more than frustrating; it really makes me angry, because you have at least two tiers of medical care again. . . . It's going back to the very old days.

Since so many private practitioners had decided that they could not or would not provide medical care for the poor, whether covered by Medicaid or utterly uninsured, the provision of AIDS care often fell to clinics, like Vaughn's, funded under the Ryan White Care Act, the federal support program for patient care, and to the wards and clinics of public hospitals. The quality of care and the extent to which medications and services were available in those settings varied greatly. Among the best was San Francisco General Hospital. Constance Wofsy was clearly proud of her institution's response.

We're a public hospital that can't turn anyone away. I really think we've been able to provide pretty much what we want. If the patient is not able to pay [for drugs], they get them. [We have to fill out] many pieces of paper and special formulary requests and all this garbage, but by and large, ultimately, the patients get most drugs they need. Once antivirals were licensed and approved by the FDA, MediCal—boom, boom, boom—put them on the formulary. . . . It's the bureaucracy, the paperwork, the absolute lack of space, the horrendous physical conditions, the intolerable waits. But if you looked at the actual patient: Did they get their lab tests? Did they get their drugs? Yes, they did.

Robert Cohen, who had been responsible for organizing the AIDS services in New York City's municipal hospitals, described a situation of considerable incongruity: devoted staff, able to prescribe the most expensive medications, working often under dreadful physical conditions.

I fought, and didn't have to fight that hard, to have AZT available in the public hospitals. It was actually a pretty easy victory. It cost a lot of money for the city, but it happened right away. At all the hospitals there were people who cared about AIDS. . . . There was a substantial effort on the part of these doctors to provide very good care for people with HIV infection. A lot of them were gay, but not all of them, and they really tried hard to do it. . . . The physical conditions at some of the hospitals—Queens Hospital Center—is just a horror: these gigantic tanks of oxygen filling up the only walk space within the facility, one sink at the end of a floor. Nobody could be cared for well in settings like that. Kings County Hospital, again, had serious problems with oxygen, dysfunctional administration; and the conditions for people were very rough. The physical plant being relatively recent in a place like Bellevue or Lincoln— even Harlem had a reasonable physical plant—people who were seen within the clinics probably got reasonable care.

And then there were hospitals that doctors viewed as awful. Eric Goosby's depiction of Washington's public hospital, D.C. General, was filled with outrage.

The pharmacy will run out of drugs every week. The vendor wasn't paid; they stopped delivering their AZT, their Septra, their ddI, their 3TC, their d4T, and therefore we can't give it to them. The patient will bring the prescription to the pharmacist—they can't go out and buy the drug because they don't have any money—and the pharmacist basically says, "We're out of this drug. See you later." . . . This is the second largest AIDS clinic in the city in terms of patients seen. The X ray department was shit—still is. Early changes for *Pneumocystis* they read as normal. Late changes for *Pneumocystis* they can read as normal. We've seen it over and over again. They have an unsophisticated radiology, who are all into private practice and are doing this to make extra money and could care less about this group. It was extraordinarily difficult; I've never practiced with this type of lack of support. This microlab is on the level of a community hospital's microlab in a rural setting. Very rudimentary, unsophisticated, using techniques that were developed and perfected in the '40s and '50s. . . . There's such an attitude of laziness and unprofessionalism that it's been difficult to maintain a quality that's acceptable.

Private hospitals, too, played a role by caring for those with Medicaid and even those without insurance protection. Many doctors with institutional affiliations and commitments believed a vast distance had been traveled since the epidemic's first years, when hospitals across the nation demonstrated a singular resistance to embracing the care of people with AIDS. Gabriel Torres was especially laudatory of his own St. Vincent's Hospital, a Catholic institution in the heart of Greenwich Village. His observations were all the more striking since, as a gay man, Torres was painfully aware of how the Church and its leadership had clashed on a regular basis with AIDS activists on matters involving AIDS education and condom distribution.

Thank God the Catholic Church has been one of the few that has actually publicly opened their arms, including Cardinal O'Connor, to immigrants in general—not HIV per se—and also to the homeless and to the poor. So I really feel happy that I'm in a Catholic institution for that reason.

Jerome Groopman was similarly enthusiastic in describing the secular Deaconess Hospital in Boston: "Everyone is taken care of. There's never been anyone that I know of who's ever been turned away or treated differently on the basis of money or status."

Not all doctors were so enthusiastic. No longer tied, in 1995, to Montefiore Hospital in the Bronx, an institution with a reputation for social responsibility, Abigail Zuger was bitingly critical. Close up, she noted, "It was really kind of an outrage."

When I made rounds in the hospital, I occasionally would see a noticeable distinction in the way [privately insured patients] got treated by the hospital. Actually, a friend of mine and I were going to do a little study comparing length of time from first cough to bronchoscopic confirmation of PCP by insurance status. People with Medicaid were usually allowed to cough for a long time and then were treated empirically with this, that, and the other thing. You know, "Give them over the weekend." And people with private insurance were brought in, were given a diagnostic test within 24 hours, and were treated for what they had.

But whether they believed that their institutions provided good or wretched care, many doctors were almost blind to the extent to which the poor with HIV infection failed to benefit from many of the therapeutic advances being heralded as transforming the nature of AIDS. They were most knowledgeable about those who became their patients, even those they referred to public institutions. What they seemed only dimly aware of was the large numbers of those who never crossed the threshold to patienthood. In New York, state officials estimated that as many as 50 percent of individuals with HIV infection were not receiving regular care for their disease. In the mid-1990s, national estimates suggested that somewhere between "37 and 64 percent of individuals with HIV infection do not see a medical care provider outside of an emergency room at least every six months."[7] Most were poor, Black, or Latino and had inadequate health insurance or none at all.

The Normalization of AIDS

Fifteen years into the epidemic, AIDS appeared to be shedding some of the features that had made it so exceptional. It was fast becoming, like most infectious diseases, a disorder of the impoverished populations in the United States. And it was beginning to bend before the force of new pharmacological interventions. The striking scientific achievements of the mid-1990s further contributed to the reintegration of AIDS care into American medicine and the erosion of the boundaries that had defined the world of AIDS doctors.

The degree to which the new drug therapies prevented HIV infection in newborns, or extended survival in those infected, tended to strengthen the growing sense that AIDS, so long a vector of dread, was on the verge of being subdued. Increasingly, physicians considered the possibility that AIDS was about to become "normalized": to lose its extraordinary status as an exceptional clinical and public health problem. With new antiretrovirals, AIDS, they predicted, would eventually join the class of chronic, potentially fatal diseases. Those physicians who treated AIDS would be reabsorbed into the hierarchies and conventions of the medical mainstream.

Many who sought an appropriate metaphor to describe AIDS in the mid-1990s found it, ironically, in cancer. AIDS doctors, predicted Arye Rubinstein, would become like successful oncologists. Oncologists provided their patients with a series of potent chemotherapies only to see them die. But powerful AIDS drugs, Rubinstein anticipated, would be different, offering a considerable measure of clinical control to their physicians.

I think we are going to be more fortunate than the oncologists. The oncologists used combined chemotherapy: You use one drug; if it doesn't work you take the next, and the next one, and at the end of the road you're just running out of chemotherapeutic agents. And you destroy the bone marrow, and that's the end of the story.

I think that with HIV, but at a major expense, you'll be able to prolong life and create new drugs that will be able to run after the virus, or even predict in which direction the virus is going to mutate and get ahead of the virus, and prevent it from replicating. And there are studies showing this already. So you'll be able to keep the AIDS virus at bay for a long time, and slow down the decay of the immune system.

Among those doctors who foresaw the normalization of AIDS, perhaps the most optimistic was Barbara Starrett, whose private practice consisted mainly of gay men and women. Always a therapeutic enthusiast, she believed that current and future clinical practice would so prolong the lives of her HIV patients that almost all, like the classic Kaposi's sarcoma sufferers before the epidemic, would die of some other cause. In her opinion, HIV disease in the late 1990s would be analogous to hypertension in the 1950s.

I think probably everybody that I take care of now is going to live, except maybe two people [I currently have] in the hospital. Live for years. They all have the potential to die of something else. It's like hypertension in the '50s, where we had diuretics, risurpine, [and other early antihypertensive medications]. Many of those people on those imperfect drugs did live complete lives. So now we're going to have patients who live complete lives on these [AIDS] drugs. But hopefully, we're going to have better drugs. My hope is, we're going to be able to lower the viral load so low that people will then be able to be on minimal treatment and live full lives.

The normalization process—the successful placement of HIV into a constellation of other medically serious disorders—was visually captured by Abigail Zuger. In a graph she had produced that traced the number of AIDS medical articles published annually in the 1980s and 1990s, she was surprised to discover that a peak was reached in the late 1980s. By 1992, the volume of articles on certain other serious disorders surpassed those on AIDS. On Zuger's graph, AIDS was midway between breast cancer and heart attacks.

These are journal articles from Medline; I just went through and enumerated them. Now it's going down. It peaks in '88, and then it starts declining relative to lung [cancer], breast [cancer], myocardial infarction, diabetes. . . . It's still fairly high, but it's heading down. It's the *normalization* of a disease. Isn't that something?

For Zuger, this was a historical juncture she had long anticipated; she had "always waited for AIDS to become medicalized." She wanted AIDS to cease being an extraordinary disease. And she wanted an end to that prolonged state of heroic doctoring associated with it. "It's a disease," she observed. "It's not a way of life."

By the mid-1990s, in fact, many physicians found that AIDS doctoring had lost its charismatic edge. Fifteen years into the epidemic, the practice of AIDS medicine was reverting to the contours and expectations of conventional medicine, including—as Constance Wofsy made clear—the traditional lines of academic power and authority. By 1995, she noted, AIDS had become "big money." A disease "owned" by young, relatively unknown doctors in the epidemic's earliest years, AIDS, as Wofsy characterized it, now had a "big national reputation. It's big egos; it's very hierarchical and very power-based."

In the traditional academic model, the professors have the most power, the associates have the next most, and the assistants are kind of hanging out there hoping they get to the next step. In AIDS it was a cowboy disease, and the assistants were the only people doing it. So they had—the word "power" is hackneyed—they had something that junior people don't usually have: they had grants, they had media visibility, they had youth and energy, and that thing that we love, you know, going through crises, carrying out war. Not power in the traditional sense, but visibility, attention, whatever all those sorts of Roget's thesaurus words are, went to young, energetic, attractive people. But in the traditional model, it's very much a pyramid that goes up, and now the pyramid goes up. The people with the most experience, money, the heads of things, on the powerful committees, are professors—just the way it always was, and, to a relative degree, I include myself.

For Peter Selwyn, a seasoned AIDS practitioner, who had begun his AIDS work at Montefiore Hospital in the Bronx before moving to Yale–New Haven Hospital with Gerald Friedland, the esprit de corps of the early years had faded. So had the old idealism. He recognized unhappily that medicalization of AIDS cut two ways, producing both the more successful management of the disease through drugs and the reassertion of that academic "business-as-usual" style he had always tried to avoid.

I've found myself sometimes in this surprisingly wistful position where the last thing in the world I would want to do would be to hark back to the days when there were no therapies that were effective for this. But there's just something about the medicalization of AIDS that I think has brought with the benefit some other consequences that I don't think are that good. For example, there's this whole world now of clinical trials which is just an incredible maze of bureaucracy. And there's a lot of personal investment; people's whole careers are now tied up in AIDS clinical trials, and there's competition for grants and renewals and which drug is going to work. Some of the early camaraderie and solidarity has been lost I think—or innocence maybe?

Consistent with his politics, Selwyn evoked the image of a romantic and youthful hero of the Left to express his sense of loss, his discomfort in a world of AIDS medicine that was perhaps all too solid, routinized, and corrupting.

I have a poster of Che Guevara up on the wall in my office here. Maybe what I'm for is some perpetual revolution or some sort of new place to go. And in fact I've found myself thinking sometimes, What other hopeless, life-threatening disease can I focus my attention on now? Because now it seems like AIDS is just becoming commonplace and treatable.

Gerald Friedland, Selwyn's colleague at both Montefiore and Yale, had often spoken with him about the normalization or formalization of the medical response to the epidemic. For Friedland, who had been a graduate student in sociology, the reestablishment of relatively conservative social institutions and norms—the transformation of "comrades-in-arms" into colleagues—was both expected and necessary. Could their independence as "AIDS people," he wondered, be salvaged, even as they were incorporated into conventional medicine?

When AIDS [programs were] a small thing with [their] own identity, apart from the rest of the system, there's a limited amount that [they could] do. There's a penalty that you pay for not being integrated into the larger system, and you need the larger system. You have to feed on it, be connected to it; you can't construct your own system. So it is right somehow or other for these AIDS programs to be integrated into the larger health care system, and the trick then—this is what we're really struggling with in this decade—is how to retain both an independence and a coherence about AIDS programs. So we're still "the AIDS people," because we like that. It's important for preventing burnout, but also delivering services, to retain that and yet to integrate into the health care system and hope that maybe it will bend a little bit towards [us]. So the trick is to somehow or other make it part of the system and yet retain its uniqueness.

But Friedland understood that many of the clinical responses and values appropriate to a period of therapeutic impotence, particularly those that had defined him and the other "AIDS people," were fast fading. The introduction of successful drug therapies made caring and closeness less necessary, even as the growing patient census made them less feasible. The new standards of AIDS medicine rested instead on the skillful introduction of multiple medications.

Peter Selwyn and I talk a lot about this, we reminisce about the good old days when you couldn't do anything. Isn't that terrible? Because you had to focus on the caring part, and the love and interaction and the arrangement of a good death. Now we're more like doctors. We write prescriptions all the time; we wind up juggling medicines and different things like that—with so much involved in the technical aspects of care that you don't have time for some of the human things; and so it has changed. On the scale of things, it's much better. People live longer, their quality of life is better, but something has been lost in the increasing complexity of AIDS care.

Concurrent with its medicalization and normalization, AIDS work was becoming increasingly complex and esoteric. And its practitioners, even those like Alvin Friedman-Kien, who had followed AIDS-related research from the epidemic's inception, were finding themselves unable to keep up with the literature, even in their specialties.

There was a time when [I could be asked,] "Where was that paper on CD4 counts dropping after three months or four months with AZT?" I remembered it like that. But now the field is gigantic, there are 10 journals, there are millions of people infected and thousands of people all over the world doing research. I can't keep up with everything. I have trouble keeping up with just skin and Kaposi's sarcoma.

When Donald Abrams could teach Richard Chaisson everything there was to know about AIDS in five minutes, treating under conditions of therapeutic ignorance was one of the principal challenges faced by physicians. By 1995, Constance Wofsy, who, like Friedman-Kien, discovered that keeping current was among her greatest burdens, recast the past to claim, ironically, that unequivocal ignorance had provided her with confidence and comfort.

You knew what there was to know, which wasn't much, but you knew that you knew what there was. And it was a great sense of confidence, not in knowing the answers, but in knowing when you could say, "The answer isn't known." That was 10 years ago. It's challenging to keep up. There is so much information, and so much opinion, that to be a general AIDS physician actually is about as challenging as being a general internist. People have become subspecialists, you know.

In the new era of complex therapies, goodwill and commitment were no longer adequate guides: A highly technical expertise was needed. This, too, signaled the normalization of AIDS. Only those trained and experienced in AIDS possessed the requisite skills and complex knowledge needed to provide adequate medical care.

AIDS Has Been Good to Us

Years of AIDS work—starting with the initial period of impotence—had fundamentally affected the professional lives of the first generation of AIDS doctors. Many had gained formidable reputations and enhanced and accelerated their careers. Others had found at last what had long eluded them: a place for themselves in medicine. Some had located in the epidemic an opportunity to express social outrage through medical action. And almost all had found a new affinity group that transcended the narrow confines of medical specialization.

Among the few physicians who, somewhat older, had already achieved some recognition before the epidemic, a number found that their AIDS work had added significant luster to their professional lives.

Alvin Friedman-Kien, who had worked at the National Institutes of Health and enjoyed prominence as a virologist and dermatologist, discovered that AIDS served to invigorate an already mature scientific career.

> Most physicians at my stage in life would have been taking a backseat in what their work was about, perhaps relaxing more and spending more time in personal things rather than keeping up with the literature and keeping up with professional awareness of the latest developments in the field. What AIDS did at a time in my life when most of my colleagues were withdrawing a bit—I found myself suddenly being more productive than I've ever been. I've probably published more papers in the past 15 years than I published earlier, and even at this very moment I probably keep up more with what's going on in the literature related to my field than most people do. And so it's kept me very acute. It's a creative moment in your life.

Marcus Conant had a well-established dermatological practice and academic status at the University of California in San Francisco; the epidemic enhanced his stature among peers with whom he shared years of epidemic struggle and within his specialty, the members of which had refused early on to acknowledge AIDS when he had first brought it to their attention.

> I guess among my peers it is important to me to be recognized as someone who is expert, who is articulate, who is knowledgeable, who is compassionate, and I have achieved that in not only my specialty, but, more importantly, in the specialty that arose after the beginning of AIDS. We now have a group of people who identify themselves as AIDS treaters. It was never a goal for me to be recognized by this group of people, but at this point in my life I am pleased and proud that I am recognized by my peers as someone who is an equal among very, very competent physicians. It's been an interesting metamorphosis because I went from a dermatologist who was well known nationally to an AIDS doctor who's well known nationally, and am now seen by my dermatological colleagues as even more prominent than I had been before the AIDS epidemic, because now I'm seen as a dermatologist who has made a contribution to another major field.

For many younger physicians, either in or barely out of medical school, whose careers and commitments were still developing, the AIDS epidemic proved formative and far-reaching. Paul Volberding had just completed his oncology fellowship when he became fascinated by a disease that was to make his reputation. He had, he admitted, no previous or competing scientific stature: "AIDS" he said, " is my career trajectory." Another prominent veteran, Sheldon Landesman, infectious disease specialist in the largest of New York City's public hospitals in the early 1980s, was both honest and ironic when he confessed, "AIDS has been very good to me. It's given me a professional career. It's given me something that is important, interesting, challenging, and intellectually stimulating, and you can't ask for anything more."

A few of the younger physicians believed that they would have achieved significant academic status without the epidemic. But AIDS allowed them to go further than they would have, or to attain their high positions at an accelerated rate. Jerome Groopman, who had been warned when he left Los Angeles for Boston that he would be wasting the professional capital he had amassed doing early AIDS work, observed,

> AIDS definitely accelerated my career. I was one of the youngest people ever promoted to full professor at Harvard. Here, they sort of take your c.v. and put it on a balance scale and see how many papers you've published. So the opportunity to publish quality papers in a very short period of time was enormous, because there was a new disease. Every three months you had information that was publishable, and even though it took awhile for the government to ramp up and get grants, if you were writing good grants and stuff you were getting funded. So I had funding and I had papers, which is the currency of academic advancement here, as in most places.

In San Francisco, Donald Abrams, who had quickly become a national AIDS figure, acknowledged, "My promotions in academia have been accelerated; I did in eight years what people do in 16 years, and, you know, obviously it's because of my work in AIDS and HIV." Finally, Howard Minkoff, when assessing his career, noted:

> To be honest with you, in the field of obstetrics, I'm known for other things. . . . I was one of the first people to point out the relationship between vaginal pathogens and preterm birth. I was already "on the circuit" in obstetrics. I think that I would have been

a tenured professor—only it probably would have taken a bit longer. But many of the academic opportunities I have would not have come my way. I don't think I would have been a distinguished professor. I don't think I would ever have had the Assistant Secretary of Health Award. And more importantly, I would not have had the richness of experience in fields beyond my own.

But many physicians were less certain that they would have achieved their medical prominence and national stature without the epidemic. Molly Cooke, whose professional recognition rested on her AIDS-related teaching and clinical and behavioral research work, admitted, " I don't know what I would be doing, but I'm sure it wouldn't be as interesting as this. . . . I'm not a bit ashamed to say that I don't think I would be anywhere near as successful in academics had it not been for AIDS." Her colleague in San Francisco, Stephen Follansbee, a prominent infectious disease specialist, recalled, "I had no status prior to HIV. The question, Would I be where I am if there weren't HIV? is a question that I'm very clear what the answer is. . . . I'd be another community physician, probably practicing internal medicine and some infectious disease. So I've benefited incredibly." In Newark's inner city, Anita Vaughn sadly recognized, "If I wasn't involved in HIV, most people wouldn't know what I do; I could be the most wonderful doctor in the world, but if my whole universe [was] the health center here, it wouldn't mean anything except to my patients."

Others found their careers enriched because AIDS offered them, in essence, a second chance to find what they had initially sought in medicine. For Carol Brosgart, who had resigned from a residency program in pediatrics to work in public health to have the time to start her family, the AIDS epidemic allowed her reentry into the world of academic medicine and research. As a leftist and a feminist, she found in AIDS a unique opportunity to join her progressive politics to what she loved in traditional but conservative medicine.

I was a very active political activist-leftist who had a little bit of a hard time figuring out where I fit in medicine. If you're an activist, you end up veering towards pediatrics or community medicine or public health; that's where a lot of more socially conscious physicians ended up. That I ended up in AIDS or gravitat[ed] towards it doesn't seem surprising to me. And I was sort of in the right place. I was in public health. And because I had made a decision to have children and family, I pulled out of academia before I was really ready to. I always wanted to go back. So [through AIDS] being able to be involved in clinical research and teaching as a community physician fulfills those sorts of academic yearnings of mine. So I kind of got to marry those things together.

For those whose careers were foundering and who might have been lost to medicine entirely, the AIDS epidemic sometimes provided something like a resurrection. John Mazzullo, for example, whose private and public life had been laced by experiences of failure and who had retreated professionally to working in a student health clinic, discovered in AIDS a galvanizing personal focus. As a gay man and internist, the epidemic renewed him and gave his medicine a purpose it had entirely lacked before.

[Without AIDS], I probably wouldn't have had a career because I was floundering. I was thinking of perhaps leaving Boston, going to New York, kind of starting anew. So I was really unhappy with general internal medicine. It hadn't gotten to me. And I certainly was floundering in clinical pharmacology. So I tried different things. I tried general medicine. I thought about rheumatology. I stopped reading the *New England Journal*. I stopped going to conferences. So AIDS gave me back my scholarliness. It gave me back a reason to read the *New England Journal*. It gave me reason to go to conferences, and it gave me a subspecialty that made primary care worthwhile.

But not all physicians saw their careers transformed or if changed, changed for the better. Donald Armstrong, an older and senior doctor, chief of infectious disease at Memorial Sloan-Kettering Cancer Center in New York, although intensely interested in AIDS, felt the epidemic had left his position and status largely unchanged. "I've been working in opportunistic infections all along, before AIDS came along, and I'm still working in them. So it really hasn't changed my career very much."

And Jeffrey Laurence, an oncologist and virologist at New York Hospital, and, like Armstrong, focused primarily on laboratory research, thought his career owed little to the AIDS epidemic. Well trained and able, a *Wunderkind* who graduated from Columbia at age 18 and medical school three years later, he might, in fact, have had a more prominent career had he grappled with other scientific matters.

I have an ego the size of the state of Texas. I was a Rhodes scholar; I graduated at some ridiculously young age. Whatever I did was going to be important. I was doing AIDS because I was really very interested in it. I have the feeling that if I'd done something more mainstream I might have been more successful.

For a few, the AIDS epidemic, far from serving to enhance or accelerate their careers, proved a sad conclusion. Doctors who treated patients with hemophilia not only saw them die of iatrogenic HIV infection, but also lost the trust and affection of many patients and families with whom they had worked for years. AIDS is a professional tragedy that casts its shadow over the hemophilia treaters, among them Margaret Hilgartner.

Because of that shadow, I'm a little bit more in a hurry to [retire] than I would be otherwise. Because I've enjoyed the work tremendously, I really have. And I've enjoyed what I've been able to do, and it's nice to be able to think of the unit that I helped develop move on as the new hospital grows. But the specter is hanging there; and it hurts to think that it's going to destroy whatever last years I've got.

In one unique example of personal sacrifice, Neil Schram, nephrologist at Kaiser-Permanente in Los Angeles, put AIDS before his own professional development. Forced to educate himself about and treat people with AIDS while simultaneously maintaining a full load of nephrology patients, Schram was unable to keep current in his specialty.

Now, [in 1995], I'm going back and trying to re-update myself. But for at least five years I could not attend any nephrology conference; I couldn't do it. Whatever time I had had to go to staying up on HIV disease. . . . And that was hard for me to accept. To be honest, I thought of myself by 1980 as probably the best nephrologist in Kaiser-Permanente in Southern California. I no longer consider myself that. Some of my best skills were lost over the years— knowledge skills. . . . It's basically having dropped out of keeping current for five years. I have now in nephrology the challenge of keeping current and learning what I missed for the five years, and that gets very difficult to do. So I accept that I will never be the quality nephrologist that I was. I'm not bad. I'm good. But I'm not as good as I was.

Even among those for whom the epidemic provided personal successes, these could have a bittersweet quality. A small number of practitioners saw their careers soar during the earliest years, only to see their prominence fade. A few of these, among them Fred Siegal and Michael Gottlieb, were in part victims of the competitive politics of major medical centers. Siegal, a young clinical immunologist, published one of the earliest articles on AIDS in the *New England Journal of Medicine*, organized the initial international conference on what came to be known as AIDS at Mt. Sinai Medical Center in New York in 1982, and wrote, with his wife, one of the first books on the disease targeted to a nonmedical audience. During those years, he, like Gottlieb in Los Angeles, became a public medical voice and face, sought after by the media hungry for AIDS stories. Perhaps his early rise to prominence, along with his refusal to collaborate with powerful figures at New York's Mt. Sinai Medical Center, fostered an environment hostile to his presence.

And in a way, I think what happened to me at Sinai is what happened to Mike Gottlieb at UCLA. With all of the surge of interest in AIDS nationally, I was always deluged by requests for lectures, requests for interviews with the press. I became a kind of high-profile person at a rather young age in this maelstrom of interest and activity. As I said to my kids at one point, the greatest moment of my life was having my picture in *Rolling Stone* magazine. And I was on committees, and I was doing all kinds of other things, and I think it was resented roundly at Sinai. . . . So I'm sort of philosophical about it, but I understand that Mike Gottlieb encountered more or less the same kind of thing at UCLA and that that's why he left, because people were jealous of him.

Moving to another New York area hospital, Long Island Jewish, Siegal increasingly devoted himself to patient care instead of research. And as many more physicians and researchers got involved in the epidemic, he increasingly became an integral—rather than prominent—part of the AIDS landscape—a reality with which he had to make his peace.

I've been diluted out. I like to call it that because it's the easiest way to describe it. There are now lots of people who know how to deal with AIDS. It's a disease that a lot of people know about, that they write about. There are some people who have remained in the spotlight from the very beginning, and probably the one who most stands out is Paul Volberding, and a few other people like him. But I think many of the early AIDS researchers have sort of faded into the background because there's been such an extraordinary outpouring of brilliant people into this area. And because, after all, to a certain extent one becomes obsolescent in science unless one is really terrific or finds the time. And so, I decided a while ago that for me the clinical part was the part that I loved. I wanted to maintain a presence in the science of AIDS, but I didn't have illusions that I could become the molecular biologist or virologist that I never was to begin with. And so my role in the scientific part has become more of a reviewer and a member of a study section [at the National Institutes of Health] for a while. I'm sort of basking in my old age, as it were, as a scientist.

But not only researchers were "diluted out." During the early phase of the epidemic, physicians, often gay doctors watching the epidemic emerge in their offices, provided a growing body of valuable clinical observations. Because of this wealth of clinical experience, they were invaluable to academic and government researchers, who invited them to local and national conferences. Within the gay communities, these physicians became known not only because they would treat people with AIDS but also because they sounded the tocsin about the new disease and its risk factors, and they wrote the first guides to treatment and prevention. Over time, many of these doctors, among them James Campbell, "faded into the background," returning to the relative obscurity of their private practices.

I think [in 1982 and 1983] I felt like I was really very much closer to the front lines of the AIDS epidemic than I do now. We were the people who were seeing the disease. [The first researchers] were the people working in labs, and together we were day to day making new observations which had never been reported. They were relying quite heavily on our input. I don't feel like I have quite the responsibility that I had then. In 1981–1985, I was one of the people formulating guidelines for the management of people who had HIV or whatever it was called then. I was also one of the few people that had seen, by the end of 1984, probably more cases of AIDS than they had reported in my home state of Indiana. I felt like I was an expert in the field due to my extensive experience. Now HIV is something that most primary care physicians see. Also, there is a "standard of care" for people with AIDS or HIV infection, and I feel I'm more or less going through a routine. And now I'm not on the cutting edge; it was exciting to be on the cutting edge.

Even those who retained a national or international reputation understood how transient were their positions and glory. Neil Schram, who, in addition to his clinical work, played a prominent AIDS political role for the Los Angeles gay community, made that point, albeit ironically. "My 15 minutes of fame lasted years. It was great. It really was. For a couple of years it was hard to get out of it. I don't have the energy for it anymore. I really don't." If fame was both an opportunity and a burden for Schram, for Gerald Friedland it was another opportunity to put himself and his work into perspective. "AIDS has been a wonderful teacher. It's certainly made me famous for a transient period of time, *Dr. Famous Fleeting*. And it continues to make me humble."

Looking Back: Life and AIDS

Years of exhaustion, the passage of time, and aging had left a number of AIDS doctors tired. For example, Peter Selwyn doubted that he could muster sufficient drive to match that of a decade earlier.

> For years I actually enjoyed staying up all night writing papers. And I would literally, one day a week, just stay up all night and write or read and then write, and so I was very productive, and I wrote many, many papers, book chapters and things. But there was just this sense of urgency that I had or a feeling that there was so much that had to be put out. [There] was the feeling, there was just so much that had to be done. I don't think that now, 10 plus years later, that I either could do that anymore or that I would want to.

Constance Wofsy, wearied by her own struggle with breast cancer, began to discover an empathy for the senior professors and researchers who had remained aloof from AIDS, those who had failed to become "gripped" by the powerful new epidemic. She had, in the intervening years, started to become like them.

> I now see on the horizon the emerging infectious diseases. The professors aren't going to roll up their sleeves and take on ebola. The Turks are going to say, "Okay, this is hot, I've got energy, I'm young, I'll do it." They're the ones. And I go, "Oh, God, you know, forget it. Just don't even talk about a new infectious disease to me; I'm exhausted. I gave at the office already; get some young person." And then the young person's on TV and getting interviews. I

think, Thank God that young energy is there. Give them the money; give them the positions. Please, do the work. I don't have the energy; he doesn't have the energy; she doesn't have it. We've done our thing. And I understand why the old-time infectious disease people now didn't look at AIDS and go, Wow! Isn't that interesting? They said, "Oh, I got my grants on rhinovirus," or e-coli or whatever. "Please, I'm tired."

Even when exhausted by the demands of years of epidemic involvement, however, many gay AIDS doctors found it difficult to step back. This was especially so for those, like Stosh Ostrow in Atlanta, who shared with their patients infection with HIV.

So I'm a doctor who's treating people with a disease that is often fatal. I have the disease myself. I'm politically involved in those aspects of the disease. I've been arrested as a result of my political involvement. I've been in the media. I've had to fight with my parents over this. It is pervasive. It involves every aspect of my life. There have been times when I've had to say, "Okay, I can't do this anymore." [But] I certainly can't pull back from my own disease— it's there! And I can't pull back from my practice—it's my living, it's my life. So sometimes I cut back on the community involvement aspects, and I'm not quite as active as I have been.

Not only had AIDS affected the professional lives of those who had been involved in providing care over the past decade and more; it had been, for many, a defining life experience. Alexandra Levine was direct in her assessment of the epidemic's impact.

There's no question that AIDS allowed my life to be bigger than it would have been otherwise. . . . I'm walking into the White House; I'm talking to the president. In a million years that would never have happened to me. . . . One of the things that is so amazing to me . . . is the unbelievable joy of having been in the middle of something that was so prominent in the lifetime in which you lived and to really understand what it was about from the inside out. . . . The other part of it, the personal part, is the whimsy of fate, how everything that I ended up doing in life would have been so much different if it had not been for that germ. It is so awesome to think about it: a germ changed my life, and I wasn't even infected by it.

For some, it was the image of war that helped to explain the all-pervading impact of AIDS. Michael Gottlieb had experienced the elation of fame when describing the first cohort of men with AIDS in 1981 and had then suffered humiliation at the hands of his academic superiors at UCLA as well as the end of a marriage. For him, Vietnam provided the metaphor.

> One of the reasons I wound up going to medical school was not to go to Vietnam. Well, AIDS has been my Vietnam. Young men went to Vietnam, and their courage and their personalities were sort of steeled for their future life. . . . What I've seen has profoundly changed my life and my outlook, and I feel much more complete as a man and a human being than I was prior to 1980.

For Donald Kotler, whose Jewish identity was so crucial to his initial commitment to AIDS, the metaphor was the Warsaw Ghetto Uprising.

> I'm an outsider and an outsider and an outsider, and I deal with very highly emotional things in a way that I'm still an outsider. . . . I'm fighting Hitler when I do this. In some way, I was cheated by being born after World War II into an environment where people just wanted to be American and move away from their heritage. It's like the Warsaw Ghetto. I'm sort of fighting but can't win. It's the fight that's the honor.

Less drawn to such public imagery, Hermann Mendez, who had cared for children and babies with AIDS in Brooklyn, focused on how AIDS had given him a sense of fulfillment.

> In many aspects it's shown me my limits, my definite limits. In many respects it has humbled me a lot. It has made me feel fulfilled also. It also allows me to feel if something happens to me now, and I'm not there tomorrow, that I lived for something that was worthwhile. It fits my ideals. It fits into my idea of helping people.

AIDS was not, however, always so deeply felt, so life defining. Abigail Zuger resisted the tendency of many to elide the worlds of work and identity. "I'm just a doctor," she said simply, "who happens to be wandering through this particular epidemic." Judith Currier, who had moved from Boston to Los Angeles, also rejected any effort to confound her work as a doctor in AIDS with the notion that her identity was synonymous with her professional commitments. She was, she said, not an AIDS doctor. To the extent that a single identity was called for, she was, referring to her son, "Andy's mom."

At times the process could take on psychologically ominous dimensions. Said Donald Kotler,

I don't have time for a boat. I don't have time for a stamp collection. I don't have time for anything. An occasional mystery novel if I'm really away and relax some. But nothing else. Aside from my family and their development I have a lot of trouble getting excited about other things. . . . There's no excitement for the simple things. I can't be interested in sports anymore or get addicted to a television program because none of that stuff really is important.

For gay physicians the epidemic, which involved friends and lovers as well as patients, had a profound and special personal significance. "AIDS has been the defining experience of my life," said Ronald Grossman. A generation younger, Howard Grossman, who had worked with Ronald at the epidemic's onset, had always wanted a "career that would be a life." And that is what he had made of his work treating friends, becoming friends with patients. It came at a price, however, because there was no separation between his professional and private worlds. Such overarching involvement is precisely what had transformed the life of John Mazzullo.

There's a group of people who really have seen me change professionally and saw me when I kind of went through the motions of my job, doing it okay but not galvanized. And I think, for those people, seeing how much I really love this job—every AIDS doctor works incredible hours, but I'm here at seven o'clock, and I go home at six o'clock, usually to another meeting that starts at seven o'clock. But I'm not tired.

With all its misery and grief, AIDS thus provided a number of gay physicians a juncture where sexual, personal, and professional identities could join, so that medicine became a more intensely meaningful vocation. Marcus Conant confessed that he had been unhappy before the epidemic despite his prominence. He had gone into medicine at the behest of a strong-willed mother and chose dermatology partly in reaction to his mentor, Dr. Eugene Stead. Stead's work life, including making

6:30 hospital rounds every day of the year, struck his student as onerous, compelling a narrow existence. Conant wanted something different.

You can do dermatology from 9:00 in the morning until 4:00 in the afternoon, make a good living, teach at a university, find a research project that's really interesting, and yet have a whole other life. You can go to the opera, you can have friends in for dinner, you can do whatever you like. And I did that from 1964 until 1981. And then AIDS came along. I became a doctor because my mother wanted me to be a doctor. I am a doctor. I get up at 5:30 in the morning now because I absolutely love what I do. It has nothing to do with my mother anymore. And I love what I do; I find it invigorating. If there is anything wrong, [it's that] I do too much of it. I do a 12- to 14-hour day seven days a week. But what an incredible joy to have something challenging, that's intellectually invigorating, that you can see growing, that's prospering, and that's doing good. So at this point—and it began shortly after the AIDS epidemic began—I suddenly found out who and what I was, or who and what I was going to be. I tried to go into dermatology to get away from this physician who had become this creature who was totally dominated by his profession, Dr. Stead. And I, in fact, became the same thing. And maybe that was one of the reasons it scared me so much to begin with. I mean, maybe at some level I realized if I'm not careful that's going to happen to me. I don't recall ever thinking that at the time, but certainly it did. And I hope Gene Stead was as happy as I am today.

Intense involvement over the years of epidemic work almost inevitably had an impact on the most intimate relationships of AIDS doctors. This was especially the case for those who were heterosexual. AIDS could be a world apart, drawing spouses away from each other, parents from children. Eric Goosby found that his commitment to AIDS and the attendant stress was a dark place in his marriage where communication and support had become impossible.

It's funny. [My wife] knew what I was going through. I would verbalize it, but there wouldn't be a long discussion around it. It was important to me to have something other than that, so I didn't really want to talk to her a lot about it. She knew what was going on and felt fairly helpless. From her perspective, I became driven, kind of obsessed. She saw it as something that she had to step back

[from] and just let me kind of go through, and realized that she didn't really have a role [in] it. I never found any satisfaction or decompression of my feelings from talking with her. It was something that she didn't share with me.

Alexandra Levine's husband, also a physician, found himself drawn to psychoanalytic training as a way of confronting the gulf.

[He] was seeing that this had invaded my soul. I was absolutely committed to something in my life other than him. And he understood that. And that was a hole. And he didn't feel good about it.

Not all AIDS doctors became as deeply involved as Alexandra Levine. Even among those who did, not all accepted the rigors of public engagements. To do so meant to face a number of difficulties, among them how to balance the demands of AIDS work with those of family life, particularly the needs of younger children. That was virtually always a woman's concern. Torn, Carol Brosgart shared her uncertainties with her close colleague and friend, Constance Wofsy.

That's a lot of what Connie and I talked about, . . . both of us figuring out how you do this job which takes—it's not a full-time job; it's a full-time life—and where do you draw the line? When do you accept a speaking engagement and when don't you? How many times can you be away in a month? How do you stay in touch with your kids and what's going on with them? We never wanted to miss a concert, a performance, a game. . . . I remember talking to Connie when I went to [the International AIDS Meeting in Stockholm in 1988]. It meant missing my oldest daughter's high school graduation and my other daughter's eighth birthday. And it was a big decision. And my kids said it was okay, and I did it, and I loved the Stockholm meeting but I felt very bad. And the year—I guess '91—which was the Italian meeting, and Connie and I had a number of things planned in and around that meeting, at the last moment I called Connie and said, "Connie, I'm not going to go. I've just been gone too much." It was a day or two before I was supposed to go, and [my daughter] burst into tears. She wanted her mommy to be there. And I canceled. . . . I think you just try to do your best, and sometimes it isn't your best and everyone's going to be a little disappointed.

Deborah Cotton was haunted by the fear that on one journey she might die.

> I don't like being away from my kids, so very often I get to the meeting late and leave early. . . . Like many women in my era, there's a lot of guilt about my profession versus my personal life. And one of my big fears is that either something would happen to one of my kids and I couldn't get back, or my other ongoing paranoia is, What if this plane crashed? Was it worth my putting myself on these planes and flying through any kind of weather when I could be leaving these children motherless?

While men evidenced little such anxiety and rarely described decisions to restrict their professional commitments because of the needs of their children, nevertheless, when looking back over the years of involvement with AIDS, some did wonder about the toll that might have been taken. "If there's a price to be paid, it may be personal," said Howard Minkoff, "in the sense that when my kids were very young I was on the road a lot."

> I spent a lot of time being in a world that I didn't have to, but you do get caught up in it. You get an opportunity to meet with a lot of interesting people. You get away from your family; you get a little bit too full of yourself. I remember I had just come back from a meeting, and I came in the house. My oldest daughter was upstairs, and my wife said to my daughter, "Come downstairs. Dad's on TV, on the national news." "I don't want to see a TV daddy; I want to see the real Daddy." But that was how it was. Kids are singularly unimpressed with any of this stuff. They just want you to be there.

In 1995, Paul Volberding, who, since the epidemic's earliest years, had been a central figure in the international AIDS arena, thought back on the previous decade and a half with mixed emotions. He had derived enormous satisfaction from his work but wondered about the costs.

> You're on the important committees. You're going to the important meetings. You're giving important [speeches]. You're testifying at important hearings. You have to do that. You can't be famous without doing that. Maybe it's not synonymous, but it's required; it's a prerequisite. And what you give up, what I gave up, [produced]

tension in my marriage, the feeling of having lost time with my family, that I've been distracted from things that I think ultimately are going to feel more important for things that are truly less important. . . . I accept what I've done. I've enjoyed it, loved it, and at the same time I regret it. It's not that I go around feeling sorry that I did what I did, but I recognize the price that I've paid for it. And I hope my marriage survives; I hope that my kids grow up healthy and loving and that they'll forgive me for being distracted.

However justified and rationalized, the toll was tellingly underscored by Deborah Cotton, who recalled her son's pointed observation.

I remember once, when my oldest was about 13, on Mother's Day, he said, "You know, Mom, you are a really great mother." And before I even had a chance to bask in that for 30 seconds, he said, "You know, for somebody who does it on the side, the way you do."

In the end, those who had chosen to work in the AIDS epidemic—whether the personal impacts were deep or more superficial, whether they had attained professional prominence or had remained clinicians known primarily to those for whom they cared—had faced the challenge of a lifetime. For Richard Chaisson, it was that collective experience that defined his generation's effort.

There was an *esprit de corps* that continues to this day. There's a very special connection there that will never erode, because we were all there together. And I think it was melded by a number of different factors: the newness and the strangeness, the stigma, that we were stepping into this epidemic that other people were condemning or walking away from or refusing to have anything to do with, that we were dealing with things that were absolutely bewildering to us but learning all the time. There's the evolution of experience that everyone shared. Everyone sort of grew up together, and I think that the war analogy really fits there, that we all trudged through the trenches together but had an experience that was different from almost anyone else in the world. When you go to medical school, or you go to your internship, you're entering a club of sorts where you suffer and you build bonds with colleagues who are going through the same thing. But generations of people have gone through it, and you get through it, and then you sort of try to go on with your life. But this was different, because there was no precedent for it. We were doing it for the first time in history.

What no one could know for certain in 1995, 14 years after the onset of the epidemic, was how profoundly the transformations in the clinical management of AIDS—the process of reintegration into medicine, the demands of specialization, the waning of the sense of epidemic crisis— would affect the world of AIDS doctors, how the ties and identities forged in the "dark years" would atrophy.

2000
AN EPILOGUE

The good news continues in the battle against
AIDS. In the United States, the age-adjusted
death rate among people with human immunodeficiency virus (HIV) in 1997 was less than
40 percent of what it was in 1995. The 16,685
deaths in 1997 represent the lowest annual total
in nearly a decade. . . . Not only has mortality
from AIDS decreased, but so has the incidence
of AIDS among those who have HIV infection.
. . . The dramatic declines in morbidity and mortality due to AIDS in Western nations are the
result of the widespread use of potent combinations of antiretroviral drugs.

The New England Journal of Medicine
December 24, 1998

The wave of therapeutic optimism that began to swell in 1995 had produced by mid-1996 a mood approaching euphoria in the world of AIDS.
The protease inhibitors and combination therapy would, it was believed,
change AIDS, transform it in a way that would subdue it for increasingly
extended periods.[1] In the next years, the hopes of the enthusiasts seemed
close to realization. In 1998, the seventeenth year of the epidemic, hospital wards were emptying; the lives of many patients had been radically
improved. Engaged since the very earliest days of the epidemic and
having experienced the optimism and then the disappointment that accompanied the introduction of AZT in 1987, Ronald Grossman had to
reach back to breakthroughs of the late nineteenth century, when the
germ theory of infection was given its initial scientific foundation, to

imagine a comparable moment: "I feel like I am living in the time of a Pasteur or Semmelweiss."

Donald Kotler had been among the most acerbic critics of the new chemotherapies. In 1995 he saw in the trumpeted hopes aroused by the protease inhibitors yet another example of the promotion of drugs that would provide greater benefit to researchers than to their patients. By 1998 he was compelled to note, if somewhat grudgingly, that progress had outstripped his expectations.

> Things are better than they were. We've gone from real despair, which I guess was Berlin, to real euphoria in Vancouver. [Now we're in the middle.] I don't want to minimize [what's gone on], having been shown to be wrong before. But it's only two years.

Richard Chaisson went further.

> My initial response was more pessimistic than the events of the last two years would warrant. The new drugs are extraordinary. They're having an extraordinary effect. It's amazing, the effect that they're having. However, they are not having the effect of curing people; and so ultimately the question is how long will this last. But the fact that people who were months away from dying are robust and healthy and enjoying life now—two, three years afterwards—is wonderful. I haven't had a patient die for 10 or 11 months. So it's gone from constant death to very infrequent death. Our memorial services are not nearly as frequent, and the numbers are quite small. And they're very often memorials for people who died of causes unrelated to AIDS. Mortality in our clinic in the last three years has fallen by about 65 percent.

For Wafaa El-Sadr, who oversaw the care of poor African-American women and men at Harlem Hospital in New York, the change could be seen in her patients.

> Before, you really had to talk about death and illness so much of the time, and now you're really talking about life. You're talking about what's happening in their life. You're managing side effects and so on, but it's very different. [One] patient told me the other day, "You know, I'm going to use this time to go to school. I'm going to go to school because I know they're going to make me go to work, so I want to get a good job."

Perhaps more striking was her characterization of her Friday clinic.

> I would walk into clinic several years ago on Fridays and just look—
> I always look—at the waiting room to see who's there. And there
> were a lot of sick people, leaning against the wall, very sick people.
> And now it's just amazing. I walk in, and it's like bubbling with
> energy and conversation, people hanging outside the door, smoking
> cigarettes, whatever; it's just filled with life and energy. I think it's
> wonderful. When I see a sick person today at that clinic it's unusual.
> The very sick people are in the hospital. It's almost like having a
> well-baby clinic. Maybe the bubble will burst, but it's wonderful.
> It's wonderful.

But even amid the excitement there was reason for concern. A few
took the occasion to focus on what the current successes suggested about
earlier efforts. Physician enthusiasm and patient desperation had con-
spired to injure the most compliant—those who embraced their doctors'
recommendations. Charles van der Horst was struck by the fact that it
was his patient Gio, who had over the years refused antiretroviral therapy, who was best positioned to benefit from combination therapy.

> Look what we did: we made terrible mistakes; and no one's written
> about that. We did sequential monotherapy [giving only a single
> drug at a time] for the last 10 years. We've got 300,000 patients
> who have had sequential monotherapy, so they're resistant to AZT,
> 3TC, ddI, ddC, d4T. And now the only thing left are the protease
> inhibitors. So we were wrong. We should have not treated it. And
> the activists were wrong.

Joseph Sonnabend, for years an outsider who had been bitterly critical
of the approval of AZT in the mid-1980s, believed the rash of enthusiasm
carried with it dangers for patients. Acknowledging that the new therapies had had a very positive effect on sicker individuals, he remained
unconvinced that early treatment of asymptomatic disease would prove
beneficial. Sonnabend was troubled by

> the incredible pressure placed on physicians and patients to start
> virtually all asymptomatic individuals on antiviral therapy, in the
> absence of any evidence, other than theoretical, that years of taking
> drugs will result in a better or worse clinical outcome or make no
> difference.

Even among those who could benefit from the new treatments, however, there were problems.[2] Many could not tolerate the drug combinations. Others found the demanding medical regimen impossible to sustain. In some studies, close to half of patients being treated, while symptom free, had virally "broken through," their virus counts rising to troubling levels. No one could tell for sure what the ultimate clinical significance of those increasing viral loads would be in such patients. Finally, there were the disturbing visible and not-so-visible side effects. As a gastroenterologist, Donald Kotler was acutely aware of the swollen bodies, the humpbacks, and the metabolic changes.

If the complications of the disorder that we're starting to see now with the high cholesterols and high triglycerides translate, and they will, into heart attacks and strokes, well then we really may have a rough road ahead of us. And we're just sort of in the eye of the storm.

Most worrisome was the fear that viral resistance would sooner rather than later render the new therapeutic regimens ineffective, once again setting the stage for the cascade of events that would make patients vulnerable, ushering in the return of death. Gerald Friedland ruefully anticipated such a possibility.

It's really been wonderful, so much so that it's almost hard to remember what it was like when everybody was dying. It's really extraordinary; it's a magical moment. [But] I think it will be transient. I've been very happy, very quick, to unlearn the death part [of my work], even though I got pretty good at it; it became incorporated into my persona. I say to a lot of my colleagues that we have to prepare ourselves because we're going to be dealing with death and dying again, because many of our patients are going to fail the therapies that they're on now. And I'm looking forward to that with a great deal of dread, and everyone is having the same feelings; [there is] almost a bit of denial. So I think the next couple of years are going to be very interesting as we almost certainly get back into where we were before, when this magical moment in the epidemic recedes again.

For James Oleske, who had cared for dying children in Newark since the early 1980s, the prospect of witnessing a resurgence in deaths of his no longer very young patients challenged the protective myths that had served him so well in previous years.

We only had one death [in 1998]. In 1996 we peaked with 34 deaths in our program, and it was devastating. Not having to go to Perry's Funeral Home is pretty nice. I know that even though I now have a big cohort that are surviving into their teenage years, there's going to come a time when they're going to start dying again. I can't believe—and maybe that's my lack of hope, and I feel bad saying this—but I just can't believe that we're not going to have a rebound, [when] my 16-, 17-, 18-year-olds hit a wall and then have another bad year. Maybe that's not going to happen; maybe with the newer drugs and the newer treatments there will be more breakthroughs, but I have to say there's sort of a hidden fear that I don't even talk about, that next year or the year after all of these kids that have survived are all going to die on us. These are kids that we've known now for 15 years, so it's going to be maybe a worse time if that happens. Maybe I should practice what I preach: I always say you should have hope and focus on the one child and do all you can and not worry about all of the things that are going to happen. But there's a part of me that dreads, possibly, the death of a lot of our older kids, when they all hit the wall together and they all get cryptosporidiosis and they all get wasting.

Not all caregivers responded to the dramatic changes of the years between 1995 and 1999 with equal enthusiasm. For some, changes in the very aspects of AIDS work that had served to draw them close presented an ironic, if unacknowledged, threat. Hermann Mendez, who, like Oleske, worked with children, was struck by the seemingly troubled response of some of his colleagues in Brooklyn.

About the switch from [threatening disease] to chronic illness, I have to say to you that, for me personally, I'm okay with it. For the staff as a whole and for the providers as a whole, I don't know. I have intuitively this notion that perhaps people that selected themselves out to come to work in this field with a dying population are finding themselves in a field where the patients won't die. Our staff find themselves dealing with people on a long-term basis when they were never prepared to deal with that. . . . I've begun to observe some uncontrolled anger on the part of the provider, [what I call] the Lazarus syndrome by proxy, a reaction to the shift from death to chronic illness. You're no longer offering comfort and quality of life to people who are going to be dying; now you have to live with people whose lifestyles maybe you can't stand, or poverty or lack of education, use of drugs, et cetera, you may not like. They are not dying, and you have to live with that.

Whether they responded like Mendez's colleagues or with great joy, whether they could acknowledge the prospect of a resurgence in deaths or not, no one involved in the care of AIDS patients could deny that 1999 was different, even if it was only an interregnum. In this period when the carnage had ended, it was possible for Carol Brosgart to announce a truce, if not a lasting peace. "It's not like war anymore."

For most of those who had committed themselves to AIDS medicine, 1999 made possible the further routinization of AIDS care, the stabilization of AIDS practices, if at a lower level of intensity. Like Donna Mildvan, they saw their professional commitments to AIDS as undiminished. "I'm here for the duration. I was there in the beginning, I want to be there when we kiss it good-bye. I want to see it sail off into the sunset."

A few, however, among them some of the most intensely involved, took the occasion to make changes that they would scarcely have considered in the grimmest years of the epidemic. Peter Selwyn, who had moved from the Bronx to Yale, and who had discovered in his AIDS work the need to care for the dying through the provision of palliation, decided to leave the Yale AIDS service. He returned to Montefiore to be the chief of the Department of Family Medicine and to direct the palliative care service. In coming back to Montefiore, Selwyn hoped to pick up, on a part-time basis, where he had left off at the hospital's AIDS clinic and in the methadone program where he had made his reputation. But the epidemic he was returning to was one that did not require his full attention. In the early 1980s, when thinking about the emerging epidemic, he had used the metaphor of an invisible, insidious but deadly monster, silently invading the neighborhoods and tenements of the Bronx. He now had a dramatically different vision, seeing the epidemic as "a sort of wounded Leviathan, kind of big and messy and having an impact all over the place, but something able to be confronted and taken on in some way, dying, but still a weighty kind of process."

Carol Brosgart, now 50, took an even more radical step. "For three years in a row we had mortality down by 70 percent, by 50 percent, and another 40 percent. Hospitalizations were down dramatically. The whole tenor had changed. It really opened the possibility to think about other things," she said. It was under those circumstances that Brosgart was approached by a major pharmaceutical firm to oversee its development of an AIDS drug.

I'm the kid who wouldn't even go to my pharmacology classes in medical school because I was against the medical/industrial complex. And now I'm going to work for industry? How does a left-wing girl from Berkeley end up in industry? I thought, What would it be like to have a day where I wasn't running from one thing to the next and running from the hospital to the clinic to the meeting? And, What would it be like to have a focus? And it started to seem very peaceful, this concept of just being able to be more focused.

With an understanding that she could preserve one day per week for her clinical work, Brosgart, who years earlier had been troubled by her move from a public health clinic to the AIDS service at a private—albeit not-for-profit—community hospital, took the job.

Richard Chaisson, who had come to AIDS as a way of fighting the forces of darkness, also took the occasion to "step away." Despairing about how managed care had altered the demands on a clinic administrator like himself, Chaisson, who had seen in AIDS in America a challenge every bit as worthy of his attention as the disease ravaging the Third World, was now drawn to the new prospect of confronting the threat to human survival abroad.

I see the big challenge, certainly for me personally, as being the challenge of doing something about HIV and TB in the rest of the world. And there it's the old-fashioned "fight the bad guys" approach. I feel as if I'm disengaging from HIV in the United States [where] my opportunity to contribute a lot and my availability as a clinician is not so important anymore.

Like Chaisson, Marcus Conant also stepped away from AIDS, but largely because of the unremitting demands of managed care plans, which had reduced the time he spent on patients in his HIV practice. Professionally unfulfilled before the epidemic, Conant had found in AIDS a passionate cause and a consuming medical challenge. Squeezed financially in recent years, he felt forced to sell his private practice and face the loss of his hard-won raison d'être. Struggling to regain the world he had lost, Conant soon turned to AIDS clinical trials in order to reengage himself intellectually and emotionally.

As a gay man, physician, and researcher, Donald Abrams had been a central a figure in the world of AIDS in San Francisco since the epidemic's first days. He, too, saw the current juncture as permitting a transition. It also made clear to him how much being on the front lines, confronting a new challenge, was integral to his identity. Thus Abrams began to consider the possibility of devoting himself to work in a new area, that of alternative therapies.

> We were pioneers and were involved in a strange new frightening, challenging problem-solving endeavor. And now it's a bit like cancer in that the research is sort of looking at three drugs compared to those four drugs, and which one gives you the marginal improvement in the surrogate marker benefit. You're not dealing with the intensities that we were dealing with previously, which were fear, contagion, death, disfigurement. A lot of the drama and the intensity of the early days of the epidemic are gone. So it seems to me that this position is a natural segue in my career into something that I think will be invigorating, because I look at the field, the science of integrative medicine, and studying these complementary and alternative therapies is a bit like where HIV was in the early '80s in that it's new and there aren't many people doing it. And it's sort of a risk, and you're a pioneer if you delve into it. Paul [Volberding] and Connie [Wofsy] and I, we were the people that were doing this here. Now you go to these AIDS conferences and there are just millions and hundreds of people doing what we used to do or what we do. I've worked in this now for 18 years, and I probably have another 18 years left in my career. I would really prefer being on the front lines again, doing something that's unique.

Finally, for Alexandra Levine, the change in AIDS opened the way to thinking about her pre-epidemic work on the lymphomas as well as about her needs as a 51-year-old woman. In 1999, she had begun her first sabbatical in more than 20 years.

> This was the time to be able to make the break. My patients weren't in the hospital. It was easy. I was seeing patients once a month, once every two months, not once a week. People weren't as needy emotionally as they had been. . . . The change in the epidemic was a tremendous factor that allowed me to interrupt [my] schedule.

If war and its demands seemed so apt an image to capture the first 15 years of the AIDS epidemic, the years since 1995 seemed to be characterized by a slow demobilization. Even the ties and identities that so defined the lives of AIDS doctors in the most desperate years had begun to attenuate. Levine noted in 1999:

> In my own experience [the relationship with other AIDS doctors has] started to become more distant. Whereas I would call somebody all the time, all over the country, "Have you ever seen this? What's this side effect? What do you recommend?" I've made one such call in the last month. I hope it won't mean we won't be friends and that we won't see each other, but it won't shock me if the meetings start to get less frequent. I'm hoping that normal life will come back at least to some extent. I can't allow myself to become so completely involved with a disease and with work that I don't know who I am anymore. I can't do that. Maybe it's because 15 years have passed and I'm truly exhausted, or maybe it's because 15 years have passed and I'm 15 years older, that [I have] a different perspective. Maybe it's simply because 15 years have passed and the epidemic has scaled down a little bit, so I'm allowed to think about other things that I couldn't do before. Whatever the cause, I hope that during this sabbatical I'll be able to teach myself that I must spend time in my own personal endeavors.

As some veterans depart the field and others begin to modulate their involvement with AIDS, the burden of caring for patients with HIV will inevitably begin to shift to a new generation. Those who come to AIDS now are, in some ways, not dissimilar from those who took up the challenge in the 1980s. They are often drawn by the desire to care for the dispossessed; they are attracted by scientific questions that demand resolution. Some find themselves drawn to the very doctors who took on AIDS in the era of clinical impotence. A young clinician at Columbia Presbyterian Hospital in New York thus noted, "They were involved in a crusade, battling an unpopular plague; they were advocates for the disempowered, outcasts; they were very romantic. I wanted to be like them."

Donna Mildvan remarked in 1995 that infectious disease was a perfect field for optimists—until AIDS. In 1999, her mood was once again informed by therapeutic promise. Nevertheless, the AIDS years had robbed her of the naive belief that epidemics of unknown origin were a thing of the past. They could happen again. And when they did, then others, perhaps the generation of doctors she was now training, would have to take up the burden. They are, she thought, primed for the next challenge. It's not going to be this one. There'll be another one. I'm not looking forward to the next one, but that won't be my fight. I don't want to be a doomsayer, but if it's happened once, it could happen again.

In Mildvan's observation there is an echo of the last pages of Albert Camus's *The Plague*. Dr. Bernard Rieux, his protagonist, had understood that in compiling his account

the tale he had to tell could not be one of final victory. It could only be the record . . . of what assuredly would have to be done again, in the never ending fight against terror and its relentless onslaught. . . . [3]

AIDS did not announce itself when the first cases of HIV-related disease began to appear in the late 1970s. And, as the most awful years of the American epidemic draw to a close, AIDS will not come to an end. With between 650,000 and 900,000 infected people and some 40,000 new cases of HIV infection each year, most among Black and Latino drug users and their sexual partners, those committed to the care of the dispossessed will have work to do. But the experience of the new generation of AIDS doctors, trained when the epidemic had already established itself, when it demanded the skills and clinical sophistication of medical subspecialists, will be fundamentally different from that of physicians who came to AIDS in the early 1980s, when there was no alternative but to return to an older tradition of caring. Whatever draws the next generation to AIDS, the world that they and their patients will inhabit will be more like the world of normal medicine. That world will have its tragic dimensions, but they will be the familiar tragedies of doctors when faced with illnesses that threaten the lives of their patients.

In memorializing those who served in the formative years of the epidemic and the uniquely sad world that is being left behind, we too have borne witness. We have rememberd the efforts of men and women, who, like those who confront AIDS in Africa and Asia still, bore witness as they sought to heal and comfort their patients in the darkest moments. It is a memory worth preserving for the next time.

Appendix 1
MAKING AN ORAL HISTORY
A Methodological Note

For those interested, we here offer greater detail concerning the selection of the doctors we interviewed, the formulation of our questions, and the conduct of the interviews themselves.

We began by asking three AIDS doctors to prepare lists of 50 others who had been involved in the care of patients since the epidemic's earliest years. On reviewing their initial rosters—which had a remarkable consistency—we came to believe that there were important gaps. We wanted more office-based practitioners to complement the many hospital-based infectious disease specialists and oncologists. We wanted more local doctors, physicians not on the original lists because they had not established reputations beyond their communities. Finally, we wanted to include some doctors who were themselves infected with HIV. And so we probed our contacts and others. We thus compiled a list of some 80 physicians. In the end, 76 agreed to participate in the creation of an oral history archive.

While it was important for us to identify physicians who cared for patients with AIDS, our goal was not to create a sample that was, in a conventional sense, scientifically representative. Rather, we sought to find physicians with broad experience who could reflect on what was common in the epidemic experience as well as what was utterly unique about caring for people with AIDS.

At the outset, we made another fundamental decision: We rejected the anthropological and sociological convention of anonymizing those with whom we spoke. Even had that been possible, given the readily recognizable roles some doctors played in the epidemic's history, we believed that much would have been lost in shrouding their identities. These were women and men who practiced in real hospitals, clinics, and offices with complex and important professional, public, and personal ties. Stripping these doctors of their identities would have necessitated stripping them of important aspects of their histories.

We knew that our decision carried a price: Without the protective shield afforded by anonymity, it was possible that some elements of candor would be sacrificed. To overcome that threat to our project, we offered each of those with whom we spoke the opportunity to review the interview transcript. Following the procedures of Columbia University's Oral History Office, we gave each doctor the option to amend or eliminate material, or to sequester from public scrutiny—and from our use— portions of the interview. Those restricted segments will only become available at a future time selected by the physician.

Our first interviews took place at the end of 1994 when clinical prospects for people with HIV were not promising, and they extended through the summer of 1997 when new therapeutic advances had begun to presage radical changes in the management of HIV disease. On average, our interviews were four hours long. The briefest lasted two hours; some were as long as eight, taking place over a number of sessions. In all, we spent more than 300 hours with those we interviewed. In 1998 and 1999, we went back to some doctors to explore with them how the changes in therapy, the improved clinical outlook, and the dramatic reduction in AIDS-related deaths, had affected their world, their commitments. In the spring of 1999, we sent a questionnaire of six items covering the same issues to the remaining doctors, over 90 percent of whom responded.

Interviewing was not new to us: Both of us have, in the course of our work, met with informants in search of data and insights for studies that relied primarily on conventional documentary material. This undertaking was, however, different in important respects. These interviews were both longer and more intense than anything we had ever done, and the results, rather than supplementing other sources, were to provide the core material for this book. In addition, they were the sole source of the archive we had decided to create (which is now deposited at the Columbia University Oral History Office, located at Butler Library, Columbia University, New York City). The burden of doing it right was thus enormous—all the more so since we demanded of those we interviewed a considerable investment of time.

Our experience of oral history is aptly characterized by Ronald Grele, who describes it as a "conversational narrative,"[1] a mutual effort by the interviewer and interviewee to tell the latter's tale. But for the conversation to work and for the narrative to emerge, it is critical for the interviewer to be steeped in the background of the person whose memories are to be probed. Only by reading what the doctors had written and what had been written about them were we able to construct the questions that would guide and shape the narrative. Our questions were further informed by our own understanding of the history of the epidemic and our sense of what was of particular salience in that history.

Although preformulated questions, which were posed to all the interviewees, drove the interview in its initial stages, our conversations often gathered an intensity that gave them a life of their own. During our interchanges, physicians often responded with unanticipated but surprisingly rich information that sparked a new set of queries. Above all, we learned to listen. And watch. As a doctor spoke, a word, a facial expression, a gesture, might offer a clue that there was something worth probing further. In the heat of our interviews, a kind of bonding would often occur, making some questions easier to ask, others more difficult. It was at such junctures that a clash of interests could emerge. We always wanted more and pushed deeper. A sense of vulnerability, a commitment to privacy, sometimes led doctors to hold back. In the end, of course, the controls were in their hands.

We cannot provide a measure of the degree to which physicians answered candidly or consciously withheld critical material. We do know that some have sequestered portions of their transcripts because they deemed those sections too sensitive. We also felt that a significant number of them spoke with amazing frankness about patients, colleagues, and administrators, and about emotions they said they had rarely shared with others.

Every story was different, a unique voice, a separate document to be remembered as such. The recorded conversations and the texts that emerged from them capture, within a story, the structure and nuance of each doctor's language, his or her use of metaphor and telling detail. Every completed interview provides a firsthand account of a professional and personal passage through the heart of a medical and social crisis.

Appendix 2
BIOGRAPHICAL NOTES ON PHYSICIANS INTERVIEWED

Abrams, Donald   Born in 1950, he completed a residency in Medical Oncology, Hematology, and Internal Medicine in 1980. At the time of the interview he was Co-Director of the AIDS Program at San Francisco General Hospital and Director of the Community Consortium, which links local physicians into a clinical trials network. In 1999 he was Professor of Clinical Medicine at the University of California, San Francisco.

Armstrong, Donald   Born in 1931, he completed a residency in Internal Medicine and Microbiology in 1961. At the time of the interview he was Chief of the Infectious Disease Service in the Department of Medicine at Memorial Sloan-Kettering Cancer Center, New York City, specializing in infectious diseases in cancer patients. He has recently retired.

Bastien, Arnaud   Born in Haiti in 1961, he completed a residency in Internal Medicine in 1997. At the time of the interview he was a resident at Cooper Hospital, University Medical Center, in Camden, New Jersey. In 1999 he was Assistant Professor of Medicine at the University of Medicine and Dentistry New Jersey.

Bolan, Robert   Born in 1946, he completed a residency in Family Medicine in 1977. At the time of the interview he was in private practice in San Francisco. During the first half of the 1980s, he participated actively in AIDS politics in San Francisco, serving, for example, as president of the Bay Area Physicians for Human Rights. In 1999, he was medical director of the Lambda Medical Group in Los Angeles.

Brosgart, Carol L.   Born in 1951, she completed a residency in Preventive Medicine in 1988. At the time of the interview she was Medical Director of the East Bay AIDS Center at Alta Bates–Herrick Hospital in

Berkeley, California. A feminist committed to the interest of the dispossessed, she came to AIDS through her work in public health. In 1999 she became Director of Clinical Research at the pharmaceutical firm Gilead Sciences.

Cade, Jerry Born in 1954, he completed a residency in Substance Abuse/Chemical Dependency in 1984. At the time of the interview he was Medical Director of the University of Nevada Medical Center's HIV Inpatient and Outpatient Clinic and was in private practice. In the first years of the AIDS epidemic in Nevada, he and his partner were the sole AIDS treaters in Las Vegas. In 1999 he was Medical Director of HIV Services at the University Medical School and Clinical Assistant Professor at the University of Nevada School of Medicine. He serves on the President's Advisory Committee on AIDS.

Calabrese, Leonard H. Born in 1949, he completed a residency in Internal Medicine, Rheumatology, and Immunologic Disease in 1978. At the time of the interview he was Head of the Section of Clinical Immunology in the Department of Rheumatic and Immunologic Disease at The Cleveland Clinic in Cleveland, Ohio. Committed to treating people with AIDS well before most other physicians in Cleveland, he was one of the first to associate rheumatic syndromes with HIV infection. In 1999 he was Vice Chairman of the Department of Rheumatic and Immunologic Disease, Head of Clinical Immunology, and R. J. Fasenmyer Chair of Clinical Immunology for The Cleveland Clinic.

Campbell, James He completed his residency in Internal Medicine in 1968. At the time of the interview he was in private practice in San Francisco. A physician with many gay patients, he became a clinical expert on AIDS during the early years of the epidemic. He is now retired.

Capaldini, Lisa Born in 1955, she completed a residency in Internal Medicine in 1986. At the time of the interview she was in private practice in San Francisco's Castro district. Her Catholic background provided her with an abiding interest in the spiritual dimensions of AIDS care. In 1999 she remained in private practice and was Assistant Clinical Professor of Medicine at the University of California, San Francisco Medical School.

Chaisson, Richard E. Born in 1954, he completed a residency in Internal Medicine and Infectious Diseases in 1985. At the time of the interview he was Director of the AIDS Service and Medical Director of the

Tuberculosis Clinic at the Baltimore City Health Department and Johns Hopkins Hospital in Baltimore, Maryland. His interest in epidemic disease in vulnerable populations led to significant public health research in the relation of HIV infection to intravenous drug use and tuberculosis. In 1999 he was Professor of Medicine, Johns Hopkins University School of Medicine, and was shifting his focus to AIDS in the less developed world.

Cohen, Mardge H. Born in 1951, she completed a residency in Internal Medicine in 1980. Her interest in the health issues facing impoverished women drew her to AIDS. At the time of the interview she was Director of the Women and Children HIV Program at Cook County Hospital in Chicago, Illinois, a position she continued to hold in 1999.

Cohen, Robert L. Born in 1948, he completed a residency in Internal Medicine in 1979. At the time of the interview he was in private practice in New York City. He entered private practice after overseeing care of prisoners in New York and indigent patients in New York's municipal hospitals. He continued in private practice in 1999.

Conant, Marcus A. Born in 1936, he completed a residency in Dermatology in 1967. At the time of the interview he was in private practice in San Francisco. Among the first to recognize Kaposi's sarcoma as a diagnostic sign of a new disease, he organized a special KS clinic in 1981 at the University of California, San Francisco, to study the new epidemic. In 1999 he was Clinical Professor at the University of California, San Francisco, and although he continued to manage AIDS clinical trials, he had left private practice.

Cooke, Mary Marshall (Molly) Born in 1951, she completed a residency in Internal Medicine in 1981. At the time of the interview she was Professor of Clinical Medicine and Director of the Introduction to Clinical Medicine Program at San Francisco General Hospital. She studied the attitude of physicians toward treating patients with AIDS and examined many other AIDS-associated ethical issues. She is currently Professor of Medicine in the Division of General Internal Medicine at the University of California, San Francisco.

Cotton, Deborah Born in 1949, she completed a residency in Internal Medicine and Infectious Disease in 1978. At the time of the interview she was Associate Professor of Medicine at Harvard Medical School. She strongly supported the inclusion of women in AIDS clinical trials. In 1999 she was Professor of Medicine, Epidemiology and Biostatistics at Boston University School of Medicine; Assistant Provost of the Medical Campus at Boston University; and Director of the Office of Clinical Research of Boston University Medical Center.

Currier, Judith Silverstein   Born in 1956, she completed a residency in Internal Medicine and Infectious Disease in 1988. At the time of the interview she was Medical Director, Rand Schrader AIDS Clinic, Los Angeles County Hospital–University of Southern California Medical Center. In 1999 she was Associate Professor of Medicine, UCLA, and Associate Director, Center for AIDS Research and Education.

Drew, William Lawrence   Born in 1936, he completed a residency in Internal Medicine, Infectious Disease, and Medical Microbiology in 1968. At the time of the interview he was Director of the Clinical Microbiology and Virology Laboratory and Associate Chief of the Department of Medicine at Mt. Zion Medical Center in San Francisco. An expert on viral diseases, he conducted pioneering studies on the efficacy of male and female condoms as barriers to the sexual transmission of viruses. In 1999 he was Director of Infectious Disease and Microbiology at the University of California, San Francisco.

El-Sadr, Wafaa   Born in 1950 in Egypt, she completed a residency in Internal Medicine and Infectious Diseases in 1976. At the time of the interview she was Director of the Division of Infectious Diseases at Harlem Hospital Center in New York City, a position she retained in 1999. She researched the natural course of, and treatment for, HIV infection, especially in intravenous drug users.

Fischl, Margaret Ann   She completed a residency in Internal Medicine in 1979. At the time of the interview she was Director of the AIDS Clinical Research Unit and Comprehensive AIDS Center and Director of the Special Immunology Clinic at Jackson Memorial Hospital in Miami. A clinical trials expert, she was among the earliest to report on the efficacy of AZT and of combination (multidrug) therapy. In 1999 she was Professor of Medicine and retained her position as Director of the AIDS Clinical Research Unit at Jackson Memorial Hospital.

Follansbee, Stephen Eliot   Born in 1948, he completed a residency in Internal Medicine and Infectious Diseases in 1980. At the time of the interview he was Medical Director of the Institute for HIV Treatment and

Research at Davies Medical Center and Assistant Director of the San Francisco Community Consortium. One of the founding members of the gay physicians organization Bay Area Physicians for Human Rights, he was a leading infectious disease consultant in San Francisco. In 1999 he was Staff Physician, Associate Director of the HIV Research Unit, and Medical Director of HIV Services, Kaiser-Permanente, San Francisco.

Friedland, Gerald H. Born in 1938, he completed a residency in Internal Medicine and Infectious Disease in 1968. At the time of the interview he was Director of the AIDS Program at Yale–New Haven Hospital in Connecticut. Drawn by his political commitments to work with impoverished patients, he pioneered in defining and treating AIDS in intravenous drug users at Montefiore Hospital in the Bronx. He was among the first researchers to demonstrate that AIDS could not be transmitted through casual, household contact. In 1999, he remained Director of the Yale–New Haven AIDS Program.

Friedman-Kien, Alvin E. Born in 1934, he completed a residency in Dermatology in 1962. At the time of the interview he was Professor of Dermatology and Microbiology at the New York University Medical Center and Consultant Physician and Director of the Dermatology Service at Goldwater Memorial Hospital. He was one of the first physicians to recognize the emergence of an epidemic of Kaposi's sarcoma in gay men in New York City and the lead author of the second *Morbidity and Mortality Weekly Report* on AIDS in July 1981, alerting physicians to this new phenomenon. In 1999, he continued as Professor of Dermatology and Microbiology at New York University School of Medicine.

Futterman, Donna Born in 1952, she completed a residency in Pediatrics in 1988. At the time of the interview she was Medical Director of the Adolescent AIDS Program and Director of Adolescent Ambulatory Care Services at Montefiore Medical Center Hospital in the Bronx, New York. In 1999 she remained the Director of the Adolescent AIDS Program and Associate Professor of Pediatrics at Montefiore Medical Center.

Goosby, Eric Paul Born in 1953, he completed a residency in Internal Medicine in 1981. An African American, he worked at San Francisco General Hospital and with intravenous drug users. At the time of the interview he was Director of the Office of HIV/AIDS Policy in the Department of Health and Human Services, Washington, D.C., a position he continued to hold in 1999.

Gottlieb, Michael S. Born in 1947, he completed a residency in Immunology and Rheumatology in 1977. At the time of the interview he was in private practice in Los Angeles and Sherman Oaks, California. As a young assistant professor at the University of California, Los Angeles, he recognized and traced the first cases of *Pneumocystis carinii* pneumonia in gay men. His published results in the *Morbidity and Mortality Weekly Report* in June 1981 marked the official beginning of the AIDS epidemic in the United States. In 1999 he continued in private practice.

Groopman, Jerome E. Born in 1952, he completed a residency in Internal Medicine, Medical Hematology, and Medical Oncology in 1978. His work with AIDS began in Los Angeles. At the time of the interview he was Chief of the Division of Hematology/Oncology at New England Deaconess Hospital in Boston. A researcher and observant Jew, he found in both science and faith a basis for working with patients with fatal diseases. In 1999 he was Chief of Experimental Medicine at New England Deaconess Hospital.

Grossman, Howard A. Born in 1954, he completed a residency in Internal Medicine in 1986. At the time of the interview he was in private practice in New York City. Politically and personally involved in the gay community, he saw himself as a "country doctor" in an urban setting. In 1999 he was an Assistant Attending Physician at St. Luke's–Roosevelt Hospital and retained a large private practice in AIDS.

Grossman, Ronald J. Born in 1939, he completed a residency in Internal Medicine in 1966. Among the first physicians to establish a practice among gay men, at the time of the interview he provided care to many AIDS patients. In 1999 he continued in private practice.

Handsfield, Hugh Hunter Born in 1943, he completed a residency in Internal Medicine and Infectious Diseases in 1971. At the time of the interview he was Director of the Sexually Transmitted Disease Control Program for the Seattle–King County Department of Health and Harborview Medical Center. He was an early proponent of viewing AIDS as a sexually transmitted disease and responding to it as a public health-STD problem. In 1999 he was Professor of Medicine at the University of Washington, and continued as Director of the STD Control Program.

Heagarty, Margaret C. Born in 1934, she completed a residency in Pediatrics in 1964. At the time of the interview she was Director of Pediatrics at Harlem Hospital Center in New York City. A dominant presence at Harlem Hospital, she struggled to fund her AIDS programs and rally her staff in a public hospital where the epidemic was only one of many serious health problems. She has retired.

Hilgartner, Margaret W. Born in 1924, she completed a residency in Pediatric Hematology/Oncology in 1958. At the time of the interview she was Vice-Chairman of the Department of Pediatrics, Director of the Division of Pediatric Hematology/Oncology, and Director of the Hemophilia Comprehensive Treatment Center at New York Hospital–Cornell Medical Center in New York City. A physician who practiced during the 1970s, when the introduction of clotting factor transformed the treatment and experience of hemophilia, she witnessed in the following decade the professional tragedy of seeing her patients become infected with HIV as a result of their therapy. In 1999 she had reduced her professional commitments.

Hirsch, Martin Born in 1939, he completed a residency in Internal Medicine and Infectious Diseases in 1966. At the time of the interview he was Professor of Medicine at Harvard Medical School and Professor of Virology and Cancer Biology at the Harvard School of Public Health and Massachusetts General Hospital in Boston, and he remains in these positions. A virologist and clinical trials expert, he was closely associated with testing the efficacy of AZT and of the use of combination therapy.

Hollander, Harry Born in 1955, he completed a residency in Internal Medicine and Infectious Diseases in 1984. At the time of the interview he was Director of the HIV Clinic at Moffitt Hospital, University of California, San Francisco. In 1999 he was, in addition, Professor of Clinical Medicine.

Holmes, King K. Born in 1937, he completed a residency in Internal Medicine and Infectious Diseases in 1969. At the time of the interview he was Director of the Center for AIDS and STD, and Section Head of the Division of Allergy and Infectious Disease at Harborview Medical Center and the University of Washington, Seattle. An internationally recognized expert on sexually transmitted disease, he described the twin epidemics of AIDS and traditional STDs, seeing their convergence as a potential catastrophe in the United States and developing nations. In 1999 he was Professor of Medicine at the University of Washington and continued as Director of the Center for AIDS and STD.

Kass, Elizabeth Born in 1958, she completed a residency in Internal Medicine in 1988. At the time of the interview she was in clinical practice in Boston. She had been the medical director of one of the first hospices for AIDS patients. In 1999 she was Medical Director of the Urban Medical Group.

Kotler, Donald P. Born in 1947, he completed a residency in Internal Medicine and Gastroenterology in 1976. At the time of the interview he was Director of the Section of GI Immunology in the Gastrointestinal Division at St. Luke's–Roosevelt Hospital Center, New York. An expert on nutrition, starvation, and wasting disease, he established that wasting disease in AIDS followed the classic model. In 1999 he was Professor of Medicine, St. Luke's–Roosevelt Hospital Center.

Landesman, Sheldon H. Born in 1944, he completed a residency in Internal Medicine and Infectious Diseases in 1976. At the time of the interview he was Director of the AIDS Study Center at the State University's Health Sciences Center at Brooklyn and of the AIDS Clinic at Kings County Hospital. He established early on that AIDS was epidemic in Brooklyn and in its Haitian community. In 1999 he was Chief of Infectious Disease at Brookdale Hospital and Professor of Medicine at the SUNY Health Science Center.

Laurence, Jeffrey C. Born in 1952, he completed a residency in Internal Medicine and Hematology-Oncology in 1979. At the time of the interview he was Director of the Laboratory for AIDS Virus Research at Cornell University Medical College and New York Hospital–Cornell Medical Center, New York. In 1999, he remained Director of the Laboratory and held the positions of Associate Attending Physician and Associate Professor of Medicine at New York Presbyterian Hospital/Cornell University.

Levine, Alexandra M. Born in 1945, she completed a residency in Internal Medicine and Hematology-Oncology in 1974. At the time of the interview she was Chief of the Division of Hematology at the University of Southern California Medical Center, Los Angeles. Drawn to AIDS early in the epidemic, despite the antipathy of her peers and administrators, she later became a strong advocate of including women in AIDS clinical trials. In 1999 she was Professor of Medicine, Chief of the Division of Hematology, and Medical Director, USC Norris Cancer Hospital.

Makadon, Harvey J.   Born in 1947, he completed a residency in Internal Medicine in 1980. At the time of the interview he was Medical Director of Ambulatory Services and Co-Director of the Division of General Medicine and Primary Care at Beth Israel Hospital in Boston. In 1999 he was Vice President for Medical Affairs at Beth Israel Hospital.

Mansell, Peter W. A.   Born in 1936, he completed a residency in Internal Medicine and Oncology in 1967. At the time of the interview he was Adjunct Professor of Internal Medicine, M.D. Anderson Cancer Center in Houston. He became Associate Corporate Medical Director of Pasteur Merieux Connaught (France). In 1999 he had retired.

Mayer, Kenneth H.   Born in 1950, he completed a residency in Internal Medicine and Infectious Diseases in 1980. At the time of the interview he was Chief of the Infectious Disease Division at The Memorial Hospital of Rhode Island and Director of the Brown University AIDS Program. In 1999 he was Professor of Medicine and Community Health at Brown University and continued as Chief of the Infectious Disease Division at The Memorial Hospital of Rhode Island.

Mazzullo, John M.   Born in 1943, he completed a residency in Internal Medicine in 1971. At the time of the interview he was practicing in Boston. In 1999 he was Attending Physician at New England Medical Center and Assistant Professor at Tufts University School of Medicine.

Mendez, Hermann   Born in 1949 in Guatemala and reared in El Salvador, he completed a residency in Pediatrics in 1983. At the time of the interview he was Director of the Brooklyn Pediatric AIDS Network at the State University of New York's Health Science Center at Brooklyn and Medical Director of the Pediatric Maternal HIV Center at Kings County Hospital Center. Immersed in the issues of pediatric AIDS once the disease was recognized in children, he struggled to find funding to develop the first treatment facilities for impoverished, HIV-infected children in Brooklyn. In 1999 he was Associate Professor of Clinical Pediatrics.

Mildvan, Donna   Born in 1942, she completed a residency in Internal Medicine and Infectious Diseases in 1970. At the time of the interview she was Chief of the Infectious Diseases Division and Director of AIDS Research at Beth Israel Hospital in New York. She was one of the first doctors on the East Coast to recognize that the unusual symptoms and diseases she was seeing in patients portended an epidemic of a new disorder. In 1999 she continued in her positions at the time of the interview.

Minkoff, Howard L. Born in 1950, he completed a residency in Obstetrics and Gynecology and Maternal-Fetal Medicine in 1979. At the time of the interview he was Director of Obstetrics and Maternal-Fetal Medicine at the State University of New York's Health Science Center, Brooklyn. Working in a medical center that drew high-risk poor populations in Brooklyn, he became one of the nation's experts on AIDS in pregnant women and on the transmission of HIV to the fetus. In 1999 he was Chairman of Obstetrics and Gynecology at Maimonides Medical Center in Brooklyn.

Mitchell, Janet L. Born in 1950, she completed a residency in Obstetrics and Gynecology and Maternal-Fetal Medicine in 1980. At the time of the interview she was Chief of Perinatology in the Department of Obstetrics and Gynecology at Harlem Hospital Center in New York. Focusing on the plight of poor, pregnant African-American women with significant health problems like drug use and AIDS, she championed their dignity and rights. In 1999 she was Acting Chairperson of OB/GYN at St. Mary's Hospital in Brooklyn, New York.

Oleske, James M. Born in 1945, he completed a residency in Allergy-Immunology and Pediatrics in 1973. At the time of the interview, he was Director of the Division of Allergy, Immunology, and Infectious Diseases at the University of Medicine and Dentistry (UMD), New Jersey, and Medical Director of the Children's Hospital AIDS Program. Among the first pediatricians to recognize AIDS in infants, he has committed himself to working with HIV-infected children from the poorest populations of Newark, New Jersey. In 1999 he was François-Xavier Bagnoud Professor at UMD and continued in the positions he held at the time of the interview.

O'Neill, Joseph F. Born in 1953, he completed a residency in Primary Care Internal Medicine in 1988. After years of caring for the most impoverished AIDS patients in Baltimore, he turned to government service. At the time of the interview he was Director of the AIDS Bureau, U.S. Health Resources and Services Administration in Washington, D.C., where he remained in 1999.

Ostrow, Stosh Born in 1948, he completed a residency in General Medicine in 1982. At the time of the interview he was in private practice in Atlanta. A vocal gay activist in Atlanta, he became the rare openly gay physician in that city who would speak to the media about AIDS and one of the few doctors who went public about his status as a HIV-infected health worker. By 1999, he had retired from the practice of medicine.

Owen, William Born in 1949, he completed a residency in Internal Medicine in 1976. At the time of the interview he was in private practice in San Francisco. In 1999 he continued in private practice.

Redfield, Robert Jr. Born in 1951, he completed a residency in Internal Medicine and Infectious Diseases in 1980. At the time of the interview he was Program Director of the Adult HIV Program and Director of Clinical Research at the Institute of Virology at University of Maryland Biotechnology Institute, Baltimore. As a military physician stationed at the Walter Reed Army Hospital, he diagnosed some of the first cases of AIDS in the armed forces. In 1999 he remained at the Institute of Human Virology as Director of Clinical Care and Research.

Rubinstein, Arye Born in 1936 in Palestine, he remained in Israel until he sought training in Switzerland. He completed a residency in Pediatrics, Allergy, and Immunology in 1967. At the time of the interview he was Director of the Center for AIDS Research, the Division of Clinical Allergy and Immunology, and the AIDS Family Care Center at the Albert Einstein College of Medicine and Montefiore Hospital Medical Center in the Bronx, New York. A prominent immunologist and clinical researcher, he observed AIDS in the infants and children he treated in the early1980s and was author of one of the first papers describing the new disease in children. In 1999 he remained in the positions he held at the time of the interview.

Schram, Neil Born in 1939, he completed a residency in Internal Medicine and Nephrology in 1969. At the time of the interview he was a nephrologist at Kaiser-Permanente in Los Angeles. The only physician at Kaiser-Permanente in Los Angeles willing to take as referrals patients with AIDS, he was a prominent AIDS political activist within the gay community and Los Angeles County. In 1999 he continued in clinical practice.

Scott, Gwendolyn B. Born in 1938, she completed a residency in Pediatrics and Pediatric Infectious Diseases in 1976. At the time of the interview she was Director of the Division of Pediatric Infectious Disease and Immunology and of the Children's Clinical Immunology Unit at the University of Miami School of Medicine. Observing the emergence of the AIDS epidemic in Haitian children and their mothers, she studied the transmission of the virus from mother to fetus and the natural history of the disease in her patients. In 1999 she was Professor of Pediatrics and Director of the HIV/AIDS Program at the University of Miami School of Medicine and continued as Director of the Division of Pediatric Infectious Disease and Immunology.

Scott, Robert Born in 1944, he completed his residency in Internal Medicine in 1977. At the time of the interview, he was in private practice in Oakland, California. Although an AIDS specialist, his primary commitment, as a physician and prominent member of the Black church, was to the health care needs of his community. In 1999 he continued in private practice.

Seitzman, Peter A. Born in 1948, he completed a residency in Internal Medicine in 1978. Prominent in gay medical groups in the epidemic's early years, he was at the time of the interview in private practice in New York. In 1999 he had retired from clinical work.

Selwyn, Peter A. Born in 1954, he completed a residency in Family Practice in 1984. At the time of the interview he was Associate Director of the AIDS Program at Yale–New Haven Hospital. Initially known for his work treating and studying HIV infection in drug users in the Bronx, he later, as a result of AIDS and the recognition of the consequences of deep grief in his own life, became an expert in death, dying, and palliative care. In 1999 he was Chair of the Department of Family Medicine at Montefiore Medical Center, Bronx, New York.

Sharp, Victoria L. Born in 1947, she completed a residency in Internal Medicine in 1987. Her initial work involved prisoners with AIDS in Albany and New York. At the time of the interview she was Director of AIDS Services at New York's St. Luke's–Roosevelt Hospital Center, a position she retained in 1999.

Sherer, Renslow D., Jr. Born in 1950, he completed a residency in Internal Medicine in 1981. At the time of the interview he was Director of the Chicago's Cook County Hospital HIV Primary Care Center. Together with Ron Sable, a gay colleague, he was instrumental in developing an AIDS program at Cook County, despite opposition within the hospital. In 1999 he was Director of HIV Coordinated Services at The Care Center at Cook County Hospital and Associate Professor of Medicine at Rush Medical Center.

Siegal, Frederick P. Born in 1939, he completed a residency in Internal Medicine, Allergy and Immunology, and Oncology in 1973. At the time of the interview he was Section Head in Hematology Research at Long Island Jewish Medical Center in New Hyde Park, New York. Early in the epidemic he organized the first conference on AIDS in New York City. In 1999 he was Medical Director of the HIV Center of St. Vincent's Hospital and Medical Center, New York.

Sonnabend, Joseph A. Born in 1933 in South Africa, he completed a residency in Infectious Diseases in 1961. At the time of the interview he was in private practice in New York and was the Medical Director of the Community Research Initiative on AIDS. A virologist and expert on sexually transmitted diseases, he was well known for challenging the view that HIV was the sole cause of AIDS and for opposing the use of AZT in the treatment of AIDS. In 1999 he was Attending Physician at St. Luke's–Roosevelt Hospital Center.

Stansell, John Dee Born in 1948, he completed a residency in Internal Medicine and Pulmonary Disease in 1988. At the time of the interview he was Medical Director, AIDS Program, San Francisco General Hospital. One of the founders of the Whitman-Walker Clinic for gays and lesbians in Washington, D.C., and strongly committed to providing appropriate health care to the gay community, he gained recognition because of his willingness to speak publicly about physician-assisted suicide. In 1999 he was Medical Director of the University of California, San Francisco, Positive Health Program.

Starrett, Barbara Born in 1940, she completed a residency in Internal Medicine in 1973. At the time of the interview she was in private practice in New York, where she served a large gay and lesbian clientele. A physician with great faith in pharmaceuticals, she treated patients with unorthodox medications like Compound Q as well as with AZT and other conventional drugs. In 1999 she continued in private practice.

Torres, Ramon A. (Gabriel)   Born in 1958, he completed a residency in Internal Medicine in 1988. At the time of the interview he was Medical Director of the AIDS Center at St. Vincent's Hospital and Medical Center of New York. He brought public attention to the problem of AIDS infection in the homeless of New York City. In 1999 he was in private practice in Manhattan.

Valenti, William M.   Born in 1945, he completed a residency in Internal Medicine and Infectious Diseases in 1975. At the time of the interview he was a physician at the Community Health Network in Rochester, New York. In 1999 he was Clinical Associate Professor of Medicine, University of Rochester School of Medicine and Dentistry.

van der Horst, Charles M.   Born in 1952, he completed a residency in Internal Medicine and Infectious Diseases in 1982. At the time of the interview he was Director of the AIDS Clinical Trials Unit at the University of North Carolina School of Medicine, Chapel Hill. A child of Holocaust survivors, he has drawn on his Jewish experience in responding to the epidemic. In 1999 he was Professor of Medicine at the University of North Carolina School of Medicine.

Vaughn, Anita   Born in 1952, she completed a residency in Internal Medicine in 1982. At the time of the interview she was Medical Director of Newark Community Health Centers, Inc. An African-American physician, she entered medicine as a way of bringing care to the most deprived. In 1999 she continued in her position at the time of the interview.

Volberding, Paul A.   Born in 1949, he completed a residency in Internal Medicine and Medical Oncology in 1978. At the time of the interview he was Director of the AIDS Program and Clinical Oncology at San Francisco General Hospital. He was the principal investigator of a trial that demonstrated the effectiveness of AZT in asymptomatic individuals. In 1999 he was Professor of Medicine at the University of California, San Francisco, and Director of the Center for AIDS Research and the Positive Health Program.

Wallace, Joyce I.   Born in 1940, she completed a residency in Internal Medicine in 1973. At the time of the interview she was Executive Director of the Foundation for Research on Sexually Transmitted Diseases in New York. Her work with female prostitutes centered on both HIV prevention and care. In 1999 she continued her work with sex workers.

Weisman, Joel Born in 1943, he completed a residency in Family Practice in 1972. At the time of the interview he was in private practice in Los Angeles. A co-author, with Michael Gottlieb, of the *Morbidity and Mortality Weekly Report* of June 1981 describing the first AIDS cases, two from his practice, he became a political activist in the gay community and was involved in the creation of AIDS Project, Los Angeles. In 1999 he had retired from the practice of medicine.

William, Daniel C. Born in 1946, he completed a residency in Internal Medicine in 1975. At the time of the interview he was in private practice in New York. Realizing from clinical care that a new epidemic disease, linked to gay sexual behavior, was emerging, he tried to warn his community, only to be treated as a Cassandra. In 1999 he was Senior Attending Physician at St. Luke's–Roosevelt Hospital and remained in private practice.

Wofsy, Constance Born in 1942, she completed a residency in Infectious Disease, Bacteriology, and Immunology in 1975. At the time of the interview she was Professor of Clinical Medicine at the University of California, San Francisco, and, with Donald Abrams and Paul Volberding, was Co-Director of the AIDS Program at San Francisco General Hospital. She died in 1996 of breast cancer.

Wolfe, Peter R. Born in 1953, he completed a residency in Internal Medicine and Infectious Disease in 1982. At the time of the interview he was in private practice in Beverly Hills. In 1999 he was Associate Clinical Professor of Medicine at the UCLA School of Medicine and remained in private practice.

Wright, David Born in 1950, he completed a residency in Family Practice in 1983. At the time of the interview he was a faculty member, Family Practice Residency Program, Austin, Texas. In 1999 he continued in his position at the time of the interview.

Zuger, Abigail Born in 1955, she completed a residency in Internal Medicine and Infectious Diseases in 1984. At the time of the interview she was Attending Physician at the Spellman Center for HIV-Related

Disease at St. Clare's Hospital, New York City. She became known early in the epidemic because of articles she wrote on the issue of whether physicians had an obligation to treat AIDS cases. Her impoverished patients became the subject of her book, *Strong Shadows*. In 1999, in addition to her clinical work, she was a medical writer for the *New York Times*.

Notes

Introduction

1. *New York Times*, July 11, 1987, 1.
2. R.M. Able, letter, *New York Times*, November 9, 1987.
3. R. Nathan Link, Anat R. Feingold, Mitchell H. Charap, et al., "Concerns of Medical and Pediatric House Officers about Acquiring AIDS from their Patients," *American Journal of Public Health* 78, 1 (April 1988): 445–459.
4. Barbara Gerbert, Bryan T. Maguire, Thomas Bleeker, et al., "Primary Care Physicians and AIDS," *Journal of the American Medical Association* 266, (1991): 2837–2842.
5. John Colombotos, Peter Messeri, Marianne Burgunder, et al., "Physicians, Nurses and AIDS: Findings from a National Study," unpublished, January 1995.
6. Cited in Abigail Zuger and Stephen H. Miles, Physicians, AIDS and Occupational Risk: Historic Traditions and Ethical Obligations, *Journal of the American Medical Association* 258 (1987): 1924–1928.
7. Abigail Zuger, "When the Patient, not the Doctor, Becomes the Hero." *New York Times* Science Section, December 15, 1998.
8. Abraham Verghese, *My Own Country: A Doctor's Story* (New York: Vintage Books, 1995).
9. Peter A. Selwyn, *Surviving the Fall: The Personal Journal of an AIDS Doctor* (New Haven, Conn.:Yale University Press, 1998).
10. Daniel J. Baxter, *The Least of These My Brethren: A Doctor's Story of Hope and Miracles on an Inner-City AIDS Ward* (New York: Harmony Books, 1997).
11. Jerome Groopman, *The Measure of Our Days: New Beginnings at Life's End* (New York: Viking, 1997).
12. Abigail Zuger, *Strong Shadows: Scenes from an Inner-City AIDS Clinic* (New York: Freeman, 1995).
13. Alessandro Portelli, *The Death of Luigi Trastulli and Other Stories: Form and Meaning in Oral History* (Albany: State University of New York Press, 1991).
14. Albert Camus, *The Plague* (New York: Vintage Books, 1972), 286–287.

Chapter 1

1. James Kinsella, *Covering the Plague: AIDS and the American Media*. (New Brunswick: Rutgers University Press, 1989), 9–10.
2. *Morbidity and Mortality Weekly Report*, July 9, 1982, 353–361.
3. *Morbidity and Mortality Weekly Report*, July 16, 1982, 365–367.

4. *Morbidity and Mortality Weekly Report,* December 10, 1982, 652–654.
5. *Morbidity and Mortality Weekly Report,* December 17, 1982, 665–667.
6. *Morbidity and Mortality Weekly Report,* January 7, 1983, 697–698.
7. James Oleske, A.B. Minnefor, R. Cooper, et al. "Immune Deficiency Syndrome in Children." *Journal of the American Medical Association* 249 (1983), 2345–2349.
8. "Acquired Immunodeficiency Syndrome (AIDS) Update-United States," *Morbidity and Mortality Weekly Report,* June 24, 1983, 309–311.
9. "Update: Acquired Immunodeficiency Syndrome (AIDS)—United States," *Morbidity and Mortality Weekly Report,* January 6, 1984, 688–691.
10. "Update: Acquired Immunodeficiency Syndrome (AIDS)—United States," *Morbidity and Mortality Weekly Report,* June 22, 1984, 337–339.
11. "Update: Acquired Immunodeficiency Syndrome (AIDS)—United States," *Morbidity and Mortality Weekly Report,* May 10, 1985, 245–248.
12. "Antibodies to a Retrovirus Etiologically Associated with Acquired Immunodeficiency Syndrome (AIDS) in Populations with Increased Incidence of the Syndrome," *Morbidity and Mortality Weekly Report,* July 13, 1985, 377–379.
13. "Update: Acquired Immunodeficiency Syndrome (AIDS)—United States." *Morbidity and Mortality Weekly Report,* January 17, 1986, 17–21.
14. "Current Trends Update: Acquired Immunodeficiency Syndrome (AIDS)—United States," *Morbidity and Mortality Weekly Report,* June 7, 1991, 358–363, 369.

Chapter 2

1. Ronald Bayer. *Private Acts, Social Consequences: AIDS and the Politics of Public Health* (New Brunswick, N.J.: Rutgers University Press, 1991); Randy Shilts, *And the Band Played On* (New York: St. Martin's Press, 1987); Dennis Altman, *AIDS in the Mind of America* (Garden City, NY: Anchor/Doubleday, 1986); Robert Padgug and Gerald M. Oppenheimer, "Riding the Tiger: AIDS and the Gay Community," in *AIDS: The Making of a Chronic Disease* ed. Elizabeth Fee and Daniel M. Fox (Berkeley: University of California Press, 1998).
2. "Acquired Immune Deficiency Syndrome (AIDS): Precautions for Clinical and Laboratory Staffs," *Morbidity and Mortality Weekly Report,* November 5, 1982, 577–580.
3. Anthony S. Fauci, "The Acquired Immune Deficiency Syndrome: The Ever-Broadening Clinical Spectrum," *Journal of the American Medical Association* 249 (1983): 2375–2376.
4. Gerald M. Oppenheimer. "In the Eye of the Storm: The Epidemiological Construction of AIDS," in *AIDS: The Burden of History,* ed. Elizabeth Fee and Daniel M. Fox (Berkeley: University of California Press, 1998), 267–300.
5. American Civil Liberties Union, *Epidemic of Fear: A Survey of AIDS Discrimination in the 1980s and Policy Recommendations for the 1990s* (New York: American Civil Liberties Union, 1990).
6. "Recommendations for Prevention of Transmission of Infection with Human T-Lymphotropic Virus III/Lymphademopathy-Associated Virus in the Workplace," *Morbidity and Mortality Weekly Report,* November 15, 1985, 681–686, 691–696.
7. "Update: Prospective Evaluation of Health-Care Workers Exposed via the Parenteral or Mucous Membrane Route to Blood or Body Fluids from Patients with Acquired Immunodeficiency Syndrome—United States," *Morbidity and Mortality Weekly Report,* February 22, 1985, 101–103.
8. *New York Times,* December 14, 1984, p. 17.
9. Ibid.

10. Michael Rogers, "Doctor Doom," *Los Angeles Times Magazine,* April 21, 1991, 20.
11. *San Francisco Chronicle,* November 13, 1989, B3.

Chapter 3

1. Margaret Fischl, G. M. Dickinson, and L. LaVoie, "Trimethoprim-sulphamethoxazole Prophylaxis for Pneumocystis Carinii Pneumonia in AIDS," *Journal of the American Medical Association.* 259 (1988): 1185–1189.
2. Peter Arno and Karyn Feiden, *Against the Odds: The Story of AIDS Drug Development, Politics and Profits* (New York: HarperCollins, 1992), 43.
3. Paul Volberding et al., "Zidovudine for Asymptomatic Human Immunodeficiency Virus Infection," *New England Journal of Medicine* 322 (1990): 941–949.
4. Gerald Friedland, "Early Treatment for HIV: The Time Has Come," *New England Journal of Medicine* 322 (1990): 1000–1002.
5. Steven Epstein, *Impure Science: AIDS, Activism and the Politics of Knowledge* (Berkeley: University of California Press, 1996).
6. Harlan Dalton, "AIDS in Black Face," *Daedalus* (Summer, 1989): 205–227.
7. Jean-Pierre Aboulker and Ann Marie Swat, "Preliminary Analysis of the Concorde Trial," *Lancet* 341 (1993): 889–890.
8. Concorde Coordinating Committee, "Concorde: MRC/ANRS Randomised Double-Blind Controlled Trial of Immediate and Deferred Zidovudine in Symptom-Free HIV Infection," *Lancet* 343 (1994): 871–881.
9. Ronald Bayer, "Beyond the Burdens of Protection," *Evaluation Review* 14 (October 1990): 443–446.
10. Epstein, *Impure Science,* chapter 6.
11. Carol Levine, "Women and HIV/AIDS Research: The Barriers to Equity," *Evaluation Review* 14 (October 1990): 447–463.
12. E. L. Kinney et al., "Underrepresentation of Women in New Drug Trials," *Annals of Internal Medicine* 95 (1981): 495–499.
13. Levine, "Women and HIV/AIDS Research," 448.
14. Cited in Epstein, *Impure Science,* 258.
15. Carol Levine, Nancy Nevaloff Dubler, and Robert Levine, "Building a New Consensus: Ethical Principles and Policies for Clinical Research on HIV/AIDS," *IRB: A Review of Human Subjects Research* 13 (January–April 1991): 1–17.
16. *New York Times,* September 2, 1990, Section I: 42.
17. *New York Newsday,* June 8, 1993, 108.
18. *San Francisco Chronicle,* March 10, 1990, A6.

Chapter 4

1. Data provided by the Centers for Disease Control.
2. "Update: Mortality Attributable to HIV Infection/AIDS among Persons Aged 25–44 Years—United States, 1990 and 1991," *Morbidity and Mortality Weekly Report,* July 2, 1993: 481–485; "Update: Mortality Attributable to HIV Infection among Persons Aged 24–44 Years—United States, 1994," *Morbidity and Mortality Weekly Report,* February 16, 1996, 121–125.
3. Fabrizio Starace and Lorraine Sherc, "Suicidal Behavior, Euthanasia and AIDS," *AIDS* 12 (1998): 339–347.
4. "Depleting the Front Lines: Medicine's Loss," *Medical World News,* April 9, 1990, 24–29.

Chapter 5

1. Edward M. Connor et al., "Reduction of Maternal-Infant Transmission of Human Immunodeficiency Virus Type I with Zidovudine Treatment," *New England Journal of Medicine* 331 (1994): 1173–1180.
2. Ronald Bayer, "Ethical Challenges Posed by Zidovudine Treatment to Reduce Vertical Transmission of HIV, *New England Journal of Medicine* 331 (1994): 1223–1225.
3. Mark B. Feinberg, "Changing the Natural History of HIV Disease," *Lancet* 348 (1996): 239–246.
4. Jesse Green and Peter Arno, "The 'Medicaidization' of AIDS: Trends in the Financing of HIV-Related Medical Care," *Journal of the American Medical Association* 264 (1990): 1261–1266.
5. Robert Steinbrook, "Caring for People with Human Immunodeficiency Virus." *New England Journal of Medicine* 339 (1998): 1926– 1928.
6. Arnold Doyle, Richard Jefferys, and Joseph Kelly, "National ADAP Monitoring Project: Interim Technical Report" (March 1998).
7. Samuel A. Bozzette et al., "The Care of HIV-Infected Adults in the United States," *New England Journal of Medicine* 339 (1998): 1897–1904.

Epilogue

1. "Highlights from the Fourth Conference on Retroviruses and Opportunistic Infections (January 22–26, 1997)," *The AIDS Reader* (Supplement, n.d.).
2. Kenneth H. Mayer, "Practical Application and Limitations of 'Eradication' Therapy," *The AIDS Reader* 7 (July-August 1997): 130–133.
3. Camus, *The Plague.*

Appendix 1

1. Ronald J. Grele, *Envelopes of Sound: The Art of Oral History,* 2nd ed. (New York: Praeger, 1991), 135.

Glossary of Medical Terms

Acquired Immunodeficiency Syndrome (AIDS)   Advanced stage of HIV disease, characterized by certain opportunistic infections and cancers and by the severe loss of CD4 cells.

Acute HIV infection   The first stage of HIV disease, when the virus invades the body, replicating and spreading rapidly.

Candida   A yeastlike fungus, commonly found in the normal flora of the mouth, skin, intestinal tract, and vagina. Generally, candida is harmless but can become clinically infectious in immune compromised people.

CD4 cell   "Helper" T-cell, a white blood cell responsible for coordinating much of the body's immune response. CD4 cells are one of the main targets damaged by HIV.

CD4 count   The number of T-helper lymphocytes per cubic millimeter of blood. The CD4 count is a good predictor of immune health. In the presence of HIV infection, a CD4 count less than 200 qualifies as a diagnosis of AIDS.

CD8 (T8)   A protein embedded in the cell surface of killer and suppressor T-lymphocytes.

CMV, CMV colitis, CMV retinitis   See Cytomegalovirus.

Cytomegalovirus (CMV)   A herpes virus that is a common cause of opportunistic diseases in people with AIDS and other people with immune suppression. While CMV can infect most organs of the body, people with

AIDS are most susceptible to CMV of the retina (retinitis) and the colon (colitis).

Colitis   Inflammation of the colon.

Cryptosporidiosis   An opportunistic infection caused by a protozoan parasite (Cryptosporidium parvum). Cryptosporidiosis causes diarrhea and abdominal pain.

Enteric   Relating to or of the intestines or gastrointestinal tract.

Encephalitis   A general term denoting inflammation of the brain.

Gastroenteritis   Inflammation of the stomach and/or intestines.

Giardia   Intestinal protozoa.

Gonococcus   A single bacterium of the species *Neisseria gonorrhoeae,* the agent causing gonorrhea.

Helper-suppressor ratio   The ratio of helper (CD4+) T-cells to suppressor (CD8+) T-cells.

Hepatitis B   A viral liver disease that can be acute or chronic and even life threatening, particularly in people with poor immune resistance. Like HIV, the hepatitis B virus can be transmitted by sexual contact, contaminated needles or contaminated blood or blood products. Unlike HIV, it is also transmissible through close casual contact.

Herpes simplex virus 1 (HSV-1)   A virus that can cause painful "cold sores" or blisters on the lips ("fever blisters") or in the mouth or around the eyes. The symptomatic disease stage occurs at unpredictable intervals of weeks, months, or years. The latent (inactive) virus can reactivate due to emotional stress, physical trauma, other infections, or suppression of the immune system. HSV-1 responds well to treatment with acyclovir.

Herpes simplex virus 2 (HSV-2)   A virus closely related to HSV-1 that causes similar lesions. However, HSV-2 is usually transmitted sexually, and its lesions generally are in the anogenital area.

Herpes zoster virus A virus that causes chicken pox in children and may reappear in adulthood as herpes zoster. Herpes zoster, also called shingles, consists of very painful blisters on the skin that follow nerve pathways.

Herpes virus A family of viruses including Herpes simplex I and II, Herpes zoster, Epstein-Barr virus, cytomegalovirus, and the newly discovered Kaposi's sarcoma and associated herpes virus.

Kaposi's sarcoma (KS) A tumor of the wall of blood vessels, or the lymphatic system. It usually appears as pink to purple, painless spots on the skin but may also occur internally in addition to or independent of lesions.

Lymphadenopathy Swollen, firm, and possibly tender lymph nodes. The cause may range from an infection such as HIV, the flu, mononucleosis, or lymphoma (cancer of the lymph nodes).

Lymphoid interstitial pneumonitis (LIP) A chronic, diffuse pneumonia, the result of a gradual building up of lymphoid and other white blood cells in the lung tissue. It occurs almost exclusively in children with HIV infection.

Lymphoma Cancers of the lymphatic system. Many lymphomas count as an AIDS diagnosis.

MAC See Mycobacterium avium complex.

Mycobacterium avium complex (MAC) A common opportunistic infection caused by bacterial organisms. In people with AIDS, it can spread through the bloodstream to infect lymph nodes, bone marrow, liver, spleen, spinal fluid, lungs, and intestinal tract. Symptoms of MAC include prolonged wasting, fever, fatigue, and enlarged spleen. MAC infection is one of the diseases making up the AIDS definition.

Mycoplasma A class of microorganism, simpler than a bacterium, but more complex than a virus. Some mycoplasma may play a role in HIV disease-related conditions.

Neuropathy An abnormal and degenerative state of the nervous system. HIV, some treatments, and other diseases can cause a peripheral neuropathy marked by burning, tingling sensations in the extremities, loss of deep tendon responses, and decrease in sensitivity to touch stimulation.

Nezelof syndrome   A group of immunodeficiency disorders. Those with the syndrome have a high susceptibility to life-threatening infections.

Nongonococcal urethritis   Inflammation of the urethra, the canal through which urine passes from the bladder to the exterior of the body, which can be caused by a number of infectious organisms. See Ureaplasma *urealyticum.*

Opportunistic infections   An infection in an immune-compromised person caused by an organism that does not usually cause disease in healthy people. Many of these organisms are carried in a latent state by virtually everyone and cause disease only when given the opportunity of a damaged immune system.

PCP   See *Pneumocystis carinii* pneumonia.

***Pneumocystis carinii* pneumonia**   An opportunistic pneumonia often seen in HIV-infected patients. Left untreated it can be fatal.

Papillomavirus   A virus associated with sexually transmitted diseases. Certain papillomavirus variants have also been associated with cervical cancer, particularly in HIV-infected women.

Peripheral neuropathy   See Neuropathy.

Persistent generalized lymphadenopathy   See Lymphadenopathy.

Pharmacokinetic   Concerning the study of how a drug is processed by the body, with emphasis on the time required for absorption, duration of action, distribution in the body, and method of excretion.

Protease inhibitor   A class of antiretroviral drugs that work by inhibiting the HIV protease enzyme. Some examples include Saquinavir, Indinavir, and Ritonavir.

Retrovirus   A class of viruses that copy genetic material using RNA as a template for making DNA. (HIV is a retrovirus.)

Reverse transcriptase   A retroviral enzyme that is capable of copying RNA into DNA, an essential step in the life cycle of HIV. AZT, ddI, and ddC act against reverse transcriptase.

Schistosomiasis   An infection caused by a type of worm (schistosomes or blood flukes) that spends part of its life cycle in humans or other mammals, another in water-borne snails.

Shigella   A genus of rod-shaped anaerobic bacteria, species of which may cause diarrheal disease.

Shingles (herpes zoster)   A skin condition characterized by painful blisters in a linear distribution on one side of the body that generally dry and scab, leaving minor scarring. Shingles is caused by the reactivation of a previous infection with the varicella-zoster virus that causes chickenpox, usually early in life. Shingles may be a symptom of HIV disease progression.

T-helper cells   Lymphocytes responsible for assisting other white blood cells in responding to infection, processing antigens, and triggering antibody production (also known as T4 cells, CD4 cells).

T-suppressor cells   T lymphocytes responsible for turning the immune response off after infection is cleared, a subset of CD8+ lymphocytes.

Thrush (or oral candidiasis)   A yeast infection (usually caused by *Candidia albicans*) of the mucous membranes of the mouth.

Total parenteral nutrition (TPN)   A type of nutritional feeding that delivers all nutrients in liquid form intravenously.

Toxoplasmosis   A life-threatening opportunistic infection caused by a parasite (Toxoplasma gondii) found in raw or undercooked meat and cat feces. Toxoplasmosis may lead to brain swelling, coma, and death in people with suppressed immune systems.

Ureaplasma *urealyticum*   A bacterium commonly found in the genito-urinary tract and associated with sexually transmitted nongonococcal urethritis.

Viral burden/load   The concentration of a virus in the body.

Viremia   The presence of virus in the blood.

Wasting syndrome   A condition among HIV-infected individuals characterized by involuntary weight loss of more than 10 percent of baseline body weight. Other symptoms may include chronic diarrhea or chronic weakness and fever for more than 30 days; a CDC AIDS-defining condition.

Index of Physicians Interviewed

Subject Index

ACTG (AIDS Clinical Trials Group): activist critique of, 149; physician critique of, 132, 137–38, 145, 222; physicians as researchers in, 148

ACTG 076, 149; protest against, 150–51, 224; significance of, 224

ACT UP (AIDS Coalition to Unleash Power), 138–40, 150–51, 166

Acyclovir, 123–24

ADAP (AIDS Drug Assistance Program), 239–40

Adolescents: AIDS in, 147–48, 162, 269; treatment of, 162

African Americans: epidemiology of AIDS in, 3; fear of AZT among, 140–41; and Kemron, 163–64; marginalization of, 151; as patients, 164, 243; as physicians, 111

AIDS activism: and clinical trials, 149–50, 156; effects on doctor/patient relationship; and opposition to AZT, 138–40, 150–51

AIDS Clinical Trials Group. See ACTG

"AIDS doctor" as an identity, 118, 248–64

AIDS Drug Assistance Program. See ADAP

Alternative therapies: patient demand for, 162–68; physician response to, 163–68; physician use of, 165–66

American Association of Physicians for Human Rights, 14

AmFAR (American Foundation for AIDS Research), 154

Antiretroviral drugs: development of, 125. See also Specific drugs

Autonomy: of patients, 157–61, 168–69; of professionals, 156

AZT (zidovudine): for asymptomatic HIV positives, 137; and ACT UP, 138–40, 150–51; and children, 136; clinical trial of, 129–33; Concorde trial, 141–44; cost of, 134–35; criticism of, 138; harmfulness of, 135, 142; ineffectiveness of, 135–36, 142–44; as prolonging life, 133, 136–37; side effects from, 135, 141

Bathhouses, 24, 61

Bay Area Physicians for Human Rights, 21, 23–24, 153

Bisexuals, 25–26

Blacks. See African Americans

Blood transfusion and HIV transmission, 21, 82

Burroughs-Wellcome, 124, 129, 134

Camus, Albert: The Plague, 8–9, 42, 274, 301 n, 304 n

Cancer, 43, 65

Candidiasis (thrush), 18, 30, 299

Catholicism, 78–79, 215–16, 242

CCC (County Community Consortium, San Francisco), 153

CDC (Centers for Disease Control), 23, 27, 89–91; on epidemiology of early cases, 30; first reports on AIDS, 14, 19–20, 28–29, 32, 79

CD4 lymphocytes. See T-cells

Chermann, Jean Claude, 159–60